**Jere R. Mitchell,** M.S.

**Gordon A. Doak,** Ph.D.

# The Artificial Insemination and Embryo Transfer of Dairy and Beef Cattle (including information pertaining to goats, sheep, horses, swine, and other animals)

## A HANDBOOK
## AND LABORATORY MANUAL

for Students, Herd Operators, and Persons
Involved in Genetic Improvement

*Ninth Edition*

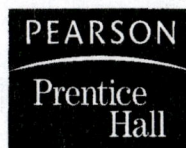

PEARSON

Prentice
Hall

Upper Saddle River, New Jersey 07458

**Library of Congress Cataloging-in-Publication Data**

Mitchell, Jere R.
  The artificial insemination and embryo transfer of dairy and beef cattle (including
information pertaining to goats, sheep, horses, swine, and other animals): a handbook
and laboratory manual/Jere R. Mitchell, Gordon A. Doak.—9th ed.
      p. cm.
  Rev. ed. of: Artificial insemination and embryo transfer of dairy and beef cattle
(including information pertaining to goats, sheep, horses, swine, and other animals)/
H.A. Herman, Jere R. Mitchell, Gordon A. Doak. 8th ed. 1994.
  Includes bibliographical references (p.).
  ISBN 0-13-112278-9
      1. Cattle—Artificial insemination—Handbooks, manuals, etc. 2.
Cattle—Embryos—Transplantation—Handbooks, manuals, etc. 3. Artificial
insemination—Handbooks, manuals, etc. 4.
Livestock—Embryos—Transplantation—Handbooks, manuals, etc. I. Doak, Gordon
Allen. II. Herman, H. A. Artificial insemination and embryo transfer of dairy and beef
cattle (including information pertaining to goats, sheep, horses, swine, and
other animals). III. Title.

SF201.5 .M57 2004
636.2' 08245—dc21

                                                          2002038124

**Editor-in-Chief:** Stephen Helba
**Executive Editor:** Debbie Yarnell
**Editorial Assistant:** Jonathan Tenthoff
**Managing Editor:** Mary Cumis
**Production Editor:** Amy Hackett, Carlisle Publishing Services
**Production Liaison:** Janice G. Stangel
**Director of Manufacturing and Production:** Bruce Johnson
**Manufacturing Buyer:** Cathleen Petersen
**Creative Director:** Cheryl Asherman
**Cover Design Coordinator:** Miguel Ortiz
**Formatting:** Carlisle Communications, Ltd.
**Marketing Manager:** Jimmy Stephens
**Cover Design:** Miguel Ortiz

Pearson Education LTD.
Pearson Education Australia PTY, Limited
Pearson Education Singapore, Pte. Ltd
Pearson Education North Asia Ltd
Pearson Education Canada, Ltd
Pearson Educatión de Mexico, S.A. de C.V.
Pearson Education—Japan
Pearson Education Malaysia, Pte. Ltd

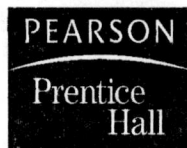

PEARSON

Prentice
Hall

ISBN: 0-13-112278-9

# Contents

## PART ONE

### The Role of Artificial Insemination and Reproduction in Livestock Improvement

## PART TWO

### Semen Evaluation; Extenders (Processing); Frozen Semen; Custom Collection

# PART THREE

## Insemination of Dairy and Beef Cattle; Insemination Training; Pregnancy Determination and Reproduction Problems

*Exercise*

# PART FOUR

## Sire Selection; Bull Health and Management; AI Organizations; Employment Opportunities

*Exercise*

# PART FIVE

## Artificial Insemination of Dairy Goats and Other Farm Animals

# Appendices

# Foreword

The main value of artificial insemination and other reproductive technologies lies in their use for the improvement of livestock. These methods make it possible to achieve genetic improvements on a large-scale basis. In this endeavor, it is important to be mindful of objectives and goals necessary for the success of individual dairy and beef producers. The following words seem to ably picture the obligation ever before us:

## THE STOCK BREEDER

Yours is the task to mate and to mould
Living things for your gain and pleasure;
To find and to fuse the purest gold
    Nature hoards as a hidden treasure.

Yours is the heritage handed down,
A trust without limit or measure;
To make, not to mar, to win renown—
    Fail not in the brave endeavor.

Yours is the art and the work to blend
Living things in beauty together;
Yours is the power to ruin or mend—
    The bonds that ye bind none can sever.

A sacred trust are these living things
To be carelessly dealt with NEVER!
And faithful stewardship surely brings
    Rich reward that shall live forever!

—Dr. A. S. Alexander

# About the Authors

## JERE R. MITCHELL

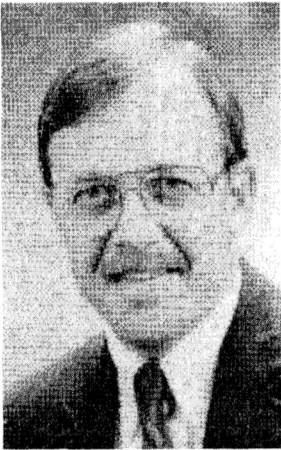

Jere R. Mitchell is Service Director for Certified Semen Services (CSS) and Technical Director for the National Association of Animal Breeders (NAAB). He conducts the national service program for the AI industry to review and audit semen production practices of participants and provides technical support to NAAB. He works closely with various NAAB committees and, in consultation with the Research Committee, coordinates the NAAB Research Program. Mitchell earned his B.S. in animal science from Kansas State University and his M.S. in dairy science from Virginia Polytechnic Institute and undertook advanced studies at Penn State University, where he was also an instructor in the Department of Dairy and Animal Science. Mitchell served for two years in the U.S. Army. Prior to joining CSS/NAAB in 1988, Mitchell worked in technical and research areas for various organizations in the AI industry. He has authored or co-authored several research publications. Mitchell is a member of the American Dairy Science Association and a member of the American Society of Animal Science and he is an associate member of The Society for Theriogenology. He is a native of Cortland, New York. Mitchell and his wife, Becky, are the parents of two grown sons, Jefferson and Wil.

## GORDON A. DOAK

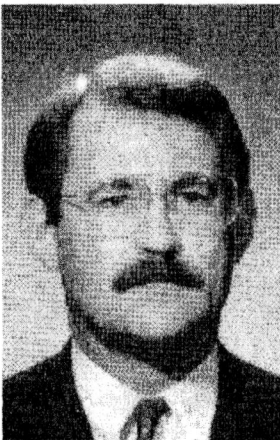

Dr. Gordon A. Doak, a native of Missouri, grew up on a diversified dairy farm. He received his M.S. in dairy husbandry and his Ph.D. in reproductive physiology from the University of Missouri in 1970 and 1974, respectively. Following two years of post-doctoral studies, he began work with NAAB and CSS in August 1976.

As NAAB Technical Director, he worked with the technical and research aspects of NAAB. Simultaneously he served as CSS Service Director, administering the programs of NAAB's subsidiary, Certified Semen Services. During his tenure at NAAB, he has worked closely with many standing committees and provided support in the technical and international areas.

Dr. Doak became President of NAAB/CSS on January 1, 1988. In this position he works closely with the Board of Directors of NAAB and CSS in formulation of objectives, goals, and policies, and he administers the association's programs and activities. He provides liaison between the Board of Directors, committees of the association, the membership, and allied industry groups.

He has served on many industry committees, including NCDHIP Policy Board, NDHIA Quality Certification Committee, U.S. Dairy Genetics Council, Foreign Agriculture Service's Agricultural Technical Advisory Committee for Trade in Livestock and Livestock Products, Joint Council on Dairy Cattle Breeding, and U.S. Livestock Genetics Export. He is a member of the American Dairy Science Association, the American Society of Animal Science, and the American Society of Association Executives.

# Acknowledgments

The late Dr. Harry A. Herman and Dr. F. W. Madden authored the first seven editions of this manual. They were assisted by many AI industry and university colleagues who are acknowledged in previous editions. The current authors first contributed to the eighth edition (1994). That this manual has received worldwide distribution is a tribute to the pioneering efforts of Dr. Herman in artificial insemination and animal breeding.

The ninth edition is the first edition without the direct involvement of Dr. Herman. However, while technology is ever changing, the history of the basics is important in understanding advances in technology.

We are grateful to Brenda Coleman, NAAB, for word processing and assistance in preparation of the manuscript.

Jere R. Mitchell
Gordon A. Doak

# How to Use this Manual

The Ninth Edition of *The Artificial Insemination and Embryo Transfer of Dairy and Beef Cattle* is a revision and updating of earlier editions.

Basic information on reproduction and the practice of artificial insemination (AI) is presented, along with an overview of embryo transfer (ET) and developments in biotechnology applicable to cattle. Artificial insemination of dairy goats and methods for genetic improvement are covered in detail. Also, techniques for AI in other farm animals are briefly described.

This is a practical handbook for AI personnel, insemination training students, herd operators, college and high school students, and other persons involved in the genetic improvement of farm animals.

The book is conveniently arranged by topics for easy and ready use of the particular information desired.

**Part One** provides information on the advantages and considerations of artificial insemination, basic livestock genetics, the anatomy and reproductive processes of the cow and bull, and semen collection methods. In addition, it relates statistics on AI usage and general information about NAAB and CSS. Persons interested in livestock improvement should study this section.

**Part Two** deals with semen characteristics, including evaluation, processing, and extension; freezing and cryogenic storage; and care of the refrigerator unit. The various tests for semen quality are discussed in detail. Custom collection of semen is described. The section is presented largely for AI center operators engaged in semen production, distribution, and sales. Also described are control measures followed by laboratory personnel at semen-producing businesses. Discussion of these quality tests also provides a means for teaching students in the classroom about semen physiology, semen characteristics, and artificial insemination.

**Part Three** explains insemination techniques for dairy and beef cattle, inseminator training, pregnancy determination in cattle, conception rates, and breeding problems. It provides essential information for the herd operator and the inseminator-technician regarding important factors contributing to a satisfactory conception rate. In addition, the exercise on "Embryo Transfer (ET) and Related Practices" explains the advances and techniques involved in the field.

**Part Four** includes an overview of sire selection, sire health, sire management, AI organizations, and career opportunities. This section provides information of value to students and others who anticipate a career in some phase of the AI industry.

**Part Five** explains the use and techniques for artificial insemination in dairy goats and other farm animals.

The **Appendices** provide a description of the NAAB uniform coding system used in North America for identifying semen, a list of uniform breed codes as used throughout the cattle industry, a list of AI equipment manufacturers and suppliers, a list of AI businesses in the United States, frozen embryo labeling requirements, a gestation table for cattle, a list of stud code numbers assigned by NAAB, CSS Guidelines for AI Center Management Practices, and the Breeder's Guide to CSS.

Questions at the end of each of exercise are principally designed to reinforce information presented in the text. However, in certain instances, other sources should be consulted to find answers to questions. The intent is to broaden knowledge through investigation of additional pertinent materials.

Also important to note are the references cited at the end of each exercise. In courses taught at the college level, adequate lecture material obtained from current reports of research and development in the field of animal reproduction and artificial insemination should be provided as appropriate background material for a scientific approach to the techniques and practices in use.

# Introduction

Artificial insemination and embryo transfer as means of livestock improvement are now accepted and utilized worldwide.[1] The increased use of outstanding proven sires to enhance production potentials, control genital diseases transmitted through natural service, and aid in animal improvement results from the expanding use of AI and other bio-techniques.

**Terminology**—The term "artificial insemination," commonly called "AI," implies the deposition of spermatozoa in the female reproductive tract by the use of artificial means (instruments) rather than by natural service involving the male. Although the term "artificial breeding" is often used to mean the same as "artificial insemination," the former is not technically correct. Thus, "artificial insemination" or "AI" is preferred.

**How Artificial Insemination Began**—The first authentic account of the use of AI was by the Italian Spallanzani, who in 1780 was successful in artificially inseminating a bitch. There is, however, some evidence that the Arabs used artificial insemination for horses during the fourteenth century. As early as 1890, the French—particularly the veterinarian Repiquet—were using artificial insemination in their horse breeding work.[2]

Much of the present stimulus for the artificial insemination of cattle traces to developments in the former Soviet Union, where as early as 1909 this method was used on mares. Around 1909, the Russians began inseminating cattle, and by 1928 they were artificially inseminating some 1.2 million cattle and 15.0 million sheep. Soviet Professor I. Ivanovich Ivanov (1870–1932) was the leading authority and pioneer investigator in the field application of artificial insemination in Europe. He was the first to artificially inseminate cattle and sheep successfully. He was using artificial insemination with horses as early as 1899, and during World War I (1914–1918), thousands of mares were inseminated.

In 1914, Professor G. Amantea, University of Rome, constructed an artificial vagina for dogs, and from 1934 to 1938, the artificial vagina for cattle was developed by European and American workers.

In 1936, a large cooperative association for the artificial insemination of cattle was organized in Denmark. It had about 200 members, and over 1,000 cows were inseminated the first year. Since 1936, the AI program has grown steadily and is now in use for livestock improvement throughout the world.

**Artificial Insemination Worldwide**—Surveys to determine the number of cattle, sheep, and swine artificially inseminated have been conducted by several investigators. One of the first was by Dr. W. Bielanski, Agricultural College, Krakow, Poland, who reported a survey completed in 1962 in which he estimated the total number of cattle in the worldwide AI program at about 60 million

---

[1]H. A. Herman. 1981. Improving Cattle by the Millions. Univ. of Missouri Press, Columbia.
[2]Ibid.

**Table 1. 1998 Estimated World Cattle and Buffalo Bred by AI[a]**

| Region | 1960 | 1973–1979 |
|---|---|---|
| Europe | 36,046,000 | 63,952,150 |
| Asia | 2,825,900 | 4,758,396 |
| North America | 8,310,000 | 10,876,000 |
| South & Central America | 528,162 | 4,533,617 |
| Australia & New Zealand | 570,000 | 2,034,000 |
| Africa | 111,654 | 343,551 |
| Total | 48,391,716 | 86,497,714 |

[a]H. A. Herman. 1981. *Improving Cattle by the Millions.* Univ. of Missouri Press, Columbia.

head.[3] More than 70 countries were indicated as using AI. In 1964, Dr. Y. Nishikawa, of Japan, assisted by Dr. H. A. Herman, made a similar survey.[4] A survey was also reported by Professor T. Bonadonna, of Italy, involving the years of 1971 to 1973 inclusive.[5] In 1979, Dr. H. A. Herman[6] updated the estimated figures, and they are shown in Table 1.

In a later study, Bonadonna and Succi[7] reported on "artificial insemination in the world," with an estimated summary of cattle, pigs, sheep, and goats serviced by AI in various countries through 1977/78. No total for animals inseminated on a worldwide basis was given in the summary, but the authors stated that artificial insemination was becoming more and more widespread all over the world, particularly in cattle, followed by pigs, sheep, turkeys, and chickens. In the 1980 summary, it was presumed that there were a total of about 150 million cows inseminated in the world. As to the females of the other species artificially inseminated, information was uncertain.

Thibier and Wagner[8] and Wagner and Thibier[9] in a 1998 survey reported the number of first inseminations for cattle, pigs, sheep, and goats. These are reported in Table 2.

These numbers point out the importance of AI for breeding in pigs. The overwhelming majority of semen used in pig AI is fresh. Very little frozen semen is used. (See Exercise 29.)

Since 1971, practically all AI activity for cattle, on a worldwide basis, has been reported in terms of units of semen. Because not all of the semen is actually utilized and because units per insemination vary, only a very rough estimate of the total world cattle serviced by AI is possible. (Refer to Exercise 2 for units of semen reported for the United States and export trade.)

---

[3]W. Bielanski. 1963. An attempt to determine the number of cows inseminated in the world. The A.I. Digest 11:6.

[4]Y. Nishikawa. May 1965. History and development of artificial insemination in the world. Bull. Dept. of Animal Science, Coll. of Agriculture, Kyoto Univ., Kitashirakawa, Japan.

[5]T. Bonadonna. 1975. The use of artificial insemination worldwide, 1971–73. Zootecnia E. Veterinaria La Fecondazione Artificiale (Milan) 30:2.

[6]H. A. Herman. 1981. Improving Cattle by the Millions. Univ. of Missouri Press, Columbia.

[7]T. Bonadonna and G. Succi. 1980. Artificial insemination in the world. Proc. 9th International Congr. Animal Reproduction and Artificial Insemination (Madrid) 5:655.

[8] M. Thibier and H.-G. Wagner. 14th International Congress on Animal Reproduction, Stockholm, 2–6 July 2000, Abstracts Volume 2, p. 76.

[9]H.-G. Wagner and M. Thibier. 14th International Congress on Animal Reproduction, Stockholm, 2–6 July 2000, Abstracts Volume 2, p. 77.

**Table 2. 1998 Estimated First Inseminations[a]**

| Region | Cattle | Pigs | Sheep | Goats |
|---|---|---|---|---|
| Africa | 870,892 | 16 | 20,400 | 920 |
| North America | 11,203,880 | 20,501,000 | 3,750 | 3,800 |
| South America | 1,366,678 | 308,336 | 0 | 0 |
| Far East | 58,181,005 | 1,999,000 | 1,308,358 | 391,514 |
| Near East | 1,068,991 | 400 | 3,792 | 1900 |
| Europe | 33,872,942 | 17,525,351 | 1,990,773 | 69,818 |
| Total | 106,564,388 | 40,334,103 | 3,327,473 | 467,952 |

[a]M. Thibier and H.-G. Wagner; Wagner and Thibier. 14th International Congress on Animal Reproduction, Stockholm, 2–6 July 2000, Abstracts Volume 2, p. 76–77.

**Table 3. 1998 Estimated World Production of Cattle and Buffalo Semen[a]**

| Region | Fresh Doses | Frozen Doses |
|---|---|---|
| Africa | 55,204 | 1,484,850 |
| North America | 0 | 43,270,500 |
| South America | 0 | 5,917,269 |
| Far East | 8,874,920 | 63,938,027 |
| Near East | 16,794 | 2,559,640 |
| Europe | 2,694,903 | 115,176,785 |
| Total | 11,641,821 | 232,347,071 |

[a]M. Thibier and H.-G. Wagner. 14th International Congress on Animal Reproduction Stockholm, 2–6 July 2000, Abstracts Volume 2, p. 76.

The most recent worldwide survey conducted by Thibier and Wagner[8] in 1998 reports the number of units of semen produced according to the major regions of the world according to FAO subdivisions (Table 3). They also reported that in 1998 one-sixth of female cattle and buffalo were serviced by artificial insemination.

It is estimated that in 2001 there were slightly over 1 billion cattle and buffalo in the world (Table 4). However, it must be realized that these total numbers do not refer to the potential animals eligible for AI service.

Of note is the large amount of semen imported by some countries (see Exercise 2). In 2001, AI businesses in the United States exported 9,731,702 units. The principal world regions leading in the importation of semen are South America and Central America, the European Community, Oceania, Asia, and Africa. Mexico has become a leading semen import country, with 1,030,004 dairy units and 10,277 beef units from the United States in 2001. It is not known the amount of imported semen used in a given year or the amount stored for future use. However, if only half of the semen

**Table 4. Cattle and Buffalo: Number in Specified Countries, 1990–2001[a,b]**

| Country | 1990 | 1995 | 2001[c] |
|---|---|---|---|
| | (thousands) | (thousands) | (thousands) |
| Argentina | 56,482 | 54,207 | 50,052 |
| Australia | 24,673 | 25,736 | 27,003 |
| Belgium—Luxembourg | 3,259 | 3,365 | 3,050 |
| Brazil | 140,400 | 149,315 | 150,853 |
| Bulgaria | 1,577 | 638 | 632 |
| Canada | 11,220 | 12,709 | 12,860 |
| China | 100,752 | 123,317 | 130,000 |
| Colombia | 16,835 | 17,556 | 22,663 |
| Costa Rica | 1,762 | 1,645 | 1,758 |
| Denmark | 2,232 | 2,082 | 1,970 |
| Dominican Republic | 1,986 | 1,984 | 1,918 |
| Egypt | 6,385 | 5,873 | 6,370 |
| El Salvador | 1,220 | 1,319 | 1,086 |
| France | 21,394 | 20,524 | 20,518 |
| Germany | 20,287 | 15,962 | 14,557 |
| Guatemala | 1,900 | 1,707 | 1,548 |
| Honduras | 2,424 | 2,205 | 1,602 |
| India | 270,070 | 293,922 | 313,774 |
| Ireland | 5,899 | 6,410 | 6,459 |
| Italy | 8,853 | 7,300 | 7,075 |
| Japan | 4,760 | 4,916 | 4,565 |
| Korea (Republic) | 2,051 | 2,945 | 2,134 |
| Mexico | 31,747 | 30,191 | 22,500 |
| Netherlands | 4,731 | 4,588 | 4,191 |
| New Zealand | 7,828 | 8,712 | 9,767 |
| Philippines | 4,395 | 4,570 | 5,472 |
| Poland | 10,143 | 7,120 | 6,000 |
| Portugal | 1,291 | 1,329 | 1,216 |
| Romania | 6,283 | 3,565 | 3,000 |
| Russian Federation | 58,800 | 43,296 | 25,500 |
| South Africa (Republic) | 13,398 | 12,632 | 13,700 |
| Spain | 5,331 | 5,252 | 6,516 |
| Turkey | 12,700 | 11,700 | 11,350 |
| Ukraine | 25,195 | 19,624 | 10,000 |
| United Kingdom | 11,922 | 11,981 | 11,100 |
| United States | 98,162 | 102,785 | 97,309 |
| Uruguay | 9,377 | 10,512 | 10,177 |
| Venezuela | 13,210 | 12,336 | 13,400 |
| Former Yugoslavia | 4,702 | 4,527 | 4,415 |
| Total | 1,025,636 | 1,050,357 | 1,038,060 |

[a]Livestock and Poultry: World Markets and Trade. USDA-Foreign Agricultural Service.

[b]Various dates of enumeration are used by the countries reporting animal numbers. Data presented in this table approximate January 1 as closely as possible.

[c]Forecast.

## Cattle

## AI activity

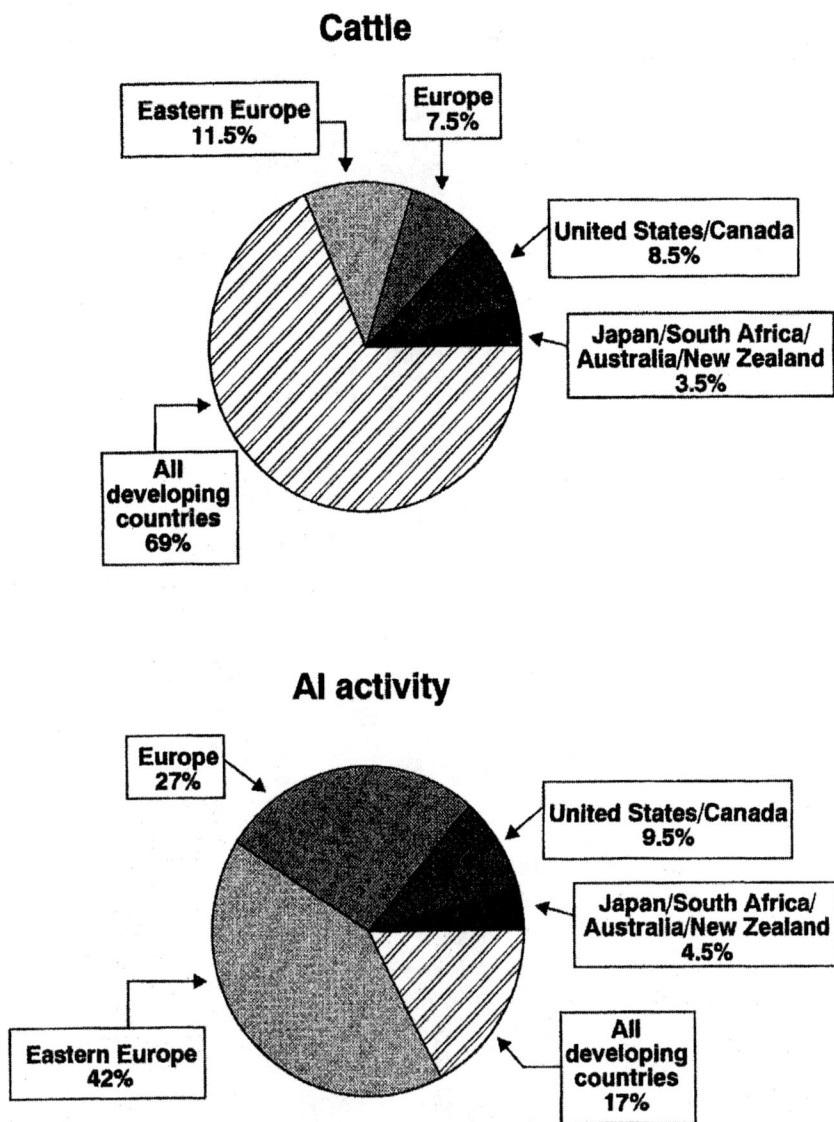

**Figure 1.** Percentage of total world cattle (upper chart) and of AI activity (lower chart) in developed and developing countries from 1980 to 1991. (D. Chupin and H. Schuh. 1993/1–2. Survey of present status of the use of artificial insemination in developing countries. World Animal Review [Rome] 74/75:26)

imported was used in 2001—possibly on the basis of two units for each animal inseminated—it could easily account for several million additional animals serviced by AI.

**Status of AI in Developing Countries**—The average person often does not realize that over two-thirds of the world's cattle and water buffalo are in what are defined as developing countries.

A survey was conducted in 1990/91 by the FAO (Food and Agriculture Organization of the United Nations, Rome, Italy)[9] to assess the AI activity in the 135 member countries in the developing countries program. Only 107 countries responded, and data from only 104 replies were used for analysis. Estimates for the percentage of cattle and AI activity in developed and developing countries are graphically indicated in Figure 1.

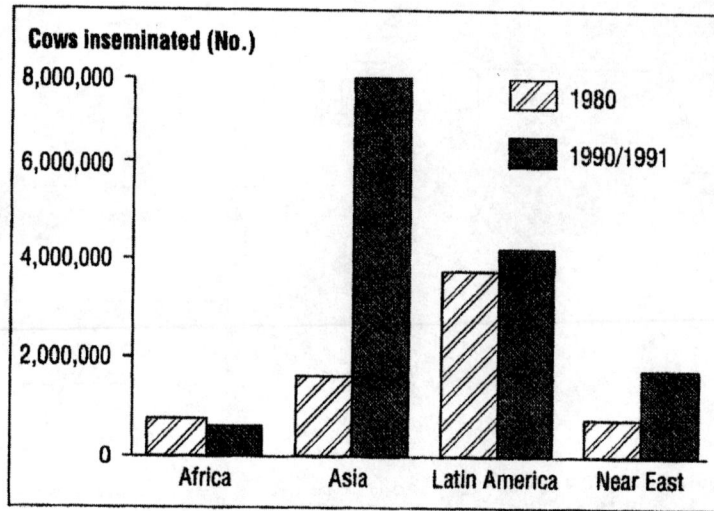

**Figure 2.** Estimated total number of cows inseminated, 1980 versus 1990/91, in developing countries, by region. (D. Chupin and H. Schuh. 1993/1–2. Survey of present status of the use of artificial insemination in developing countries. World Animal Review [Rome] 74/75:26)

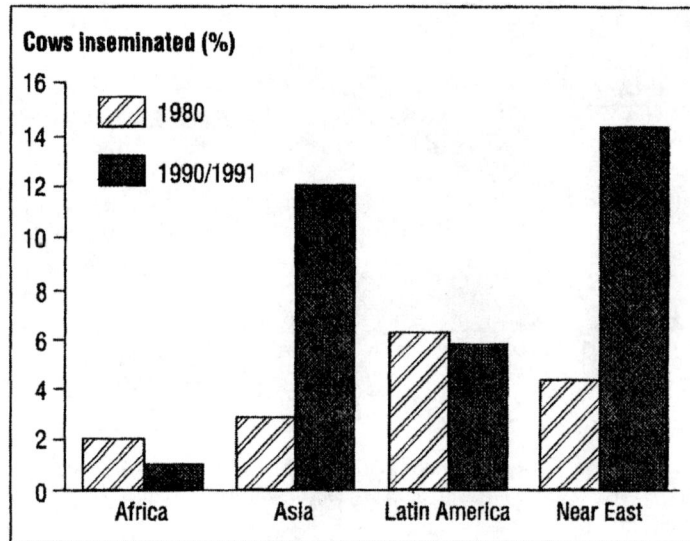

**Figure 3.** Estimated percentage of cows inseminated, 1980 versus 1990/91, in developing countries, by region. (D. Chupin and H. Schuh. 1993/1–2. Survey of present status of the use of artificial insemination in developing countries. World Animal Review [Rome] 74/75:26)

The estimates of total cattle by region illustrate the immense numbers of cattle in developing countries. The figures for percentage of cows inseminated is an estimated measure of AI activity in the world. Figure 2 indicates the number of cows inseminated in 1980 and 1990/91, and Figure 3 indicates the percentage of cows inseminated. The increase in numbers for Asia, Latin America, and the Near East is noteworthy.

About 70 percent of the developing countries replying had AI processing facilities of some kind and produced much of the total semen used. Some 12 to 15 percent of the total semen utilized was imported. Dairy breeds supplied 88 percent of the imported semen, beef breeds 9.5 percent, and tropical breeds 2.1 percent.

Most imported semen is used for crossbreeding and is an important step in increasing the production of offspring for milk and meat. In most developing countries, crosses to native and the European breeds are made to take advantage of the disease-, parasite-, and insect-resistant qualities of the local cattle. Fresh semen (unfrozen) is used in some 5 to 10 percent of the countries because liquid nitrogen, freezing procedures, and freezing equipment are not available. Constrictive breeding programs, feeding and husbandry limitations, and communication and transportation problems are deterrents to the success of AI in the same developing countries; but the potential for improvement is challenging for the entire AI industry.

**Growth in the United States**—Widespread use of artificial insemination in the United States developed largely through research and extension efforts at the land-grant colleges. Early workers in this field included college personnel at the University of Minnesota, Cornell University, New Jersey Agricultural College, The Pennsylvania State University, University of Missouri, University of Illinois, University of Nebraska, and The University of Wisconsin, to name a few.

The early AI organizations in America were largely farmer-owned cooperatives. The first such cooperative in America was organized at Clinton, New Jersey, through efforts of Enos J. Perry, Extension Dairyman, Rutgers University, New Brunswick, New Jersey. It began operations May 17, 1938, with 102 members and 1,050 cows enrolled. New York and Missouri established several small AI centers about the same time. Not to be overlooked, however, is the organization in 1937 of an AI breeding ring, on an experimental and demonstration basis, by Dr. C. L. Cole[10] at the North Central Station, University of Minnesota. Seven herds, located 1 to 10 miles from the station, were involved.

Artificial insemination in the United States has grown steadily. During 1939, there were 7 AI businesses with 33 sires involving 7,359 cows in 646 herds enrolled in the program. By 1950, the number had increased to 97 AI businesses, 2,104 sires, and services in 409,300 herds, with 2,619,555 cows involved. Because of consolidations, mergers, and federations, there are now about 5 major semen-producing businesses. By 2001, a rough estimate indicated that *7.5 million dairy cows and heifers,* Figure 4, *as well as some 2.9 million beef cows and heifers,* were serviced by artificial insemination, Figure 5 (see Exercise 2).

In 2001, there were some 33 AI businesses in the United States. About 8 were centers producing and selling semen, with some providing on-the-farm AI service. Some operators were strictly sales and service oriented. The majority are businesses that provide custom semen-freezing services (see Appendix D for list).

Expansion in the application of artificial insemination continues throughout the world. No other program in agriculture, except the use of hybrid seed and the utilization of fertilizers, has been so widely adopted. Much improvement in the methods used for collection, processing, and storage of semen and for insemination has been made since 1936.

There are still challenges with respect to improvement in the evaluation and processing of semen as well as the age-old problem of subfertility in cows. This situation has stimulated much excellent research on the physiology of the reproductive processes in both the cow and the bull. The

---

[10]C. L. Cole. 1938. Artificial insemination of dairy cattle. J. Dairy Sci. 21:131 (Abstr.).

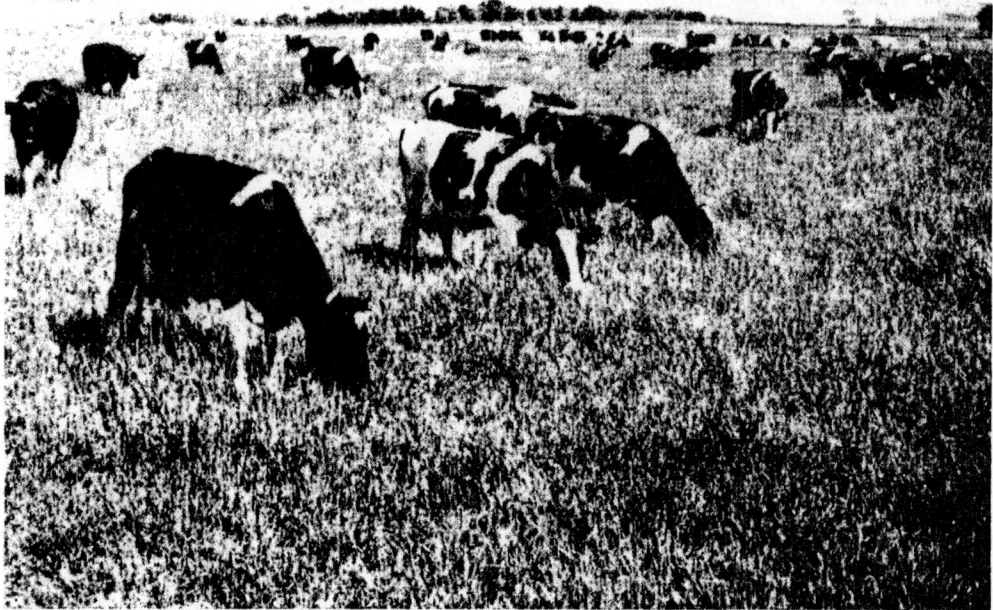

**Figure 4.** Artificial Insemination is used in both large and small dairy herds, as well as beef herds. Herd size may range from a few cows to as many as 5,000 or more. Both registered and grade cows are inseminated artificially. Above is a part of the 175-cow registered herd at Yankton State Hospital, Yankton, SD. Many cows and heifers in this herd result from selected matings using the best sires available through artificial insemination.

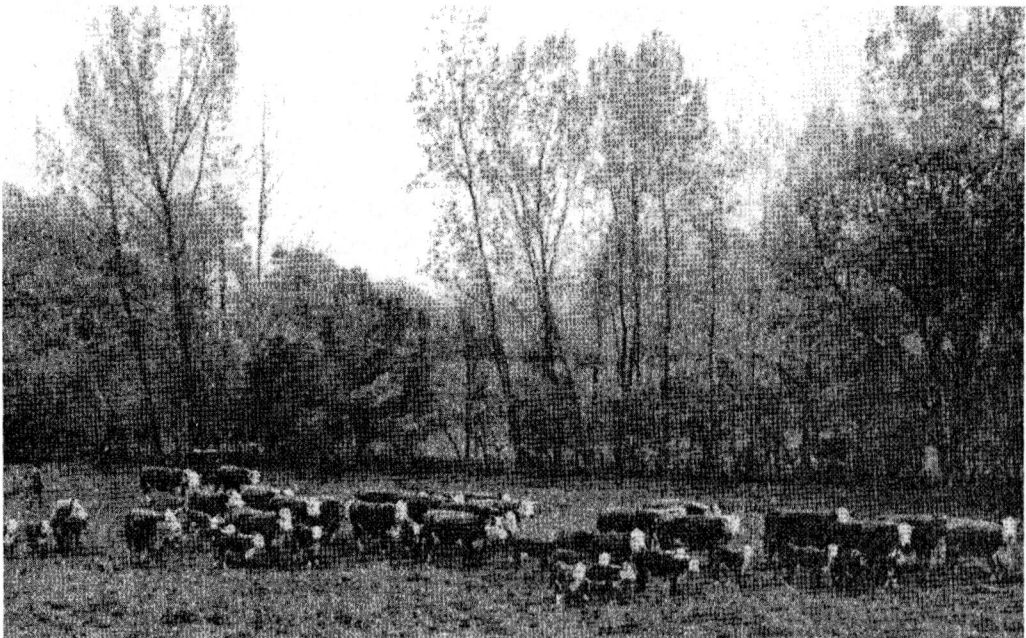

**Figure 5.** An Ohio beef herd with AI calf crop. (Courtesy, Harold Johnson, COBA/Select Sires, Columbus, OH)

development of AI has been responsible for much new knowledge relative to reproduction and fertility levels in the male and female in all species of farm animals and even in humans.

There is a continuing need in agricultural and veterinary colleges for knowledgeable persons to teach courses dealing with artificial insemination and to train high school and college students and producers to inseminate cows. Likewise, there is a demand for individuals versed in artificial insemination and livestock improvement to provide a work force for the AI centers and custom collection businesses. The need for trained personnel has inspired the preparation of this manual. The first draft was begun in 1941, when Dr. Harry Herman developed a college-level course in the artificial insemination of dairy cattle and milk goats at the University of Missouri. It is hoped that the pages that follow will serve a useful purpose in bringing together the essential information and describe the techniques necessary to conduct an AI program. Also included is pertinent information on techniques in embryo transfer and related practices.

## WEB SITES

Livestock and Poultry: World Markets and Trends—Livestock Summary Tables
   *http://www.fas.usda.gov/dlp/pubs.html*

Statistical Databases
   *http://www.fao.org/*

# PART ONE

# The Role of Artificial Insemination and Reproduction in Livestock Improvement

# EXERCISE 1

# Advantages and Considerations of Artificial Insemination

## OBJECT

To become knowledgeable regarding the advantages and considerations of artificial insemination.

## DISCUSSION

Following are some of the primary advantages of artificial insemination:

1. ***Increases production***— AI is a proven and economical means of enhancing the genetic potential for economic traits in cattle when superior, production-proven sires are utilized in the herd. In natural use, only one or two dairy sires are used in herds and rarely service over 50 cows per year. In beef herds, particularly under range conditions, a beef bull usually will not sire more than 25 to 30 calves in a season; however, through artificial insemination and the use of frozen semen, a bull may sire several hundred or even thousands of calves a year. If the bull so used has been progeny tested, the genetic gain, as well as profit from the herd, is increased.

2. ***Proves more sires***— The transmitting ability of a bull may be determined quickly and effectively. Modern sire-proving methods require many progeny be tested in many herds. It has been well demonstrated that the genetic evaluation of an AI-proven sire is highly reliable. Young, unproven bulls should be used sparingly until their transmitting ability has been shown. This is easily accomplished through the use of artificial insemination, and no one dairy herd will have more than a few daughters of unproven bulls.

3. ***Eliminates danger and expense of keeping a bull***— The danger and nuisance of keeping a bull around the farm is removed. At one time (1961), bulls killed on the average of one American farmer every four days. This number has been reduced drastically because of AI. The number of farmers injured by bulls is not recorded. Most studies indicate that using AI costs less per cow serviced than maintaining a really meritorious sire (or sires) in which the investment is substantial.

4. ***Reduces number of bulls needed***— Cattle producers who would, of necessity, have to own one or more bulls (often of average genetic merit) may dispense with keeping a bull or, in the case of beef cattle producers, with keeping so many bulls. Through the use of artificial insemination, cattle producers can participate in the use of herd improving sires at a cost lower than that of keeping a bull. This practice, among other advantages, makes utilizing genetically superior bulls for crossbreeding in beef cattle both practical and economical.

5. **Controls diseases**— The danger of spreading diseases such as campylobacteriosis (vibriosis), trichomoniasis, leptospirosis, brucellosis, tuberculosis, bovine viral diarrhea, and other diseases that can be transmitted by the bull in natural service is materially reduced. It is important that only disease-free bulls be used to produce semen for AI use. Most AI businesses marketing semen comply with the "CSS Minimum Requirements for Disease Control of Semen Produced for AI." Through Certified Semen Services (CSS), a subsidiary of the National Association of Animal Breeders, regular inspections of participating AI centers are conducted for semen and sire identification and for sire health testing.

6. **Increases sire life**— Valuable sires that because of injury are unable to serve cows may be continued in service. Also, semen can be collected, frozen, and stored while a bull is active, thus providing insurance against death or injury. Good quality bull semen may be frozen and stored indefinitely with little decline in fertility.

7. **Reduces injuries**— Yearling heifers and small cows may be mated with older, heavier bulls without the danger of injury. Bulls in AI use now are being evaluated so that the average birth weight of their calves is known. This aids in selecting which bulls are to be mated to which heifers so as to reduce difficult calving.

8. **Aids fertility control**— Infertile bulls are likely to be detected earlier with regular examination of the semen than with natural breeding. Likewise, abnormalities of a cow's genital tract (which may lead to shy breeding) may be dis-

covered earlier. As a rule, artificial insemination will equal or exceed the natural breeding conception rate.

9. **Provides for better identification of animals**— More accurate identification of cows and calves in the herd and better-kept breeding and calving records usually result.

10. **Aids special matings in crossbreeding**— Crossbreeding and linebreeding (closebreeding) may be effectively done at minimum cost for quality sires. The matings often produce outstanding individuals, especially future sires for AI proving.

11. **Reduces sire costs**— For the average dairy owners who might keep two bulls for a 50- to 75-cow milking herd, one extra cow kept instead of a bull will pay the cost every year of owning a bull, as far as herd services (compared to natural use of bulls) are concerned, and the dairy owners will be using better sires than they could afford to own.

If good herd management is carried out properly, there are few disadvantages of artificial insemination. This is particularly true when the dollar gains in improved production are considered. Some of the early objections voiced against artificial insemination were:

1. "Too much trouble to check cows for heat several times a day," and "Can't catch heifers in heat."

2. "Too much trouble to keep the cow up and call the inseminator," or, for herd operators inseminating cows under their control, "Too tired at the end of a long day and easier to use the bull."

3. "Artificial insemination has ruined the bull market."

4

4. "Too much trouble to identify cows and keep all those records."

5. "Can't get cows settled on time."

6. "Don't like the bulls used in artificial insemination."

7. "Takes too much time and labor."

8. "Can spread disease from herd to herd."

9. "May increase number of inherited or lethal defects transmitted by a 'carrier' sire."

10. "Get too many bull calves."

The early objections to artificial insemination came mostly from dairy producers but are seldom heard today. Beef cattle producers, due to range conditions and topography of the land, find artificial insemination impractical in some cases.

We mention, but do not endorse, those objections originally raised against artificial insemination. When one considers the adoption of any program for herd improvement, the problem arises as to matters of comparison involving present and past established procedures. Improvement or progress does not come without changes in practices. In view of the worldwide expansion in the use of artificial insemination, any comparison becomes one of the flexibility of a producer to adjust operations to utilize a program that will improve the herd from the standpoint of genetic potential. That is, the producer must decide to use better sires that will increase the milk check or the beef, swine, goat, or sheep income.

Artificial insemination has been in wide usage for over 60 years. It is well documented that most of the objections to AI are without basis. For example, the sex ratio of calves resulting from AI is the same as for natural service. Actually, both the spread of disease and the inheritance of defects are better controlled than where natural service is used.

## Some Considerations for Producers

In any well-managed herd, adequate records of breeding, calving, disease, injury, and abnormalities are necessary. Practical and accurate identification of each animal is a must for good management. In a healthy, well-managed herd, a high percentage of the females, if properly inseminated at the correct state of heat, can settle on the first service. The direct herd semen sales program ("do-it-yourself" system) is in wide use in America and has proved satisfactory when the inseminator is well trained and the herd is properly managed.

*Does artificial insemination discourage breeders of registered cattle to produce sires?* No, not if they desire to meet the challenge of producing proven or promising young sires in the top 5 to 10 percent of the breed in terms of performance records. Never has the opportunity been so promising nor the demand for superior seed stock so great.

There are few, if any, disadvantages of artificial insemination for the individual who desires to improve a herd so as to enjoy more income and to attain the satisfaction that comes from breeding superior animals.

AI brings these opportunities to producers:

1. Producers can use almost any leading dairy or beef bull, based on performance, from any of 5 or more AI centers. They don't have to guess. Records of milk, fat, and protein production, calving ease, and conformation are available on most dairy sires in AI use. Likewise, producers don't have to guess about beef sires in AI

use, because records for weaning weight, yearling weight, and other important traits are available from the breed associations.

2. Frozen semen, with its adequate shipping accommodations, makes any bull used in artificial insemination in the United States available almost anywhere in the world where suitable facilities exist for handling and utilizing frozen semen.

3. Today any producer can secure a choice of superior dairy or beef bulls.

4. If high-production, proven sires are used for artificial insemination, as is true of nearly all dairy sires in regular use in America, decided improvement in milk production can be made. Artificial insemination furnishes the sires to transmit the *genetic potential for improved production*. When adequate feed and management are supplied to cattle, the inherited ability is expressed in terms of pounds of milk or pounds of beef or both.

A good example of improved genetic potential for high milk yield is indicated by the increase in average annual production per cow in the United States between 1940 and 2001 (Table 1.1).

Note that in 1940, the average yield for cows in the United States was 4,622 pounds of milk. By 1970, 30 years after the AI program in America began, the average milk yield was 9,751 pounds, over twice that in 1940. By 2001, the average milk yield per cow was 18,139 pounds—an increase of more than 13,500 pounds of milk per cow per year for the 60-year period. It is also interesting to note in Table 1.1 that 9.115 million cows in 2001 produced nearly 56 billion pounds more milk than the 24.94 million cows reported for 1940. As is well known in dairy circles, the income per cow is closely correlated with the level of milk production.

However, all of the above-reported increase in milk production per cow cannot be attributed solely to artificial insemination. Dairy herds have become larger (an average of 25 cows in 1940 and 119 in 2001), dairy farms are more specialized, and management is much improved. Yet if the genetic potential

**Table 1.1.** Milk Production from U.S. Dairy Cows, 1940–2001[a]

| Year | Milk Cows[b] | Milk Production per Cow | Total U.S. Milk Production |
|------|------------|------------------------|---------------------------|
| | *(thousands)* | *(lbs.)* | *(million lbs.)* |
| 1940 | 24,940 | 4,622 | 109,412 |
| 1950 | 22,000 | 5,314 | 116,602 |
| 1960 | 17,650 | 7,029 | 123,109 |
| 1970 | 12,091 | 9,751 | 117,007 |
| 1980 | 10,758 | 11,891 | 128,406 |
| 1990 | 10,015 | 14,782 | 147,721 |
| 2001 | 9,115 | 18,139 | 165,336 |

[a]USDA/NASS. February 2002. Milk Production.

for which artificial insemination can claim much credit had not been provided, the high yield per cow could not have been attained.

In beef cattle, the use of superior, performance-tested sires by means of artificial insemination, in many cases involving crossbreeding, results in calves with a heavier weaning and yearling weight. In addition, greater pounds of gain per day in the feedlot result.

These developments have written a new chapter in the history of agriculture. Artificial insemination is available today for improvement in dairy cattle, beef cattle, goats, swine, horses, turkeys, sheep, honey bees, dogs, and other animals. It is also used in humans to combat low fertility.

Artificial insemination and embryo transfer provide the tools for mass improvement of livestock. Technological refinements in the use of AI and breeding programs will be made continually. We urge every breeder to keep abreast and take advantage of all developing information.

There are advances being made in molecular biology, including in-vitro fertilization, cloning, and the production of transgenic animals—advances that could change many concepts in animal genetics.

## QUESTIONS

1. What are six of the chief advantages of artificial insemination for dairy cattle? For beef cattle?

2. Are there any disadvantages of artificial insemination for dairy cattle? For beef cattle? Explain.

3. Why does the use of artificial insemination generally result in better record keeping and improved herd management?

4. How does artificial insemination aid in reducing diseases that can be spread by the bull in natural service?

5. Why is the use of artificial insemination very important in sampling and obtaining a progeny proof on sires?

6. Has artificial insemination aided in increasing milk production per cow in America? Explain.

7. How does the use of artificial insemination aid in detecting bulls of low fertility?

8. In which species of farm animals is artificial insemination most practical and in general use at the present time?

## REFERENCES

Ensminger, M. E. 1992. The Stockman's Handbook (7th Ed.). Interstate Publishers, Inc., Danville, IL.

Foote, R. H. 1999. Artificial insemination from the origins up to today. Proc. Int. Symposium: Artificial Insemination to the Modern Biotechnologies. V. Russo, S. Dall 'Olio, L. Fontanesi. eds. Reggio Emilia, Italy, October 8–9, 1999.

Herman, H. A. 1981. Improving Cattle by the Millions. Univ. of Missouri Press, Columbia.

Olson, K. E., 2001. Dairy Farm Numbers Drop to 76,630, Hoard's Dairyman, October 25, 2001.

## WEB SITES

Dairy industry
   *http://www.hoards.com*

U.S. cattle numbers and production
   *http://www.usda.gov/nass/publications*

# EXERCISE 2

# Status and Development of AI in the United States

## OBJECT

To become familiar with the growth, development, and present-day activity of AI in the United States.

## DISCUSSION

There have been many changes in AI since it began in 1938. The trend since 1950 has been toward fewer and larger AI centers. Due to economic pressure and changing technology, the number of AI centers (semen-producing businesses) declined from 97 in 1950 (Table 2.1) to 5 in 2001. The reduction in the number of AI centers resulted from mergers, consolidations, and the federation of many businesses founded between 1938 and 1950. One of the largest federated AI centers is Select Sires, Inc., of Plain City, Ohio, a cooperative formed by the union of 12 farmer-owned cooperative AI centers. Cooperative Resources International is a holding cooperative, with subsidiaries that include AI cooperatives, a dairy record provider cooperative, and a livestock auction cooperative. The AI subsidiary is a consolidation of five farmer-owned AI cooperatives.

The large AI organizations (AI centers), because of a greater volume of business, are able to make more efficient use of semen, breed more cows per sire, maintain more high-production, transmitting sires, and carry on constructive "young sire sampling" programs. Also, there is more efficient use of housing, equipment, laboratory facilities, and human resources. The result is greater production per employee and higher utilization of the best-proven sires. These factors account for the cost of semen, or AI service in America, being highly competitive and very reasonable.

The development and widespread use of frozen semen materially paved the way for fewer but larger AI centers and greater use of the best sires. Because it is possible to store frozen semen for years, distribution of semen and supplies to technicians and regional areas is simplified as compared to distribution of liquid semen, for which time and distance are factors. Using frozen semen, an AI center at any given location can distribute semen to all 50 states and to any place else in the world where transportation is available. With liquid nitrogen as a dependable refrigerant, semen is safely stored at $-320°$ F $(-196°$ C) in the AI technician's container for use over an indefinite period. Frozen semen also may be stored on the farms and ranches of herd owners for use in "do-it-yourself" programs.

Frozen semen makes possible the exchange, or transfer, of semen among AI centers. This advance encouraged some of the smaller AI centers facing high overhead costs to merge or dispose of their bulls and become inseminating businesses. This step is progressive, for in most cases more desirable sires are used, and the overhead cost of semen per unit is less when semen is fully utilized.

One of the factors contributing to larger and fewer AI centers is the marked decline in the number of dairy cows and dairy herds beginning in 1946, when there were nearly 27 million milk cows in the United States. For

9

**Table 2.1.** Early Growth and Development of the AI Program in the United States, 1939–1971, Inclusive

| Year | AI Centers | Sires in Service | | | | Herds[a] | Dairy Cows Bred to | | Beef Cows Bred to Beef Bulls | Total Cattle Bred | Cows Bred per Sire |
|---|---|---|---|---|---|---|---|---|---|---|---|
| | | Dairy | Beef | Total | Avg. per Center | | Dairy Bulls | Beef Bulls | | | |
| 1939 | 7 | | | 33 | 4.7 | 646 | | | | 7,359 | 228 |
| 1940 | 25 | | | 138 | 5.5 | 2,971 | | | | 33,977 | 246 |
| 1941 | 35 | | | 237 | 6.8 | 5,997 | | | | 70,751 | 299 |
| 1942 | 46 | | | 412 | 9.0 | 12,118 | | | | 112,788 | 274 |
| 1943 | 59 | | | 574 | 9.7 | 23,448 | | | | 182,524 | 318 |
| 1944 | 56 | | | 657 | 11.7 | 28,627 | | | | 218,070 | 332 |
| 1945 | 67 | | | 729 | 10.9 | 43,998 | | | | 360,732 | 495 |
| 1946 | 78 | | | 900 | 11.5 | 73,293 | | | | 537,376 | 597 |
| 1947 | 84 | | | 1,453 | 17.3 | 140,571 | | | | 1,184,168 | 815 |
| 1948 | 91 | | | 1,745 | 19.2 | 224,493 | | | | 1,713,581 | 982 |
| 1949 | 90 | | | 1,940 | 21.6 | 316,177 | | | | 2,091,175 | 1,078 |
| 1950 | 97 | | | 2,104 | 21.7 | 409,300 | | | | 2,619,555 | 1,245 |
| 1951 | 94 | | | 2,187 | 23.3 | 548,300 | | | | 3,509,573 | 1,605 |
| 1952 | 94 | | | 2,324 | 24.7 | 671,100 | | | | 4,295,243 | 1,848 |
| 1953 | 96 | | | 2,598 | 27.1 | 755,000 | | | | 4,845,222 | 1,865 |
| 1954 | 93 | | | 2,661 | 28.6 | 805,000 | | | | 5,155,240 | 1,937 |
| 1955 | 79 | | | 2,450 | 31.0 | 845,900 | | | | 5,413,874 | 2,210 |
| 1956 | 79 | | | 2,533 | 32.3 | 900,400 | | | | 5,762,656 | 2,257 |
| 1957 | 75 | | | 2,651 | 35.3 | 946,000 | | | | 6,055,982 | 2,284 |
| 1958 | 71 | | | 2,676 | 37.7 | 975,372 | | | | 6,645,568 | 2,483 |
| 1959 | 64 | | | 2,460 | 38.4 | 930,059 | | | | 6,932,294 | 2,816 |
| 1960 | 62 | | | 2,544 | 41.0 | 910,000 | | | | 7,144,679 | 2,808 |
| 1961 | 56 | 2,036 | | 2,486 | 44.4 | 863,781 | 7,047,148 | 435,592[b] | | 7,482,740 | 3,010 |
| 1962 | 56 | 2,158 | 420 | 2,456 | 43.9 | 862,150 | 6,837,681 | 911,006[b] | | 7,748,687 | 3,155 |
| 1963 | 51 | 2,140 | 401 | 2,559 | 50.2 | 621,141 | 6,468,545 | 969,748 | 235,289 | 7,673,582 | 2,999 |
| 1964 | 50 | 1,867 | 398 | 2,538 | 50.8 | 654,311 | 6,165,599 | 1,117,395 | 464,959 | 7,747,953 | 3,053 |
| 1965 | 46[c] | 1,949 | 449 | 2,316 | 50.3 | 591,859 | 6,301,178 | 963,657 | 615,147 | 7,879,982 | 3,402 |
| 1966 | 44[c] | 2,012 | 439 | 2,388 | 54.3 | 540,265 | 6,413,453 | 873,127 | 695,181 | 7,981,761 | 3,342 |
| 1967 | 35 | 2,028 | 364 | 2,376 | 67.9 | 458,782 | 6,259,425 | 788,933 | 672,819 | 7,871,265[d] | 3,313 |
| 1968 | 33[c] | 1,955 | 352 | 2,380 | 72.1 | 407,375 | 6,423,786 | 714,850 | 695,242 | 7,933,878 | 3,334 |
| 1969 | 30[c] | 1,911 | 390 | 2,345 | 78.2 | 387,979 | 6,590,147 | 694,916 | 924,381 | 8,209,444 | 3,501 |
| 1970 | 31 | 1,958 | 364 | 2,275 | 73.4 | 369,197 | 6,693,216[e] | 615,322 | 1,258,446[e] | 8,566,984 | 3,641[e,f] |
| 1971 | 24[f] | 2,167 | 349 | 2,307 | 96.1 | 350,611 | 6,759,215 | 525,956 | 1,357,918 | 8,643,089 | 3,620[f] |
| | 26[f] | | 347 | 2,514 | 96.7 | | | | | | |

[a] Prior to 1963, number of herds largely reflected membership, rather than those actually serviced.

[b] Probably includes some beef-to-beef inseminations.

[c] Includes one all-beef AI center.

[d] Total cattle bred in 1967 includes 150,088 first services, by state only, where breakdowns were not reported.

[e] Corrected figures.

10

2001, cows in milk totaled about 9.12 million head, a decrease of 17.88 million milk cows.

Dairy herds, while less numerous, are much larger and more widely scattered in rural areas. In 1940, there were 4.6 million farms reporting milk cows. In 1992, the number was only 131,535 and in 2001 only 76,630 herds. The number of cows per herd increased 62% from 72 in 1992 to 119 in 2001[1]. These developments brought about many adjustments in AI. In some cases, local AI technicians found their business disappearing as herds dispersed. The "do-it-yourself" program became a part of the answer for dairy operators, as will be discussed later.

In 2001, the organized AI centers in the United States furnished most of the semen for the insemination of between 9 and 10 million dairy and beef cows and heifers. In addition, over 8.7 million units of dairy bull semen and 806,000 units of beef bull semen were exported. Note in Table 2.2 that more than 1.9 million units of beef semen were custom collected. This semen either was used in 2001 or was stored for future use.

## Beef AI Developments

Beginning about 1950, many AI centers that previously had only dairy sires added beef bulls. Thousands of dairy producers converting to beef over the past 50 years have successfully used beef bulls. Many dairy owners, particularly in the western states, breed first-calf heifers to Angus bulls so as to obtain a smaller calf and to avoid calving troubles. Some dairy owners in less-intensely populated dairy cattle areas, with grazing land available, inseminate their lower-producing cows to beef bulls and sell the resulting offspring for slaughter purposes. In general, the first beef

bulls utilized by AI organizations were not the kind to excite a dyed-in-the-wool beef cattle breeder. For the most part, dairy producers wanted a "black calf" or "whiteface calf." As commercial beef producers have turned to artificial insemination, the caliber of beef bulls used by the AI organizations has improved steadily.

For many years the anti-AI policy of beef registry associations served as a deterrent to the use of artificial insemination between herds, except that several herd owners could own a bull jointly. Fortunately this picture changed as more beef registry associations, spurred by the "new breeds" or "exotics," adopted an "open AI policy." The result is an increasing number of carefully selected, above-average beef bulls being added to AI centers.

In 1963, the first year "beef-to-beef" matings were tabulated separately, a total of 235,289 beef cows were reported. In 1971, the total was 1,357,918, not including the use of artificial insemination in private herds. (See Table 2.1, which is presented only to show gains in AI by years before growth was measured in semen units.) In 2001, it is estimated that some 2.9 million beef cows were bred by AI.

Beginning in 1961, dairy cows inseminated to beef bulls were tabulated separately. That year, 435,592 milk cows were bred to beef bulls. In 1964, with the number of dairy herds declining rapidly, a total of 1,117,395 milk cows were bred to beef bulls (Table 2.1). Since that time, the number of dairy cows bred to beef bulls by artificial insemination has declined. The use of artificial insemination in beef cattle is increasing gradually and is expected to continue. Improved estrus and ovulation synchronization programs will have the biggest impact on AI use in commercial beef operations. Artificial insemination of beef cattle will be discussed in one of the exercises to follow.

---

[1] Kenneth E. Olson, Dairy Farm Numbers Drop to 76,630, Hoard's Dairyman, October 25, 2001, p. 663.

## Increase in the Number of Cows Inseminated

In 1950, when 97 AI centers were in operation in the United States, 2,619,555 milk cows in 409,300 herds were inseminated.

The average AI center maintained 21.7 sires, and 1,245 cows were bred per sire. In 1971, with 24 AI centers reporting, a total of 8,643,089 dairy and beef cows were inseminated at least once. The average AI center maintained about 96 sires, some of them

**Table 2.2.** Units of Semen Sold for Domestic Use, Exported, and Custom Frozen, United States, 1971–2001[a]

| | Dairy Semen Units | | | |
|---|---|---|---|---|
| Year | Domestic | Export | Custom | Total |
| 1971 | 10,876,840 | 467,989 | 336,314 | 11,681,143 |
| 1972 | 11,817,867 | 654,162 | 421,060 | 12,893,089 |
| 1973 | 11,338,980 | 682,307 | 534,972 | 12,556,259 |
| 1974 | 10,887,456 | 761,756 | 616,104 | 12,265,316 |
| 1975 | 9,760,054 | 979,850 | 613,164 | 11,353,068 |
| 1976 | 10,753,149 | 1,389,921 | 570,241 | 12,713,311 |
| 1977 | 10,907,322 | 1,448,140 | 573,607 | 12,929,069 |
| 1978 | 11,858,425 | 1,630,677 | 587,463 | 14,076,565 |
| 1979 | 12,467,351 | 1,836,000 | 681,563 | 14,984,914 |
| 1980 | 13,337,420 | 2,135,106 | 758,886 | 16,231,412 |
| 1981 | 13,331,748 | 2,233,413 | 979,465 | 16,544,626 |
| 1982 | 12,767,925 | 2,616,184 | 1,240,959 | 16,625,068 |
| 1983 | 12,857,323 | 2,763,497 | 921,709 | 16,542,529 |
| 1984 | 12,426,650 | 2,787,803 | 864,698 | 16,079,151 |
| 1985 | 12,813,645 | 2,523,673 | 641,633 | 15,978,951 |
| 1986 | 12,269,830 | 3,338,068 | 613,162 | 16,221,060 |
| 1987 | 12,929,684 | 3,680,110 | 735,314 | 17,345,108 |
| 1988 | 12,994,438 | 4,276,541 | 694,512 | 17,965,491 |
| 1989 | 12,769,532 | 4,306,906 | 760,796 | 17,837,234 |
| 1990 | 13,272,003 | 4,633,885 | 863,504 | 18,769,392 |
| 1991 | 12,637,925 | 4,660,559 | 736,317 | 18,034,801 |
| 1992 | 13,117,391 | 5,131,450 | 642,693 | 18,891,534 |
| 1993 | 12,957,368 | 6,307,345 | 711,308 | 19,976,021 |
| 1994 | 12,608,523 | 6,942,871 | 736,789 | 20,288,183 |
| 1995 | 12,787,192 | 8,149,238 | 713,890 | 21,650,320 |
| 1996 | 12,677,139 | 8,144,036 | 638,410 | 21,459,685 |
| 1997 | 12,389,241 | 8,756,759 | 637,220 | 21,783,220 |
| 1998 | 12,711,670 | 8,789,700 | 642,615 | 22,143,985 |
| 1999 | 13,621,160 | 8,420,685 | 637,755 | 22,679,600 |
| 2000 | 13,387,523 | 8,177,628 | 699,432 | 22,264,583 |
| 2001 | 14,423,416 | 8,775,424 | 826,151 | 24,024,991 |

*(Continued)*

**Table 2.2.** (Continued)

| | Beef Semen Units | | | |
|---|---|---|---|---|
| Year | Domestic | Export | Custom | Total |
| 1971 | 2,076,778 | 159,121 | 1,055,409 | 3,291,308 |
| 1972 | 2,382,955 | 213,590 | 1,144,903 | 3,741,448 |
| 1973 | 2,719,052 | 348,733 | 1,092,334 | 4,160,119 |
| 1974 | 2,869,569 | 385,153 | 1,675,843 | 4,930,565 |
| 1975 | 1,712,264 | 167,938 | 1,425,958 | 3,306,160 |
| 1976 | 1,368,618 | 179,110 | 1,273,946 | 2,821,674 |
| 1977 | 1,109,291 | 204,210 | 1,014,015 | 2,327,516 |
| 1978 | 1,019,945 | 149,399 | 1,019,984 | 2,189,328 |
| 1979 | 1,086,339 | 240,032 | 1,124,586 | 2,450,957 |
| 1980 | 1,034,166 | 253,950 | 1,472,521 | 2,760,637 |
| 1981 | 972,556 | 175,617 | 1,651,212 | 2,799,385 |
| 1982 | 863,603 | 152,096 | 1,567,507 | 2,583,206 |
| 1983 | 885,938 | 102,811 | 1,757,284 | 2,746,033 |
| 1984 | 811,306 | 159,034 | 1,927,399 | 2,897,739 |
| 1985 | 754,570 | 143,794 | 1,400,342 | 2,298,706 |
| 1986 | 694,625 | 143,642 | 923,578 | 1,761,845 |
| 1987 | 709,627 | 161,882 | 729,111 | 1,600,620 |
| 1988 | 780,844 | 244,159 | 1,086,160 | 2,111,163 |
| 1989 | 822,204 | 242,512 | 1,069,476 | 2,134,192 |
| 1990 | 880,935 | 268,471 | 1,257,196 | 2,406,602 |
| 1991 | 1,017,026 | 304,695 | 1,320,524 | 2,642,245 |
| 1992 | 1,074,645 | 451,158 | 1,522,314 | 3,048,117 |
| 1993 | 1,117,798 | 393,365 | 1,747,424 | 3,258,587 |
| 1994 | 1,156,635 | 596,412 | 2,116,399 | 3,869,346 |
| 1995 | 997,131 | 490,076 | 1,882,121 | 3,369,328 |
| 1996 | 903,224 | 438,430 | 1,762,140 | 3,103,794 |
| 1997 | 918,455 | 869,306 | 1,967,313 | 3,755,074 |
| 1998 | 907,251 | 848,677 | 2,160,216 | 3,916,144 |
| 1999 | 898,382 | 771,410 | 2,304,367 | 3,974,159 |
| 2000 | 995,211 | 733,718 | 2,304,787 | 4,033,716 |
| 2001 | 926,872 | 806,030 | 1,995,721 | 3,728,623 |

[a]Data provided by the National Association of Animal Breeders, Inc., P.O. Box 1033, Columbia, MO 65005.

young sires being sampled for proving and an average of 3,620 cows per sire were inseminated (Table 2.1). The organized AI centers do not account for all of the semen produced or all of the cows inseminated. Since the introduction of frozen semen, beginning in 1953, an increasing number of dairy cattle breeders and beef cattle operators have had semen from their bulls custom frozen. Some of this semen enters trade channels; however, much of it is used in the sire owners' herds, furnished to cooperating breeders who may have had part ownership of the bulls, or stored for future use. During 2001, there were 1,995,721 units of beef semen and 826,151 units of dairy semen reported custom frozen (Table 2.2). There is no way to determine how much of the custom frozen semen is actually utilized to breed cows.

## Growth of the AI Program—Units of Semen

The progress of AI from 1939 to 1971 is shown in Table 2.1. These data were compiled by the USDA and the NAAB. Semen sold and custom frozen from 1971 to 2001 inclusive is indicated in Table 2.2.

## Estimated Volume Based on Units

Since 1971, the volume of AI business in the United States has been estimated in terms of "units of semen." (A unit of semen is designated as the amount needed for one insemination.) This reporting of units became necessary because of changes in methods of distributing semen by AI organizations and ways of reporting its usage. Since much semen is sold directly to herd operators through distributors, who may or may not provide insemination services, it is impossible to determine accurately the number of first services. In many cases some of the semen is stored for future use; in some cases it is resold. The custom freezing businesses generally do not know

how much of the semen frozen from a given bull is used or how much is stored and then sold to other breeders. Accurate records of units of semen produced and sold are maintained and reported by all established AI centers and most custom freezing businesses.

The disadvantage of estimating AI volume in terms of units of semen is that the number of cows bred by AI cannot be accurately determined; however, it is better to estimate volume on reliable figures rather than on speculation. In general, it requires 1.6 to 2.2 units of semen to get a dairy cow in calf. In beef artificial insemination, where clean-up bulls are used, about 1.3 to 1.5 units of semen are utilized per cow settled. This figure, of course, applies only to those cows that settle on the first, or in some cases the second, service.

The estimates, in terms of units of semen sold by AI centers and custom frozen as reported for 1971 through 2001, are listed in Table 2.2.

## Registered Livestock and Artificial Insemination

In the early days of artificial insemination, there was a clamor that AI would ruin the bull market. This has turned out to be far from factual, if cattle improvement is the objective.

Progressive purebred beef and dairy breeders often work closely with AI centers. Proven dairy sires, available through artificial insemination, are genetically superior to those most breeders own. These sires are mated to outstanding cows in breeders' herds to produce sires for the future. In many cases, the calves, if bulls, are optioned to the AI organization when the cows are inseminated. Dairy cattle breeders cooperate in "young sire sampling" programs and often own an interest in such bulls. Although fewer bulls are now sold by breeders, only the most promising bulls, backed by high production and good conformation, are selected, and the selling price is usually several times that of bulls sold for natural breeding. The same type of sire procurement and breeder co-operation for beef sires is developing.

About 75 to 80 percent of the 12.8 million milk cows and heifers of breeding age are bred artificially, but only 5 to 10% of the 38.5 million beef cows and heifers of breeding age are bred artificially.

At the present time, animals registered as a result of artificial insemination, by the various breeds, on a percentage basis, are:

### Dairy

| | |
|---|---|
| Brown Swiss | 78 percent |
| Jersey | 81 percent |
| Holstein | 81 percent |
| Guernsey | 81 percent |
| Milking Shorthorn | 45 percent |

### Beef

| | |
|---|---|
| Angus | 45 percent |
| Charolais | 14 percent |
| Hereford | 10 percent |
| Red Angus | 14 percent |
| Simmental | 50 percent |

For the most part, AI offers a challenge to breeders of registered cattle because they have the opportunity to produce sires that can improve thousands of cattle rather than 100 or 200 as provided by natural service. An ever-increasing number of key purebred breeders utilize AI in their own herds to produce matings from outstanding sires proven in artificial insemination.

Young dairy sires being sampled in the United States are of high genetic merit for desired traits and are in demand throughout the world.

The number of cows inseminated per bull is largely a matter of semen utilization and demand for key production sires. Those sires with a good conception rate, 60 percent or better on first service, tend to be utilized more heavily. Frozen semen and the direct sale of semen to herd operators' "do-it-yourself" programs are responsible for an increased number of cows serviced per sire. It is not unusual to find some of the AI organizations selling from a few thousand to over 30,000 units of semen annually from a bull in high demand. Sales and custom freezing of semen by breeds in 2001 are shown in Table 2.3.

## The National Association of Animal Breeders, Inc. (NAAB)

In the United States, livestock improvement utilizing AI is strictly a free enterprise. Artificial insemination in America is unique because it receives no direct federal aid. In a few instances, there is limited state aid to support livestock improvement programs. The organizations supplying semen, insemination service, and custom freezing service are banded together in the National Association of Animal Breeders, Inc. (NAAB), to promote and carry out a program of quality service with high professional and ethical standards.

The National Association of Animal Breeders, Inc., whose headquarters are at 401 Bernadette Drive, P.O. Box 1033, Columbia, MO 65205, grew out of a series of "managers' meetings," beginning late in 1946 in Tiffin, Ohio. The official name "National Association of Artificial Breeders" was adopted in 1948. In 1964, the name "National Association of Animal Breeders, Inc.," was adopted in deference to better English. The association is supported entirely by its members on an assessment basis. It is a non-profit organization dedicated to mass livestock improvement through the use of AI. Its functions are services to the industry, education, regulation, research, public relations, and promotion. The Articles of Incorporation, as amended in 1976, state:

> The principal business and purpose of this association shall be to unite those individuals and organizations engaged in the artificial insemination of cattle and other livestock into

**Table 2.3.** Units of Semen Sold for Domestic Use, Exported, and Custom Frozen, by Breed, 2001[a]

## Dairy Breeds (Units of Semen)

| Breed | Domestic | Export | Custom | Total |
|---|---|---|---|---|
| Ayrshire | 37,385 | 20,084 | 2,933 | 60,402 |
| Brown Swiss | 134,584 | 334,600 | 52,412 | 521,596 |
| Guernsey | 52,425 | 13,915 | 4,419 | 70,759 |
| Holstein | 13,346,991 | 7,897,295 | 710,363 | 21,954,649 |
| Jersey | 828,754 | 507,148 | 53,209 | 1,390,111 |
| Milking Shorthorn | 15,621 | 1,937 | 2,815 | 20,373 |
| Other Dairy | 6,656 | 445 | 0 | 7,101 |
| Total | 14,423,416 | 8,775,424 | 826,151 | 24,024,991 |

## Beef Breeds (Units of Semen)

| Breed | Domestic | Export | Custom | Total |
|---|---|---|---|---|
| Angus | 651,508 | 248,622 | 608,739 | 1,508,869 |
| Beefmaster | 216 | 860 | 55,690 | 56,766 |
| Belgian Blue | 500 | 1,445 | 1,164 | 3,109 |
| Brahman | 14,146 | 66,078 | 27,248 | 107,472 |
| Brahmental/Simbrah | 357 | 0 | 4,268 | 4,625 |
| Brangus | 6,812 | 9,806 | 84,800 | 101,418 |
| Braunvieh | 284 | 520 | 9,076 | 9,880 |
| Charolais | 18,805 | 14,963 | 78,868 | 112,636 |
| Chi-Angus | 163 | — | 18,516 | 18,679 |
| Chi-Maine | 1,006 | 0 | 44,657 | 45,663 |
| Chianina | 806 | 10 | 12,288 | 13,104 |
| Gelbvieh | 9,466 | 4,207 | 54,537 | 68,210 |
| Hereford | 4,020 | 305 | 46,837 | 51,162 |
| Limousin | 10,639 | 14,690 | 77,275 | 102,604 |
| Longhorn | 954 | 52 | 5,007 | 6,013 |
| Maine-Anjou | 4,154 | 42 | 94,818 | 99,014 |
| Nellore | 80 | 0 | 23,049 | 23,129 |
| Piedmont | 1,170 | 80 | 12,171 | 13,421 |
| Polled Hereford | 37,560 | 49,331 | 61,824 | 148,715 |
| Red Angus | 81,665 | 338,714 | 169,635 | 590,014 |
| Red Brahman | 618 | 1,950 | 3,517 | 6,085 |
| Red Brangus | 38 | 3,730 | 22,962 | 26,730 |
| Romagnola | 121 | 21 | 3,199 | 3,341 |
| Salers | 278 | 0 | 16,039 | 16,317 |
| Santa Gertrudis | 135 | 0 | 4,729 | 4,864 |
| Senapol | 27 | 4,270 | 54,759 | 59,056 |
| Shorthorn | 2,374 | 1,761 | 18,851 | 22,986 |

*(Continued)*

**Table 2.3.** (Continued)

| Beef Breeds (Units of Semen) | | | | |
|---|---|---|---|---|
| Breed | Domestic | Export | Custom | Total |
| Shorthorn (Scotch) | 826 | 20 | 44,302 | 45,148 |
| Simmental | 70,779 | 40,425 | 55,716 | 166,920 |
| South Devon | 16 | 0 | 5,337 | 5,353 |
| Wagyu | 11 | 1,915 | 70,672 | 72,598 |
| Other Beef | 5,863 | 728 | 156,632 | 163,223 |
| Total | 925,397 | 804,545 | 1,947,182 | 3,677,124 |

[a]Data provided by the National Association of Animal Breeders, Inc., P.O. Box 1033, Columbia, MO 65205.

an affiliated federation operating under self-imposed standards of performance and conduct and to promote the mutual interests and ideals of its members and to develop and recommend procedures to protect users of semen, and persons and corporations utilizing artificial insemination to the extent technically feasible. The Association shall not, in any manner, engage in a regular business of a kind ordinarily carried on for a profit.

Many years ago, a "Code of Ethics" was adopted stipulating the manner in which members and associate members shall conduct their affairs and practices to carry out the aims and objectives of the association. While revised to keep pace with changes within the industry, this code has served a very useful purpose.

There are two classes of NAAB membership:

1. **Regular member—** Any individual or business who is engaged in the collection, processing, and freezing of semen for the artificial insemination of livestock or holds equity in a member organization in a ratio approximating the proportionate usage of semen produced by said organization may be admitted to membership as a regular voting member of the association.

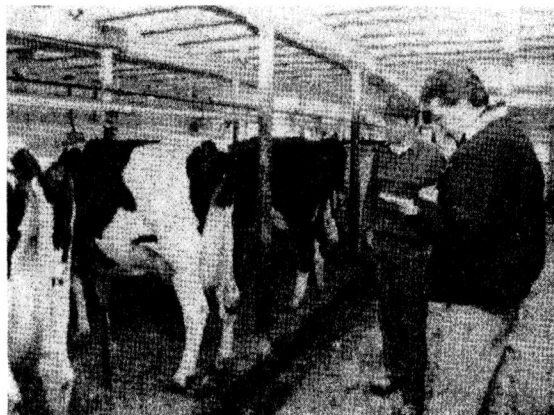

**Figure 2.1.** Evaluating young sire daughters in an AI progeny test herd. (Courtesy, Eastern AI Cooperative, Ithaca, NY)

2. **Associate member—** Any individual or business that has established interest in the purposes of the association may become a non-voting member of the association.

Included among members and associate members are all major AI centers and most custom freezing businesses in the United States.

The association, with the support of its members' organizations, encourages and promotes an extensive research program in reproductive physiology, genetics, and sire health.

The slogan of the NAAB, "Better Cattle for Better Living," along with the adopted insignia, is copyrighted.

A magazine, *Advanced Animal Breeder* (previously *The A.I. Digest*), was published until January 1, 1986. This publication carried information on new developments in AI and news concerning member organizations. It circulated throughout the United States, Canada, Mexico, and overseas countries.

A convention is held each year during which association business is conducted and the latest developments in the AI program are reviewed.

Every two years, the NAAB Technical Conference on Artificial Insemination and Reproduction is held. This conference brings together technical workers in the AI field, university professors, research workers, veterinarians, and equipment manufacturers. It has proved to be an effective means of disseminating technical information, and the proceedings of each conference are an important resource for AI workers and reproduction specialists. The NAAB Technical Committee has the responsibility for this conference.

In addition to proceedings of its conferences, which are sold, the NAAB has informational materials available on beef artificial insemination, technician training, sire health,

careers in AI, its cross-reference program, sire evaluation, and other AI-related topics.

The NAAB also works closely with the Purebred Dairy Cattle Association. The NAAB has the cooperation of many federal agencies and dairy and beef organizations, as well as other farm organizations.

**Export Semen Sales—** One of the most pronounced and successful developments of AI in the United States is global marketing.

Since the early 70s, the volume of semen exported has grown steadily. In 1975, only about 1 million units of semen were exported, but in 2001, over 9 million units of semen, with a value of over $52 million, were sold to 85 overseas countries. (See Tables 2.2, 2.3, and 2.4.)

The export market has been developed by the combined efforts of the NAAB staff, government agencies, and individual NAAB members. The export market, which has grown and is still expanding, is the result of the sire-proving program carried out by the AI organizations, cattle breeders, the breed registry organizations, and cooperating agencies. At present, the United States can claim most of the highest-ranking, production-tested bulls in the world.

**Table 2.4.  Semen Export Sales[a]**

| | Dollar Value of Export Sales[b] | |
| --- | --- | --- |
| | **2000** | **2001** |
| Dairy | $ 49,902,173 | $ 50,055,918 |
| Beef | $ 2,198,928 | $ 2,127,481 |
| Total | $ 52,101,101 | $ 52,183,391 |

[a]Data provided by the National Association of Animal Breeders, Inc., P.O. Box 1033, Columbia, MO 65205.

[b]Based on quarterly survey of semen sold for export.

## Certified Semen Services, Inc. (CSS)

In February 1976, the NAAB, so that AI in America could be effectively self-regulated, created a wholly-owned subsidiary, Certified Semen Services, Inc. (CSS). Its purpose is to establish rules and procedures for certification of businesses processing livestock semen. CSS is the service arm of the NAAB, which is the trade association for the AI industry.

The initial primary objective of CSS was to provide an auditing program for the procedures related to identification of bulls and semen used in AI. Each NAAB member AI center is visited by the CSS director at least yearly, all procedures and records are checked, and a semen identification audit is made. However, activities have been extended to the checking and certification of sire health standards as set forth in the "CSS Minimum Requirements for Disease Control of Semen Produced for AI." Thus, a sire health audit as well as a semen identification audit is a part of this progressive program.

All NAAB members are required to participate in CSS. Non-member AI centers and custom freezing businesses can participate in the CSS program by entering into an agreement for services with CSS. Also, semen distributors who purchase semen for resale only from a CSS-approved semen producer are eligible to participate and use the CSS-exclusive distributor logo. CSS is now international in scope, with four centers in three different countries participating.

The livestock breeder must have confidence in the supplier of semen, related AI services, and the product (unit of semen) purchased. CSS aids in furthering the integrity and accuracy of artificial insemination.

## PROCEDURE

If you have not already done so, read the Introduction and Exercise 1. Try to visualize the evolution of AI, and ask yourself why the growth has been steady.

## QUESTIONS

1. When was artificial insemination (AI) first employed for domestic livestock?

2. When did AI in America begin? Briefly outline the early developments.

3. What percentage of the milk cows and heifers in America are artificially inseminated on an annual basis?

4. How many beef cattle of breeding age are there in America? Approximately what percentage are artificially inseminated?

5. How many AI centers are there in the United States? Why has the number decreased since 1950? What are the advantages of consolidated, or larger, AI centers?

6. Does AI aid or hinder the registered livestock business?

7. Are there limitations to increased utilization of AI for dairy and beef producers? Explain.

8. What are the advantages of having semen custom frozen? What are the disadvantages?

9. How are the regulations governing AI in the United States developed and enforced?

10. What is the National Association of Animal Breeders, Inc. (NAAB), and what are its functions? What are the functions of CSS?

## REFERENCES

Herman, H. A. 1981. Improving Cattle by the Millions. Univ. of Missouri Press, Columbia. (Chs. 1, 2.)

Perry, E. J. (Ed.). 1968. Artificial Insemination of Farm Animals (4th Ed.). Rutgers Univ. Press, New Brunswick, NJ.

Salisbury, G. W., N. L. Van Demark, and J. R. Lodge (Eds.). 1978. Physiology of Reproduction and Artificial Insemination of Cattle (2nd Ed.). W. H. Freeman, San Francisco.

Proceedings Annual Conventions, 1950–2001, National Association of Animal Breeders, Inc., P.O. Box 1033, Columbia, MO 65205.

Also, selected readings, as assigned, from current breed journals and farm publications.

## WEB SITES

Dairy Breed Registry Associations—See Exercise 26
Beef Breed Registry Association—See Exercise 17
NAAB/CSS and U.S. Semen Sales
*http://www.naab-css.org/*

# EXERCISE 3

# Basic Genetics of Cattle Breeding

## OBJECT

To become familiar with the more important genetic principles influencing inheritance.

## DISCUSSION

The chief objective of AI is to improve the economic traits of livestock. Artificial insemination offers unique opportunities by increasing the number of progeny from the best sires and by producing superior sires for future use. Thus, any bull heavily utilized for AI purposes should be well above the breed average as measured by the production or performance of his offspring.

*The basic idea in improving a cattle population or an individual herd is to carry out a selection and breeding program that enables the best animals to produce the most offspring.* For a better grasp of how animals inherit traits, both desirable and undesirable, a few basic genetic principles must be understood.

### Mendelian Principles of Inheritance

In 1865, the Austrian monk Gregor Mendel, while experimenting with garden peas, discovered the genetic principles that today are recognized as applicable to all plants and animals.

The animal body is made up of millions of microscopic cells. In biological terms, the cell is the basic functional unit of living matter. From a genetics viewpoint, there are two kinds of cells: (1) *somatic* or body cells, such as tissue, bone, and blood; and (2) *germ* or *sex* cells, which produce the sperm from the male and the egg of the female, whose union is necessary for perpetuation of the species. In very general terms, a cell has two principal components, the *cytoplasm* and the *nucleus*. A typical cell is pictured in Figure 3.1.

The cytoplasm occupies the area between the cell membrane and the nucleus and contains numerous organelles that are necessary for the function of the cell. In this discussion,

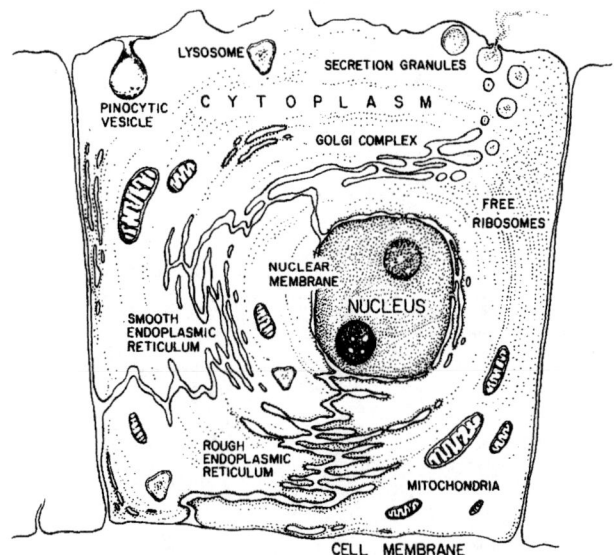

**Figure 3.1.** A typical cell showing some of the structural components that most cells have in common. (M. E. Ensminger. 1991. Animal Science [9th Ed.]. Interstate Publishers, Inc., Danville, IL. p. 57)

21

however, we are mainly concerned with the contents of the cell nucleus.

In the nucleus there are *chromosomes,* composed of deoxyribonucleic acid (DNA) molecules that contain genes in a linear sequence. Chromosomes occur in pairs. There are 30 pairs, or 60 chromosomes, in cattle. The number of chromosomes is constant for each species of animal (see Table 3.1).

Genes are segments of a DNA molecule and are the carriers or determiners of inheritance. They are commonly cited as the smallest units of inheritance containing the necessary information for synthesis of a polypeptide chain (protein). They also occur in pairs. Thousands of genes are arranged in linear fashion at fixed locations (loci) on each chromosome.

In animals the body cells have one pair of chromosomes known as sex or germ determiners in the process of inheritance. These are referred to as the X and Y chromosomes. In mammals, including humans, the male's chromosome pair is XY and the female's is XX.

### Table 3.1. Typical Number of Chromosomes in Selected Animals

| Animals | Chromosome Numbers (Full Complement) |
|---|---|
| Cattle | 60 |
| Goats | 60 |
| Horses | 64 |
| Swine | 38 |
| Sheep | 54 |
| Dogs | 78 |
| Humans *(Homo sapiens)* | 46 |
| Mules | 63 |
| Donkeys | 62 |
| Cats | 38 |

Chromosomal DNA molecules represent a "blueprint" for all the heritable characteristics of a particular cell or animal. The DNA substance of the chromosomes exists almost entirely in the cell nucleus and, through complex biochemical processes, instructs each cell what to do and when. Strands of DNA double helix replicate themselves and also serve as templates for the formation in the nucleus of messenger and transfer RNA's (ribonucleic acids). The RNA's move into the cytoplasm and influence the types of proteins (polypeptide chains) synthesized by the cell.

It is now recognized that the mitochondria of the cell also contain a small amount of DNA and can synthesize some protein. In fact, recent studies in mice[1] have demonstrated the existence of maternal lineage effects ("cytoplasmic inheritance") attributable to mitochondrial DNA.

When the somatic cells divide as a part of body growth and maintenance, the number of chromosomes stays the same. When the germ or sex cells divide to form sperm or ova, the male or female gametes, the number of chromosomes in each is only one-half that normally found in the species. When fertilization occurs by union of the sperm and the egg, the full complement of chromosomes is restored.

The inherited characteristics of an animal are determined at the time an egg (ovum) of the female and a spermatozoon from the male unite. Thus, when a bull produces a sperm, a duplicate of one or the other of each pair of genes is carried by that sperm and passed on to the resulting offspring. The same procedure, with respect to one of each pair of genes being present, applies in the production of an egg. Since a sample of semen from a bull con-

---

[1] U. Gyllensten, D. N. Wharton, and A. C. Wilson. 1985. Maternal inheritance of mitochondrial DNA during the backcrossing of two species of mice. J. Hered. 76:321.

tains millions of sperm, each representing a sample of the genes the bull carries, it becomes a matter of chance which sperm fertilizes the egg and hence the kinds of genes transmitted to the offspring. The best bulls have a high proportion of desirable genes but also some less desirable ones. No sire has all good or all bad genes. This sampling process accounts for the great variation in inherited ability and explains how an offspring can be much better or much poorer than its parents. Each gene acts independently; there is no blending of genes, but each adds to or deducts from the inherited potential of an individual animal. *Thus, the whole scheme of cattle improvement is aimed at having a high preponderance of "desirable" genes in the animals being mated.* It must be understood that the chances that any one gamete (egg or sperm) will carry a particular gene are equal to the frequency of that gene in the cattle population being mated. For example, if a given sire has 70 percent genes desirable for a given trait and 30 percent undesirable, on the average, the odds of getting a desirable gene are 7 times out of 10.

In summary, a calf receives (1) a sample half of its sire's genes and (2) a sample half of its dam's genes. The inherited potential is thus fixed. How well the animal performs (expresses its inheritance) depends upon its environment (feeding and management). Artificial insemination makes it possible for a sire to have many progeny. As a result, geneticists are able to predict fairly accurately the expected performance of future offspring.

## Selecting the Dairy Sire for Herd Improvement

No bull has all high- or all low-producing daughters. There is considerable variation in production. If we should group a bull's daughters that average 15,000 pounds of milk on a mature 2- ×305-day milking basis, a normal distribution would indicate one-half the daughters above and one-half below the 15,000-pound average. A hypothetical distribution would be much along the lines illustrated in Figure 3.2.

It should be noted that about two-thirds, or 68 percent, of the records are from 12,000 to 18,000 pounds of milk. About 14 percent are from 9,000 to 12,000, or 3,000 to 6,000 pounds below the average, and about 14 percent are from 18,000 to 21,000, or 3,000 to 6,000 pounds above the average. On the extremes, about 2 percent

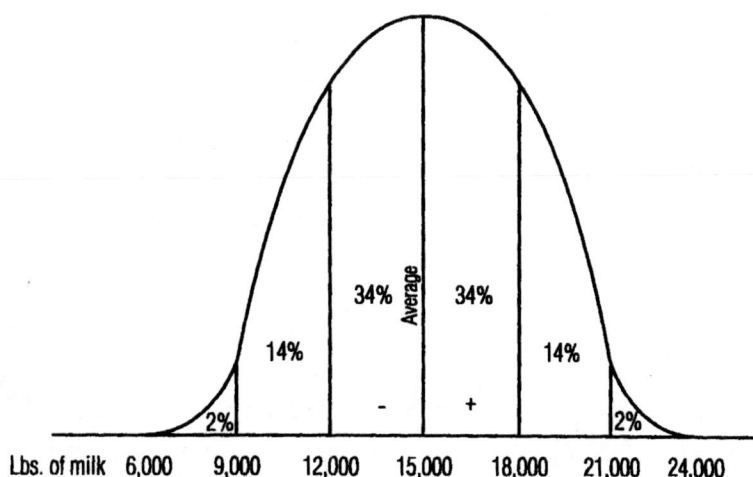

**Figure 3.2.** Distribution of milk production records by 1,000 daughters of a sire.

23

produce at the 6,000- to 9,000-pound level, and another 2 percent produce in the 21,000- to 24,000-pound range. The goal in selecting sires for herd improvement is to use as many sires as possible in the very top level of the breed, say, the upper 5 to 10 percent.

In selecting sires for herd improvement, a dairy producer should utilize semen from bulls on the basis of genetic measurements available on their economic traits, as discussed in the following sections.

## Predicted Transmitting Ability (PTA)

Sires in AI use are ranked on the basis of their predicted transmitting ability (PTA) for the various economic traits by the USDA, the National Association of Animal Breeders, Inc., and the breed associations. PTA's are the best estimate of the sire's ability to transmit superior performance to his daughters. PTA's for milk, fat, and protein are expressed in pounds. PTA's for somatic cell score (SCS) are expressed in somatic cell score units. PTA's for productive life (PL) are expressed in months a cow is in production before she reaches seven years old. For milk, fat, protein, and productive life, selecting sires with the highest PTA's will result in the most genetic progress. For somatic cell score, the lower evaluations are better.

Bulls are typically ranked on the basis of Predicted Transmitting Ability for *pounds of milk, fat,* and *protein.* Rankings may also include economic indexes, type rating, and calving ease.

In sire summaries the following information is usually recorded:

**Name of the bull, registration number, and NAAB sire code**—The code identifies the center processing the semen, the breed, and the number assigned the bull by the center.

**Sampling codes**—*Standard Sampling (S)* indicates that a bull is sampled by distribution of semen to a minimum of 40 herds, whose records qualify for USDA genetic evaluations for Holsteins and Jerseys and at least 20 herds whose records qualify for USDA genetic evaluations for the other breeds. *Other Sampling (O)* includes bulls enrolled in the Cross Reference Program of the NAAB but not accurately described by the above definitions or not assigned a sampling code by three years of age.

**Reliability (Rel.)** is a measure of the accuracy of PTA's. Reliabilities are expressed as percentages and range from 1 to 99. They increase as information on more daughters becomes available and as the amount of information on relatives increases. PTA's of sires with high reliabilities are less apt to change substantially in future evaluations. Reliabilities help determine how much semen of a particular sire should be used.

**Genetic Base 00**—PTA's are calculated relative to the average genetic ability of cows born in 1995. For somatic cell score, the deviations from the genetic base are added back to the breed average first lactation somatic cell score of cows born in 1995. Because the genetic base was last updated in 2000, the PTA's are called PTA 00.

**Lifetime Net Merit** are the economic indexes calculated by USDA to rank AI sires based on their daughters' profitability. These indexes use the national average prices for milk, fat, and protein.

**Net Merit (NM$)** ranks profitability based on PTA's for milk, fat, protein, productive life, somatic cell score, udder conformation, feet and legs conformation, and body size. Thirty-six percent of the index comes from protein, 21% from fat, 14% from productive life, 9% from somatic cell score, 7% from udder, 5% from milk, 4% from size, and 4% from feet and legs. The weights for the milk components are calculated based on the milk prices received under a typical component pricing scheme.

**Fluid Merit (FM$)** ranks profitability similar to Net Merit, except that the milk components are weighted based on pricing of milk used for fluid consumption.

**Cheese Merit (CM$)** ranks profitability similar to Net Merit, except that the milk components are weighted based on cheese yield pricing. For a detailed explanation of the USDA Lifetime Net Merit values, see http://aipl.arsusda.gov/memos/html/nm2000.html.

**PTAT—Predicted Transmitting Ability for Type** measures the expected difference in final type score between daughters of a bull and the breed average.

**Type Production Index (TPI)** is a formula or method of ranking bulls on overall merit, calculated by the Holstein Association USA, Inc., with a weighting of 2.9 for PTA protein, 1.1 for PTA fat, 1 for PTA type, .65 for Udder Composite, .35 for Feet & Legs Composite, .9 for PTA productive life, and .1 for PTA somatic cell score. Only the TPI index calculated by the Holstein Association is considered official.

**Production Type Index (PTI)** is an index developed by the respective breed association (except for Holstein) to summarize the overall lifetime performance differences between sires' daughters.

**Calving Ease** is an estimate of the Percent of Difficult Births (%DB) in heifers when they calve the first time. This should be used to decide which bulls to use when breeding virgin heifers. The NAAB is the chief sponsor of Calving Ease summaries.

In 1991, the Interbull Center was established in Uppsala, Sweden to conduct research and produce international genetic evaluations. The first global evaluations for production traits were produced in 1994. These evaluations are calculated using a Multiple-trait Across Country Evaluation (MACE) procedure. Interbull combines sire evaluations from 25 different countries then returns the combined evaluation to the participating country ranking all bulls on the receiving country's evaluation scale. Some type evaluations are MACE for type traits calculated by Interbull. Interbull type combines conformation information from 17 countries. In the United States, the Interbull MACE proof is considered the official evaluation when it includes both U.S. and foreign daughters. If the Interbull MACE proof contains foreign daughters only, then the Interbull MACE proof will be official if it has a higher reliability than the domestic evaluation. In all other cases, the domestic evaluation will be official. Interbull evaluations for production and type can provide more complete information for sires with additional daughters outside of the U.S.A.

Interbull allows producers to fairly and objectively compare the genetic merit of bulls from different countries. However, the system is not perfect because of low genetic correlations between different countries and other unresolved issues. Research is being conducted to develop methodologies to overcome low genetic correlations to allow increasingly accurate comparisons of bulls with daughters in different countries.

Sire summaries for AI bulls are published at regular intervals by the NAAB, the USDA, and the breed associations. All AI businesses publish sire summaries in their sire booklets and in advertising.

A summary of active AI sires in February 2002 is presented in Table 3.2.

The active sires in artificial insemination are much superior to non-AI sires, as shown by a comparison of Tables 3.2 and 3.3.

It will be noted in comparing the average milk production of daughters of the active Holstein AI sires and those of the non-AI Holstein sires that there is a difference of 960 pounds in favor of the AI Holstein sires. The average Holstein AI sire in this summary increased milk production 1,206 pounds above average,

**Table 3.2.** Production of Daughters of Active AI Sires, Summarized February 2002, USDA

| Breed | Number of Sires | PTA[a] Milk (lbs.) | PTA[a] Fat (lbs.) | PTA[a] Protein (lbs.) | NM ($) |
|---|---|---|---|---|---|
| Ayrshire | 22 | 836 | + 27 | + 24 | + 232 |
| Brown Swiss | 50 | + 1,076 | + 48 | + 36 | + 342 |
| Guernsey | 19 | + 1,259 | + 44 | + 33 | + 277 |
| Holstein | 636 | + 1,206 | + 37 | + 38 | + 335 |
| Jersey | 92 | + 1,067 | + 38 | + 36 | + 319 |
| Shorthorn | 9 | + 738 | + 19 | + 22 | + 197 |
| Red & White | 40 | + 971 | + 21 | + 25 | + 218 |

[a]PTA = Predicted Transmitting Ability.

**Table 3.3.** Production of Daughters of Non-AI Sires, Summarized February 2002, USDA

| Breed | Number of Sires | PTA[a] Milk (lbs.) | PTA[a] Fat (lbs.) | PTA[a] Protein (lbs.) | MFP ($) |
|---|---|---|---|---|---|
| Ayrshire | 34 | + 324 | + 9 | + 9 | + 82 |
| Brown Swiss | 50 | + 273 | + 13 | + 11 | + 97 |
| Guernsey | 51 | + 154 | + 6 | + 6 | + 52 |
| Holstein | 3,718 | + 246 | + 9 | + 9 | + 82 |
| Jersey | 360 | + 234 | + 8 | + 10 | + 88 |
| Shorthorn | 23 | + 133 | 8 | + 3 | + 53 |
| Red & White | 41 | − 169 | + 2 | − 3 | − 34 |

[a]PTA = Predicted Transmitting Ability.

whereas the non-AI Holstein sire's daughters produced an average of 246 pounds of milk above the average. The daughters of the active AI Holstein sires produced $253 more gross income per lactation than the non-AI-sired daughters.

More details on sire selection for AI use appear in Exercise 25.

## Why AI Must Utilize the Top Performing Sires

The success of AI in making possible the immense gains in the average production of milk and its components is largely due to the development and utilization of above-average sires. The importance of sire selection and development on a continuing basis is well documented by Lerner and Donald (1966, see Ref.), who state: "Unless each generation of bulls for artificial insemination is the product of the previous generation on which money has been spent, the profit from all the work on improvement through breeding is limited to expanding the use of good bulls in commercial herds and reducing the use of poor bulls." This observation illustrates the importance of each succeeding generation of sires being superior to the previous generation.

## Beef Sire Selection

The same basic genetic principles apply to herd sire selection in beef cattle. Traits of economic importance to the beef producer are evaluated through performance records programs of the beef breed associations. The associations summarize and publish genetic evaluations for these traits on a regular basis for their respective breeds. These sire evaluations compare bulls based on expected progeny differences (EPD's), which are a measure of the expected differences in performance of a sire's progeny when compared to the average progeny performance of all the sires for that breed. EPD's also incorporate performance information on the individual sire and his relatives.

Beef breed sire summaries typically evaluate birth weight, weaning weight, yearling weight, maternal milk, and maternal weaning weight. These EPD's are expressed in pounds. Additional traits, such as calving ease, yearling hip height, and scrotal circumference, are evaluated in some of the breeds. Each EPD has an accuracy (ACC) value that indicates the reliability of the genetic evaluations. Accuracy ranges from 0.00 to 1.00.

The beef cattle producer, after considering the strengths and weaknesses of the cow herd, can consult the sire summaries and then select the sires that will help reach herd production goals.

## Undesirable Genetic Defects

In recent years, certain economically harmful genetic defects have been the subject of serious concern to responsible cattle breeders. Defects such as syndactylism, limber leg, porphyria, congenital dropsy, white heifer disease, recto-vaginal constriction, Weaver syndrome, bovine leukocyte adhesion deficiency, and complex vertebral malformation in dairy cattle and dwarfism, osteopetrosis, double muscling, hydrocephalus, arthrogryposis, porphyria, white heifer disease, and syndactylism in beef cattle are of importance. In dairy cattle, Deficiency of Uridine Monophosphate Synthase (DUMPS) is a genetic defect considered to be of lesser economic importance.

It is urged that all organizations encourage the users of their semen to report the occurrence of unusual calves and that each AI organization maintain a file of the descriptive reports in order that patterns of appearance of similar defects can be established. When it is reasonably clear that a given bull is a carrier of an undesirable genetic defect, an action appropriate should be taken. New biotechnologies, such as DNA-based tests for genetic defects, likely will result in discovering new and previously unknown conditions, as well as providing an opportunity for their control.

Many undesirable defects are controlled by a single gene and are the result of autosomal recessive inheritance. A recessive gene is one whose phenotypic expression is masked by its own dominant allele. In this typical situation, the defect can occur only when both parents are carriers (heterozygous) of the recessive gene. When the individual receives a copy of the defective (recessive) gene from each parent for the particular trait, the undesirable defect manifests itself. Bovine leukocyte adhesion deficiency (BLAD) is an example of a lethal autosomal recessive disorder that occurs in Holstein cattle.[2] BLAD is a condition that impairs the ability of a type of white blood cell (neutrophil) in calves to fight infections, resulting in an animal's death several months after birth. Figure 3.3 illustrates the manner in which BLAD is believed to be inherited.

The B Allele represents normal functioning leukocytes (neutrophils), while b represents the defective leukocyte condition.

---

[2] M. E. Kehrli, D. E. Shuster, and M. R. Ackermann. 1992. Leukocyte adhesion deficiency among Holstein cattle. Cornell Veterinarian 82:103.

DAM

| | B | b |
|---|---|---|
| **B** | BB<br>(homozygous-normal) | Bb<br>(heterozygous-normal) |
| **b** | Bb<br>(heterozygous-normal) | bb<br>(homozygous recessive-BLAD) |

SIRE

**Figure 3.3.** The manner in which BLAD is believed to be inherited.

Theoretically, 25 percent of the offspring of heterozygous (Bb) carrier parents will receive the bb genotype, resulting in BLAD, and 75 percent of the offspring will be phenotypically normal (25 percent homozygous BB and 50 percent heterozygous Bb). One-half of all the offspring of heterozygous matings also will be carriers of the defective condition. Fortunately, in the BLAD situation, an accurate DNA-based test has been developed so that carrier animals can be easily identified. The NAAB and the Holstein Association of America implemented a comprehensive control program to substantially reduce the gene frequency of the BLAD condition. This has included identifying carriers, labeling current AI bulls, and eliminating carriers from progeny test programs.

## How the Sex of a Calf is Determined

Two important facts to remember in animal reproduction and genetics are (1) chromosomes are present in pairs, as are the genes, in body cells and one-half pairs in the gametes (eggs and sperm); and (2) there are 30 pairs of chromosomes in cattle. Each body cell contains one pair of chromosomes known as sex chromosomes because they are the determiners of the sex of an individual.

The female has two like chromosomes called "X" chromosomes. The male has one X chromosome and another called the "Y" chromosome. The female produces only one type of gamete or germ cell, and it contains only the X chromosome; however, the male produces two types of germ cells, one-half containing the X chromosome and the other half the Y chromosome. A sperm cell, carrying either an X or a Y chromosome, unites with the egg, which always bears an X chromosome. Thus, the new individual (zygote) can have either XX or XY chromosome composition. The XX is a female, and the XY a male. So on the average, the population has a sex ratio of 1:1 at birth.

The X chromosome is larger and heavier than the Y (male-producing) chromosome. Efforts have been made to separate the X- and the Y-bearing spermatozoa by gravitational methods, thus influencing the sex ratio by making a larger number of X-carrying sperm available for insemination purposes. This and dozens of other methods attempting to influence the sex ratio in cattle have not achieved desired results. Research conducted by Johnson,[3] however, demonstrated that in rabbits and pigs, X- and Y-bearing sperm cells could be successfully sorted by DNA content using flow cytometry techniques. In that study, surgically inseminated "sorted" sperm resulted in the proportion of male and female offspring closely paralleling the proportions predicted. It was the first known account of sex separation attempts being scientifically validated. Currently it is possible to accurately sex the sperm of most mammals. However, efficiency of the process is low. Studies are continuing, and someday a livestock producer may be able to designate the desired sex of a calf, lamb, or piglet. More details on sexing semen appear in Exercise 21.

---

[3] L. A. Johnson. 1989. Progress toward achieving sex pre-selection in farm animals. J. Anim. Sci. 67 (Suppl. 1): 342 (Abstr.).

## Importance of Selection

Selection is the most important tool a breeder has in shaping animals for the future. Selection occurs when certain animals are chosen to remain in the herd and reproduce while other animals are culled. In general, there are two kinds of selection: natural, which is due to natural forces in the environment, and artificial, which is controlled by the human element.

The basic law of natural selection is "survival of the fittest." In wild animals, and even in domesticated animals, there is a tendency for the weaker, low fertility, and undesirable recessive gene carriers to be eliminated. Most of the selection in domesticated cattle is artificial and controlled by humans.

Most selection by humans is on the basis of quantitative traits. Such traits are affected by the environment and the many pairs of genes acting simultaneously. Selection is based on traits that are both phenotypic (related to an animal's outward appearance and performance) and genotypic (related to an animal's breeding value as measured by the performance of its progeny). An animal's own record of production means little unless compared to that of other animals in the herd or breed. The true measure of an animal's breeding value, or genotypic traits, comes when the progeny are ranked with other animals in the population. The dairy sire summaries computed by the USDA and the beef sire summaries computed by performance and progeny test programs provide such information. They are the most dependable sources of information a breeder can use in selecting for production.

Usually dairy cattle breeders will select animals for milk production as a first priority. About 90 percent of the returns from a dairy herd are based on milk sales. Type or wearability of the animals is important and should be a part of the selection process. Beef producers who are seeking to improve economic traits will base selection largely on weaning weight, yearling weight, and average daily gain in the feedlot. The greatest progress in improvement is made when selection emphasis is placed on one trait.

For further information on the selection and application of the various biometric measures available, refer to the references at the end of this exercise.

## QUESTIONS

1. What is a chromosome? A gene?

2. What is the significance, in animal reproduction and inheritance, of chromosomes and genes always occurring in pairs?

3. How many chromosomes are there in the somatic (body) cells of cattle?

4. What is meant when we say that a calf receives half of its genes from the sire and half from the dam?

5. How would you explain a very inferior calf being produced by an outstanding production-proved sire and a high-producing cow from a good family?

6. What do we mean by the term "gene frequency"? Why is gene frequency stressed in modern breeding concepts?

7. How would you explain the fact that a red-and-white Holstein calf can be born to black-and-white parents?

8. When is the inheritance of an individual determined?

9. How can inheritance be improved for any given trait in a cattle population?

10. How does selection modify gene frequencies in a cattle population?

11. Why do some bulls sire more bulls than heifers? How is the sex ratio controlled in nature? Can the sex ratio be altered by humans? Explain.

12. What are the most important traits to select for in breeding dairy cattle? In breeding beef cattle?

## REFERENCES

Campbell, J. R., M. D. Kenealy and K. L. Campbell. 2003. Animal Sciences: The Biology, Care and Production of Domestic Animals (4th Ed.). McGraw-Hill, New York.

Lasley, J. F. 1986. Genetics of Livestock Improvement (4th Ed.). Prentice-Hall, Englewood Cliffs, NJ. (Chapters on inheritance.)

Lerner, L. M., and H. C. Donald. 1966. Modern Developments in Animal Breeding. Academic Press, London and New York.

## WEB SITES

Current Literature
*http://www.hoards.com*

Dairy Sire Summaries
*http://aipl.arsusda.gov/*

*http://www.naab-css.org/*

*http://www-interbull.slu.se/*

# EXERCISE 4

# Reproductive Organs of the Cow and Their Functions

## OBJECT

To become familiar with the anatomy and the physiological functions of the reproductive organs of the cow.

## DISCUSSION

The female reproductive tract is very complex. It not only produces ova, or female germ cells, but also it provides for the growth and nourishment of the developing fetus and later, by the act of parturition, expels the fully developed fetus.

The reproductive organs of the female, like those of the male, are controlled by an integrated endocrine system. A knowledge of the anatomy and the physiological functions of the reproductive organs of the cow is necessary for successful AI. The essential organs of reproduction in the cow are the ovaries, fallopian tubes (oviducts), uterus, cervix, vagina, vestibule, and vulva, as shown in Figure 4.1. Figures 4.2 through 4.5 depict greater detail of some anatomical features important to artificial insemination.

The two ovaries of the cow produce the reproductive cells (ova, or eggs). Normally one or more ova are shed by the sexually mature bovine, preceded by estrus, or heat, every 18 to 24 days, with 21 days being the average. In addition to their development of ova, the ovaries produce hormones (estrogens, progesterone, relaxin, inhibin) that are concerned with the processes of reproduction and growth of the mammary gland.

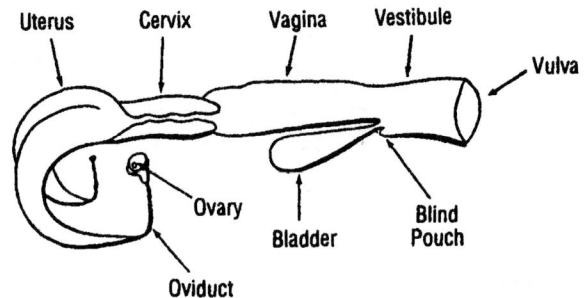

**Figure 4.1.** Reproductive organs of the cow.

The fallopian tubes, uterus, cervix, and anterior portion of the vagina are embryologically derived from the Müllerian ducts of the sexually undifferentiated embryo. They are formed as paired and entirely separate structures. In farm mammals, the Müllerian ducts become fused in a caudo-cranial manner to eventually form a single uterus, cervix, and anterior part of the vagina. The degree of fusion determines the morphological type of uterus. For example, the cow has a bipartite type of uterus. The urogenital sinus, which is derived from the embryologic cloaca, gives rise to the vestibule, the labia of the vulva, and the clitoris. The fallopian tubes, suspended in the broad ligament, open at the fimbriated end near the ovaries. These convoluted tubes serve to conduct the ova from the ovaries to the uterus. Fertilization of an ovum by the sperm of the bull usually takes place in the upper or ampullar region of a fallopian tube. The fallopian tubes, or oviducts, join the uterine horns at the utero-tubal junction. The uterus is a tubular organ composed of an inner glandular lining (endometrium) and outer smooth

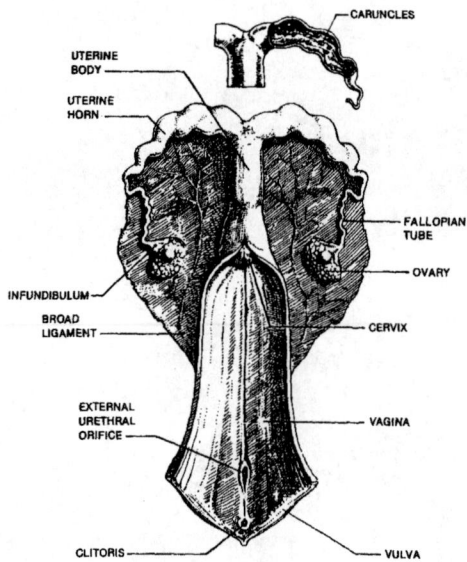

**Figure 4.2.** Diagrammatic view of the genital organs of the cow. (Adapted under the direction of M. E. Ensminger from an original illustration by the authors)

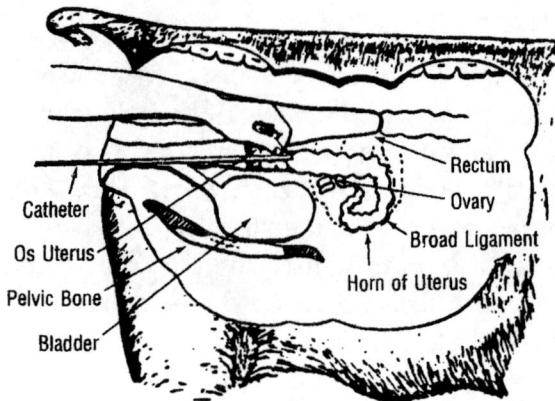

**Figure 4.3.** Schematic showing the reproductive organs of the cow and insemination.

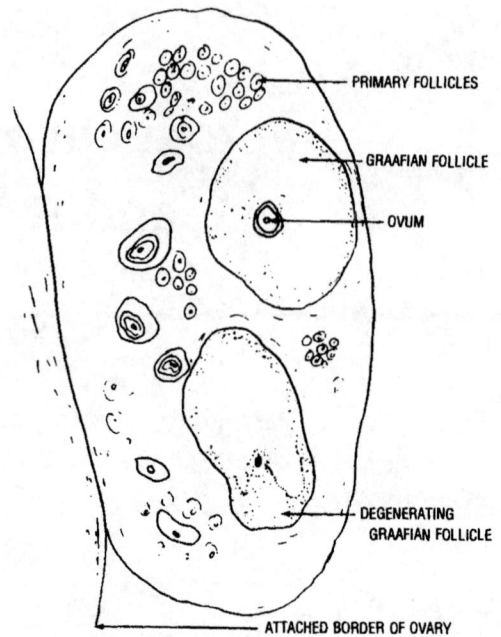

**Figure 4.4.** A cross section of the ovary of the cow. Pictured is a Graafian follicle containing an ovum, primary follicles, and a degenerating Graafian follicle that has shed its ovum.

### Ovary of Cow During Heat

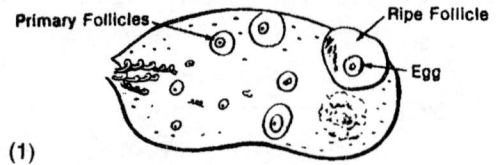

(1)

### Ovary of Cow Not in Heat

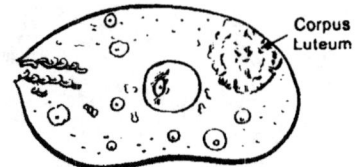

(2)

**Figure 4.5.** (1) Ovary of cow in heat showing follicle and egg and (2) ovary of cow non-estrus showing corpus luteum. (Adapted under the direction of M. E. Ensminger from an original illustration by the authors)

muscle layers (myometrium). The two horns of the uterus, right and left, are really continuations of the fallopian tubes but are much larger and thicker walled. The horns join to form the main body of the uterus. Although outwardly the main body of the cow uterus is several inches long, internally the body of the uterus, which is typically the target area for semen deposition in artificial insemination, is only about an inch in length. The uterus, in pregnancy, contains the developing fetus and, because of its muscular elasticity, is capable of changing its size with the growth of the young.

The uterus opens posteriorly into the cervix, or *os uteri*. The cervix of the cow is about three inches long and three-quarters to one inch wide. It is quite thick walled, and the cervical canal has many folds, which makes the introduction of any instrument somewhat difficult. During heat, the cervix relaxes slightly, but at parturition it relaxes a great deal to permit expulsion of the fe-

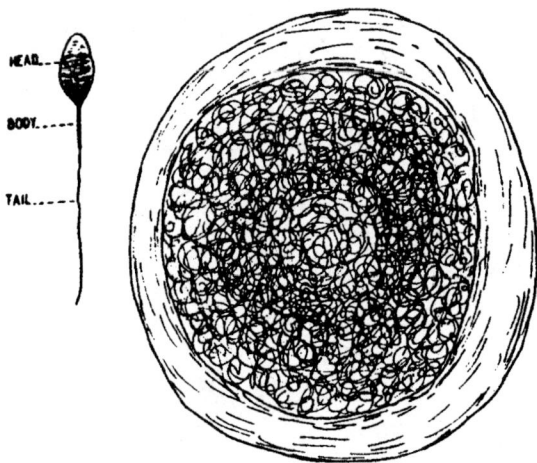

**Figure 4.6.** Comparative size of the cow's ovum and the bull's spermatozoon. In pregnancy, the cervix is sealed with a mucus plug, thus guarding the developing embryo and the uterus from microbial invasion.

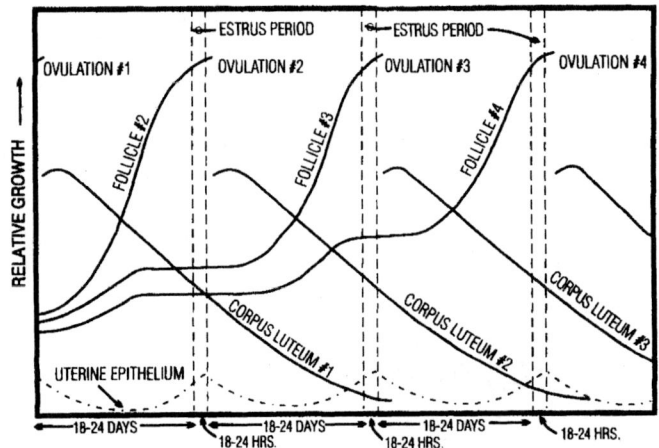

**Figure 4.7.** Recurring estrous cycles; development of Graafian follicles; formation, growth, and regression of the corpus luteum; and proliferation of the uterine epithelium in anticipation of pregnancy.

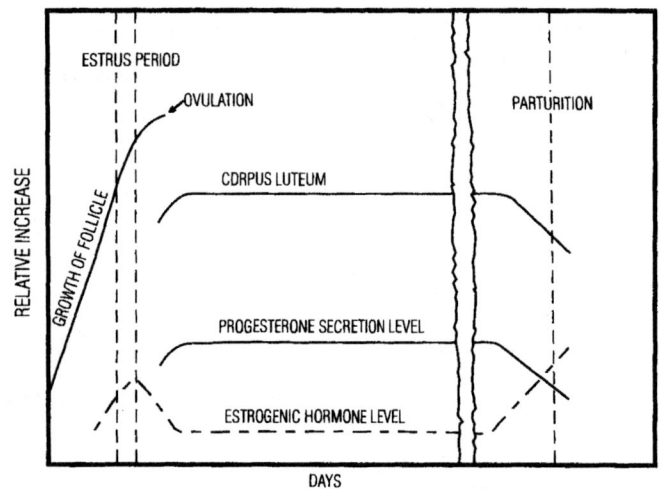

**Figure 4.8.** Relative changes in the follicle, in the corpus luteum, and in the levels of estrogenic and progesterone hormones during estrus and pregnancy and following parturition.

tus. In pregnancy, the cervix is sealed with a mucus plug, thus guarding the developing embryo and the uterus from microbial invasion.

The cervix opens posteriorly into the vagina. The vagina is strictly an organ of copulation and extends from the vestibule to the cervix. It is from 10 to 12 inches long in the cow. In copulation, the small depression just in front of the cervix apparently aids in the collection of some of the semen near the opening of this organ. The vagina is somewhat constricted at its posterior end where it joins the vestibule. The vestibule is located between the vagina and the vulva and is about three to four inches in length. It is common to both the reproductive and urinary tracts and has several sphincter muscles. The vulva or the external opening of the genital tract is composed of the labia and clitoris.

Cows, unlike some animals in their domesticated state, are not seasonal breeders and may normally be expected to come into heat about every 18 to 24 days until settled in calf. Occasionally irregular heat periods due to abnormal conditions of the ovaries are experienced, and such conditions usually call for treatment by a skilled veterinarian.

The cow's ovum, or egg, is fertilized by a single sperm from the male, and growth begins at once by a series of divisions. Figure 4.6

shows the relative size of the bovine egg and sperm cell. The single fertilized ovum divides to make two cells, then four, then eight, etc.

The reproductive system of the cow is regulated by a complex endocrine system. The functions of the reproductive organs, occurrence of estrus, conception, pregnancy, parturition, and lactation are all regulated and coordinated by the hormones of the hypothalamus and pituitary, the ovarian follicle, the corpus luteum, and the placenta. The cyclic ` nature of these phenomena is shown in graphic form in Figures 4.7 and 4.8.

The endocrine coordination of the reproductive system of the cow is indicated in Figure 4.9. A comprehensive discussion of the interrelationships can be found in the references listed at the end of this exercise.

## PROCEDURE

Study Figures 4.1 through 4.9. Become familiar with the reproductive organs of the cow and their functions. Also, observe the reproductive organs displayed in the laboratory. Note carefully the size and position of each of the various organs. (It is desirable that reproductive tracts be displayed from cows slaughtered while in various stages of pregnancy as well as from several cows slaughtered while not pregnant.)

By the rectal method, locate and "get the feel" of the reproductive organs in live cows.

Locate and observe the structure and relative size of:

1. Ovary.
2. Fallopian tube (oviduct).
3. Infundibulum.
4. Uterus (body and horns, externally and internally).
5. Cervix.
6. Vagina.
7. Vestibule.
8. Vulva.
9. Clitoris.
10. Broad ligament.

## QUESTIONS

1. What are the functions of each of the parts of the female reproductive system listed above?
2. What are the functions of releasing hormones, follicule-stimulating hormone, luteinizing hormone, estrogen, and progesterone?
3. What is the average time between estrus periods? Average length of estrus? Average length of gestation?
4. What are the basic hormonal changes that occur at estrus, during pregnancy, and at parturition? Explain.
5. Diagram the changes that occur in the sex chromosomes during formation of the ovum (oogenesis).
6. What are the changes that occur in the ovum during and after fertilization?
7. What are some of the ovarian malfunctions that result in (a) estrus periods every 12 to 15 days, (b) continual estrus, or "nymphomania," and (c) failure to come into heat (anestrus)?

## REFERENCES

Hafez, E. S. E. (Ed.). 1987. Reproduction in Farm Animals (5th Ed.). Lea & Febiger, Philadelphia. (Chs. 3, 5, 7.)

Senger, P. L. 1999. Pathways to Pregnancy and Parturition. First revised edition. Current Conceptions, Inc., Moscow, ID, Mack Printing Group - Science Press, Ephrata, PA.

Sorenson, A. M., Jr. 1979. Animal Reproduction: Principles and Practices. McGraw-Hill, New York.

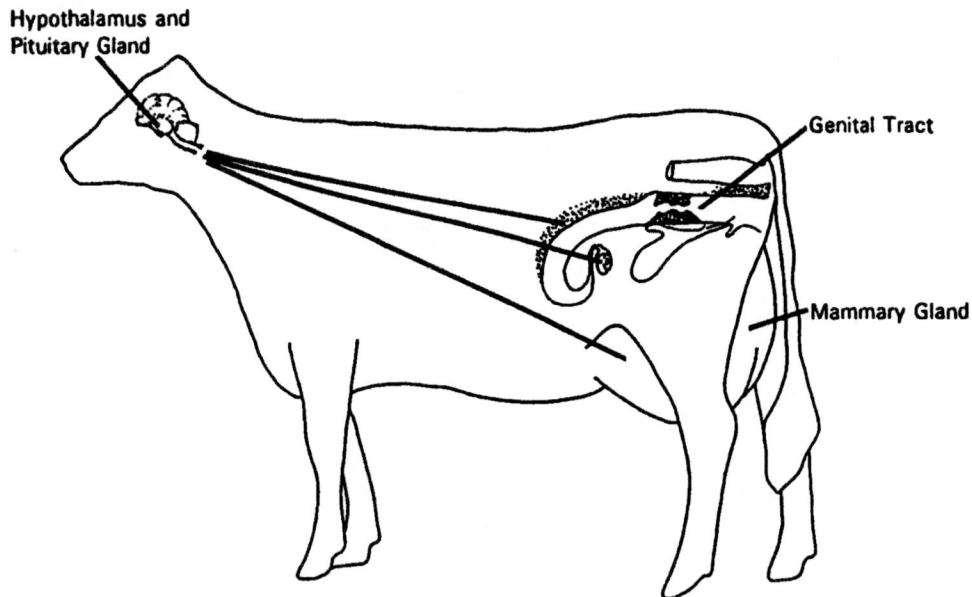

Diagram showing hormonal relationships in the cow. The gonadotrophic hormones released from the pituitary flow through the blood stream to the ovary, where they stimulate follicle development, ovulation, and formation of the corpus luteum (yellow body). Other pituitary and gonadal hormones have effects on the genital tract and mammary gland, coordinating reproductive events.

## Glossary of Endocrine Terms

**Glands** are composed of groups of cells that have the ability to manufacture or secrete certain products.

**Glands of external secretion** (exocrine) discharge their products to the outside or inside surfaces of the body. Examples: sweat, sebaceous, salivary, digestive.

**Glands of internal secretion** (endocrine) discharge their products directly into the blood stream. Examples: pituitary, ovary, thyroid, adrenal.

**Hormones** are the secretion products of the endocrine glands. After flowing into blood, the hormones stimulate the action of other glands or tissues in various parts of the body. Most hormones are composed of proteins, steroids, or fatty acids.

**Releasing hormones** produced in the hypothalamus are substances that control the release of pituitary hormones. These neurohormones are transported to the anterior pituitary gland via a unique vascular connection (hypothalamo-hypophyseal portal system).

**Luteinizing hormone-releasing hormone** (LH-RH) stimulates the release of FSH and LH from the anterior lobe of the pituitary gland.

**Gonads** are the principal male and female reproductive organs—the testicles in the bull and the ovaries in the cow.

**Gonadotrophic hormones** of the pituitary stimulate the action of the testicles and the ovaries.

**Follicle-stimulating hormone** (FSH), a gonadotrophin, stimulates growth and maturation of the mature follicle in the ovary. The follicle is fluid filled and contains an egg, or ovum.

**Luteinizing hormone** (LH), a gonadotrophin, acts in conjunction with FSH to induce estrogen secretion from ovarian follicular cells. It is responsible for the rupture of the ovarian follicle and for ovulation.

**Prolactin** (PRL) is produced in the anterior pituitary and promotes lactation and maternal behavior.

**Oxytocin** is produced in the hypothalamus and stored in the posterior lobe of the pituitary gland. It causes contraction of smooth muscle in the uterus and oviducts and is responsible for milk let-down (secretion) from the mammary gland.

**Estrogenic hormone,** secreted by granulosa cells of the follicle, has a wide range of activity. Estrogen acts on the central nervous system of the cow to induce behavioral estrus ("heat"). It also stimulates reproductive tract tissues, mammary gland development, and calcium uptake. It is responsible for female secondary sex characteristics.

**Corpus luteum** (CL), or yellow body, develops in the collapsed cavity of the mature ovarian follicle after ovulation. This glandular tissue rapidly increases in size and secretes progesterone. If the cow conceives, the CL remains in the ovary during gestation. In the non-pregnant cow the CL begins to regress about 14 to 15 days after estrus.

**Progesterone,** produced mainly by the CL, prepares the uterus for implantation and maintains pregnancy. It also acts synergistically with estrogen in promoting estrous behavior. Progesterone controls gonadotrophin secretion.

**Relaxin** is also produced by the CL during pregnancy. It causes dilation of the cervix and vagina before parturition.

**Prostaglandins** are fatty acid hormones produced in the uterus and other tissues. They cause uterine contractions and regression of the corpus luteum (i.e., luteolysis).

**Figure 4.9.** Endocrine coordination of the cow reproductive system.

# EXERCISE 5

# Reproductive Organs of the Bull
# and Their Functions

## OBJECT

To become familiar with the anatomy and the physiological functions of the reproductive organs of the bull.

## DISCUSSION

The male's role in animal reproduction is largely concerned with fertilization of the female ova. The production of fertile spermatozoa by the bull used in AI is certainly a requirement of high priority. You should develop a general understanding of the formation of spermatozoa and their part in the reproduction process.

A knowledge of the anatomy of the male reproductive organs and their functions is essential for the proper management of bulls and the collection and handling of semen for AI. A diagrammatic view of the bull's reproductive organs is shown in Figure 5.1. When learning about reproductive anatomy and physiology, it is important to bear in mind that the brain, the nervous system (through innervation of the reproductive tract structures), and the neuroendocrine system are critical in the control and modulation of reproductive function.

The principal organs of reproduction in the bull are the two testes, which are situated outside the body wall within the scrotum. The testes have at least two functions: the production and release of spermatozoa (male germ cells) and the production and secretion of testosterone, the predominant male hormone,

which markedly affects development and behavior of the male. Closely attached to each testis is an epididymis, which extends down the outside of the testis to its base. The epididymis is divided anatomically into three parts: the head (caput), the body (corpus), and the tail (cauda). The head of the epididymis contains 10 to 15 highly-coiled efferent ducts leading from the upper pole of the testis proper; these fuse to form the main epididymal duct. This single duct is highly folded (in some bulls it may attain an overall length of 45 yards) and continues in a torturous route along the caudo-medial aspect of the testis as the head, body, and tail of the epididymis.

Functionally, the epididymides have both resorptive and secretory roles. As spermatozoa traverse the epididymal ducts (a period of approximately seven to nine days in the bull), they undergo a maturation process, acquiring the capability for motility and fertility. The tail of each epididymis is largely a repository for matured spermatozoa. The number of spermatozoa in the tail of each epididymis is greatest in sexually rested bulls and is reduced proportionally based on the frequency of ejaculation.

Thermoregulation of the testes is critical for normal function. In the bull, testicular temperature is maintained at 7° to 9° F (4° to 5° C) below "core" body temperature. This cooler testicular temperature for optimal spermatogenesis is maintained by an elaborate thermoregulation system. The system consists of (1) evaporation from the scrotal skin, (2) a counter-current heat exchange mechanism in the spermatic cord (pampiniform plexus), and

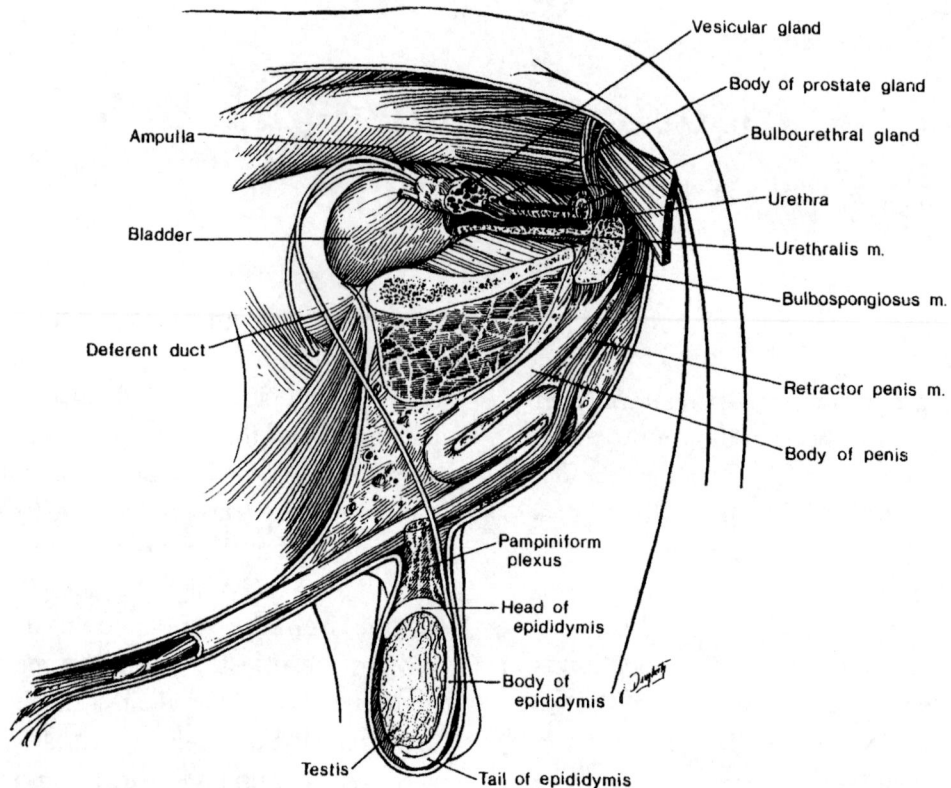

**Figure 5.1.** Anatomy of the reproductive organs of the bull. (R. P. Amann. 1986. How a bull works. Proc. 11th Tech. Conf. on Artificial Insemination and Reproduction. NAAB. p. 6)

(3) involuntary muscular control affecting both (a) the thickness and the surface area of the scrotum (tunica dartos muscle) and (b) the closeness of contact of the testes to the body wall (cremaster muscles in the spermatic cord).

Continuous with the epididymides are the deferent ducts, which run from the tail of the epididymides through the spermatic cord to the pelvic urethra. These muscular-walled ducts provide passageways to the exterior for ejaculation of the spermatozoa. The deferent ducts enlarge in diameter to form the glandular ampullae. The ampullae are located just above the anterior part of the pubis, where they join the pelvic urethra.

Lying on either side of the ampullae are the vesicular glands. In the bull, these are the largest of the accessory glands, being about two to three inches long and about one inch wide. They secrete approximately 30 to 50 percent of the fluid volume of semen. Vesicu-

lar gland secretions contain numerous proteins and a high content of fructose. Each vesicular gland opens into the pelvic urethra via an ejaculatory duct in common with the opening from the respective deferent duct.

Other accessory glands include the prostate and bulbourethral glands. In the bull, the prostate gland consists of two parts: the body of the prostate and the disseminate prostate. The former is located near the neck of the bladder, and the latter surrounds the urethra. Prostatic fluid contributes 25 to 40 percent of the semen volume. It is high in sodium and citrate and is a major source of zinc. The bulbourethral, or Cowper's, glands, are paired glands located on either side of the urethra near the ischial arch. They are covered by skeletal muscle (bulbospongiosus muscle), and each has a duct opening into the pelvic urethra. Their secretions tend to be

38

more alkaline than those of the other accessory glands.

Functions of the accessory gland secretions are not well understood. However, these fluids serve as a vehicle for the transport of spermatozoa.

The urethra is the mucous tube extending from the urinary bladder to the glans of the penis. The urethra is a joint canal for the excretion of urine and the expulsion of semen.

The penis is the male copulatory organ. It serves to introduce spermatozoa into the vagina of the cow.

Semen is the normal discharge of the male at mating or during the collection process for AI. It is whitish, somewhat thick, and composed of rete testis fluid, spermatozoa, and the secretions of the vesicular, prostate, and bulbourethral glands. The volume of semen ejaculated by a bull at a single service or collection normally varies from approximately 2 to 15 ml. The number of sperm per milliliter of bull semen usually ranges from a few hundred million to well over two billion, varying with the weight, age, and ejaculation frequency of the bull.

## PROCEDURE

Study the diagram of the reproductive organs of the bull, and become familiar with the names, locations, and functions of the various parts. Make use of organs displayed in the laboratory as well as diagrams, slides, etc.

Be able to locate and describe the function of each of the following parts:

Primary Reproductive Organs:

1. Testis.
2. Epididymis.
3. Deferent duct.
4. Ampulla.
5. Penis.

Accessory Organs/Related Genital Organs:

1. Bulbourethral glands.
2. Vesicular glands.
3. Scrotum.
4. Sheath/prepuce.
5. Spermatic cord.
6. Retractor penis muscles.
7. Prostate gland.
8. Urethra.

Study the functions of the male reproductive tract with reference to spermatogenesis.

The testes are ovoid in shape, and in the mature bull each may weigh up to 350 g. Testicular size is an important indicator of sperm production capacity. Several AI centers routinely screen entering young bulls for sperm production capacity by measuring scrotal circumference, which reflects a bull's total testicular mass. Bulls found to be below normal limits are poor sperm production prospects and are candidates for culling. The testes are made up of connective, interstitial, and spermatogenic tissue. They are richly vasculated and have intricate nervous innervation. The spermatogenic, or sperm-forming, tissues are found in the tubular compartment of the testes, which contains the convoluted seminiferous tubules. The interstitial compartment of the testes (between tubules) contains the testosterone-producing Leydig cells, blood vessels, nerves, and lymphatic vessels. The seminiferous tubules are coiled, convoluted structures with tremendous surface area. Figure 5.2 is a simplified schematic diagram demonstrating the organization of the seminiferous tubules of the bull testis and the tubular pathway for formed sperm to enter the epididymis.

Spermatogenesis, or sperm production, is a complex process that has been studied extensively. (For an in-depth account of spermatogenesis in the bull, consult the references

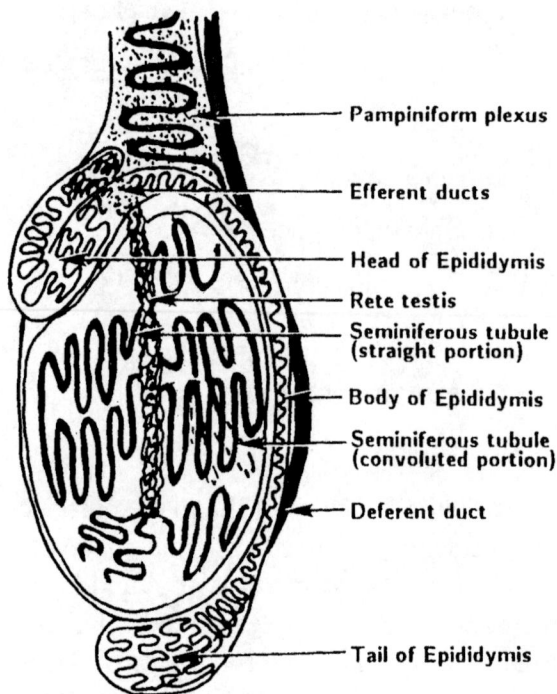

**Figure 5.2.** Spermatozoa are produced in the convoluted portion of the seminiferous tubules; are washed into the straight tubules and through the rete testis and efferent ducts; and then are transported by muscle contractions through the head and body of the epididymis, where they undergo maturation, to the tail of the epididymis, where they are stored as fertile sperm. (R. P. Amann. 1986. How a bull works. Proc. 11th Tech. Conf. on Artificial Insemination and Reproduction. NAAB. p. 6)

at the end of this exercise.) Spermatogenesis represents the sum of all the cell divisions and cell differentiations occurring in the formation of spermatozoa from spermatogonia (germinal stem cells). Spermatogenesis takes place in the germinal epithelium of the seminiferous tubules. The germinal epithelium contains the Sertoli cells, which are nondividing in adult animals, and the germ cells (spermatogonia, primary and secondary spermatocytes, and spermatids). The Sertoli cells provide a supporting framework in which spermatogenesis occurs. They line the basement membrane of the seminiferous tubule, have an endocrine function, and are believed to play a prominent role in coordinating spermatogenesis. The junctional complexes between adjoining Sertoli cells create a compartmentalization in the tubule referred to as the "blood-testis barrier." This is important because germ cell types undergoing meiosis are not recognized as foreign by the host immune system and are relatively isolated from certain substances in the circulation. The spermatogonia, which are interspersed between Sertoli cells along the basement membrane, divide mitotically to form more differentiated types of spermatogonia and primary spermatocytes. Because not all of the spermatogonia that are produced commit to the process of forming spermatozoa, there is a continuous renewal or replenishment of these cells along the basement membrane. The primary spermatocytes pass through the blood-testis barrier into the adluminal compartment (toward the lumen) of the seminiferous tubule. Figure 5.3 shows a schematic view of the cellular associations and compartmentalization in a portion of the seminiferous tubule. The primary spermatocytes then begin the process of meiosis (reduction division). It is during this period that the interchange of chromatin occurs and is of considerable interest from the standpoint of heredity. Each primary spermatocyte divides, forming two secondary spermatocytes, and each of these subsequently divides, forming two round spermatids. Each of the spermatids contains one-half the number of chromosomes for the species. Although the production of four spermatids is possible from each primary spermatocyte, it is likely that some of these cells degenerate.

The differentiation of spermatids from round cells with considerable cytoplasm to cells with a highly condensed nucleus, a small amount of cytoplasm, and a flagellum results from a process called "spermiogenesis." During this process the acrosome is also formed.

40

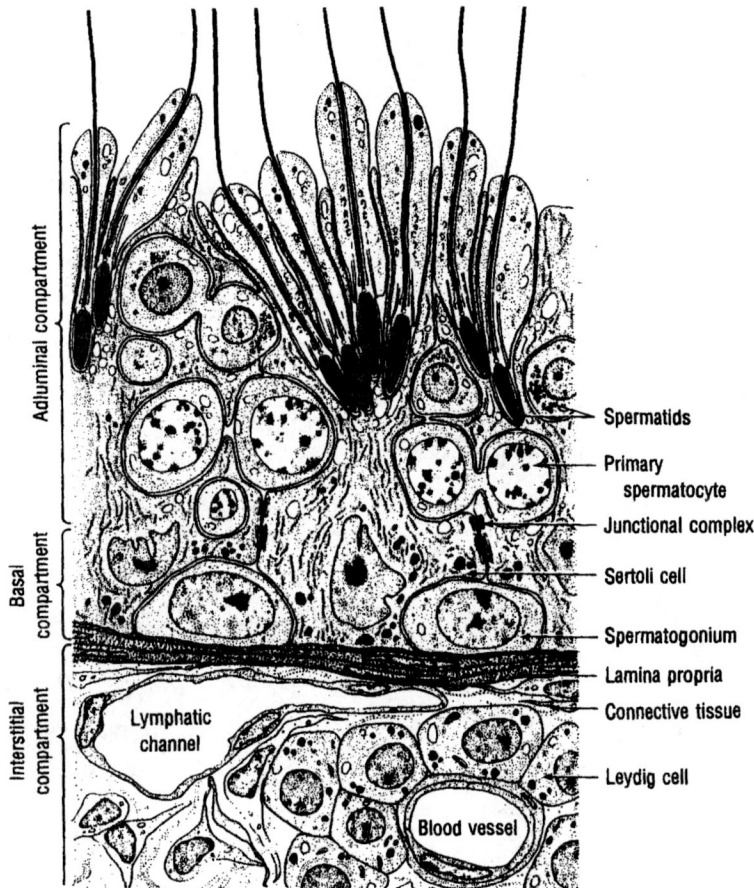

**Figure 5.3.** Drawing of part of a bull seminiferous tubule showing the relationship of the germ cells to the adjacent Sertoli cells. Formation of a spermatozoon starts near the basement membrane when a spermatogonium divides to form other spermatogonia and ultimately primary spermatocytes that are moved to a position away from the basement membrane but below the junctional complex between adjacent Sertoli cells. Later, the primary spermatocytes are moved from the basal compartment, through the junctional complexes, into the adluminal compartment, where they eventually divide to form secondary spermatocytes (not shown) and round spermatids. The spermatogonia, primary spermatocytes, secondary spermatocytes, and round spermatids all develop in the space between two or more Sertoli cells and are in contact with them. During elongation of the spermatids, they are repositioned by the Sertoli cells to become embedded within long pockets in the cytoplasm of an individual Sertoli cell. (R. P. Amann. 1986. How a bull works. Proc. 11th Tech. Conf. on Artificial Insemination and Reproduction. NAAB. p. 6)

During spermiogenesis, the elongating spermatids are embedded into pockets of Sertoli cellcytoplasm. At the completion of spermiogenesis, the spermatids are released or "spermiated" into the lumen of the seminiferous tubule. They are then called "spermatozoa." Figure 5.4 shows the pattern of spermatogenesis in the bull.

In the bull, the interval from the appearance of the stem spermatogonium (at any one location in the seminiferous tubules) to the release of spermatozoa produced from it is approximately 61 days. Spermatozoa are released sequentially at different locations along the lengths of the seminiferous tubules. This results in a continuous output of spermatozoa over time. Mature Holstein bulls are capable of producing 7 billion spermatozoa per day.

As shown schematically in Figure 5.5, the bull spermatozoon is made up of three major parts: the head, the middle piece of the tail,

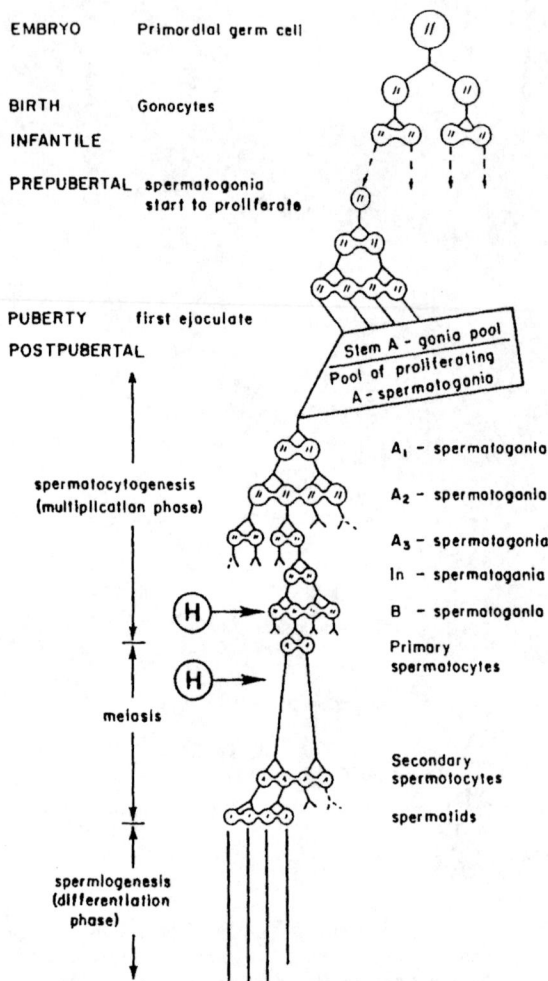

| EMBRYO | Primordial germ cell |
| BIRTH | Gonocytes |
| INFANTILE | |
| PREPUBERTAL | spermatogonia start to proliferate |

Stem A – gonia pool
Pool of proliferating A – spermatogonia

| PUBERTY | first ejaculate |
| POSTPUBERTAL | |

spermatocytogenesis (multiplication phase)

A₁ – spermatogonia
A₂ – spermatogonia
A₃ – spermatogonia
In – spermatogonia
B – spermatogonia
Primary spermatocytes

meiosis

Secondary spermatocytes

spermatids

spermiogenesis (differentiation phase)

Figure 5.4. The pattern of spermatogenesis in the bull during development of spermatogonia to form primary spermatocytes, secondary spermatocytes, spermatids, and spermatozoa. The horizontal connections between adjacent germ cells in a cohort depict the intercellular bridges that connect the germ cells. The vertical lines show the pattern of cell division, and the broken lines designate that some potential germ cells degenerate. The exact pattern of spermatogonial division or the number of different types of spermatogonia is uncertain; the pattern depicted is a hypothetical possibility. The letter "H" designates the germ cell types (B-spermatogonia and pachytene spermatocytes) especially sensitive to heat. (R. P. Amann. 1986. How a bull works. Proc. 11th Tech. Conf. on Artificial Insemination and Reproduction. NAAB. p. 6)

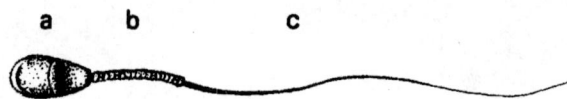

Figure 5.5. Drawing of typical bull spermatozoon: (a) head, (b) middle piece of tail, (c) principal and end piece of tail.

and the tail proper. The head is a flattened structure containing the nucleus and is about 8 to 10 microns long, 4 to 5 microns wide, and about 0.5 micron thick. The middle piece, or that portion of the tail surrounded by a mitochondrial sheath, is about 8 to 10 microns in length. The remainder of the tail (principal and end piece) is some 45 to 50 microns long.

Become familiar with the following terms concerned with spermatogenesis and be able to discuss them accurately:

1. Spermatogonia.

2. Primary spermatocyte.

3. Secondary spermatocyte.

4. Spermatid.

5. Spermatozoon.

6. Period of multiplication.

7. Meiosis.

8. Period of differentiation.

## QUESTIONS

1. What are the functions of GnRH, LH, FSH, androgen-binding protein (ABP), testosterone, and inhibin in spermatogenesis and male functions?

2. What is the function of (a) testes, (b) epididymis, (c) deferent ducts, (d) ampullae, (e) penis, (f) urethra, (g) bulbourethral and prostate glands, (h) vesicular glands, (i) retractor penis muscles, tunica dartos, and cremaster muscles?

3. What is the average volume of ejaculate and the average number of spermatozoa per milliliter of semen in bulls?

4. What factors influence spermatogenesis in the bull?

5. What are the changes in the number of chromosomes during spermatogenesis and during the fertilization process? Explain.

## REFERENCES

Amann, R. P. 1986. How a bull works. Proc. 11th Tech. Conf. on Artificial Insemination and Reproduction. NAAB. p. 6.

Coulter, G. H., and R. H. Foote. 1979. Bovine testicular measurements as indicators of reproductive performance and their relationship to productive traits in cattle: A review. Theriogenology 11:297.

Hafez, E. S. E. (Ed.). 1987. Reproduction in Farm Animals (5th Ed.). Lea & Febiger, Philadelphia. (Chs. 2, 3, 7.)

Hueston, W. D., et al. 1988. Scrotal circumference measurements on young Holstein bulls. J. Am. Vet. Med. Assoc. 192:766.

Johnson, L.A., et al. 1994. Spermatogenesis in the bull. Proc. 15th Technical Conf. on Artificial Insemination and Reproduction. NAAB. p. 9.

Miller, D. J., and R. L. Ax. 1988. Seminal plasma: What is it and why is it important? Proc. 12th Tech. Conf. on Artificial Insemination and Reproduction. NAAB. p. 97.

Salisbury, G. W., N. L. Van Demark, and J. R. Lodge (Ed.). 1978. Physiology of Reproduction and Artificial Insemination of Cattle (2nd Ed.). W. H. Freeman, San Francisco. (Chs. 8, 9, 10.)

Senger, P. L. 1999. Pathways to Pregnancy and Parturition. First revised edition. Current Conceptions, Inc., Moscow, ID. Mack Printing Group - Science Press, Ephrata, PA.

Sorenson, A. M., Jr. 1979. Animal Reproduction: Principles and Practices. McGraw-Hill, New York.

# EXERCISE 6

# Collection of Semen from the Bull

## OBJECT

To become familiar with the methods and the equipment used in the collection of semen and to practice the proper method of collecting semen from the bull.

## DISCUSSION

One of the primary requirements for the successful use of AI is a supply of fertile semen. Fertile bulls and proper management are essential. The correct technique in the collection of semen is necessary so that maximum efficiency can be obtained. Measures, or evaluations, of semen and semen processing will be taken up in later exercises.

There are basically four methods of collecting semen from the bull: (1) using an artificial vagina—the preferred method for artificial insemination; (2) using an electro-ejaculator—for impaired bulls that are unable to mount and for bulls that are not accustomed to being handled; (3) massaging the pelvic accessory genital organs (ampullae) per rectum; and (4) recovering semen from the vagina of a cow that has been naturally serviced. The last method was used in the early days of AI. It is not recommended but included here for general information.

Normally, the collection of semen is best accomplished by a work team consisting of the semen collector, the bull handler, and sometimes a mount handler. These individuals work together to provide for and control the appropriate stimulus situation(s) for the bull.

*Semen collector* — Manages the artificial vagina and performs the actual collection of semen. This person is usually the leader of the team and determines when the bull is properly prepared and when the seminal collection can be taken safely. In addition, the collector must insure that procedures are hygienic and that the semen is accurately identified.

*Bull handler* — Handles the bull using a lead rope. This person must be responsible for keeping the bull under control and safely away from other persons and bulls in the collection arena. This person is also responsible for appropriate mount animal restraint unless that animal is managed by a separate handler.

*Mount handler* — Handles the mount animal using a lead rope or halter. This person is responsible for keeping the mount animal under control while the bull is being prepared for collection.

## PROCEDURE

Seminal collection procedures normally include sexual stimulation, sexual preparation, and collection of the semen.

### Sexual Stimulation

Providing a stimulus situation that elicits mounting behavior in the bull is termed "sexual stimulation." The stimulation process starts by exposing the bull to a mount animal in a

**Table 6.1.** Techniques to provide novelty and obtain a sexual response[a]

---

- Move the teaser forward and backward in small increments.
- Remove the bull from the teasing position by walking the bull in a circle behind the mount and reintroduce the bull to the original teasers.
- Move the bull and teaser to an area of isolation where he can work alone.
- Briskly walk the teaser with the bull following in a straight line, or at a leisurely pace, or in tight or large circles.
- Slowly circle the teaser around the bull. End the movement by positioning the back of the teaser under the bull's chin.
- Allow the teaser to mount other teasers, or mount the bull.
- Change to a teaser of different size, shape, or color pattern.
- Present two teasers side by side.
- Adequately control the bull and position him near, but a safe distance away from another bull who is mounting, giving him the feeling of competition.
- Tease the bull outside rather than inside.
- Tie the bull on a long lead behind a tethered mount and move away, but continue observing for any sexual activity from the bull, quickly moving in to deflect the penis.
- **Only as a last resort,** use a bull rather than a steer as a mount, making certain that both bulls are under control and that potential risk of injury to both the collection team and bulls is minimized.
- Talk kindly to the bull and coax him to mount.
- Sexual arousal of a bull may require a combination of all the suggestions mentioned.

---

[a]J. L. Schenk. 1998. Bull semen collection procedures. Proc. 17th Tech. Conf. on Artificial Insemination and Reproduction. NAAB. p. 48.

collection environment. The presence of other animals in this environment and various visual, olfactory, and auditory stimuli sexually arouse the bull. When the bull is sexually aroused he will have an erection of the penis and will want to mount other bulls and/or a mount animal. (A mount animal or teaser is a steer or another bull whose purpose is to sexually stimulate the bull and stand in a sturdy position as the bull mounts him, as if in a natural breeding situation.) Novelty in a stimulus situation is an important component for successful semen collection. Table 6.1 lists various techniques that may be used to provide novelty and obtain a sexual response from the bull. Cows are not excluded as mount animals, but their use is not advocated. Depending upon the libido of the bull and the frequency of collection, the stimulation may be accomplished in a matter of minutes or it may take much longer.

**Sexual Preparation**

Sexual preparation is the intentional prolongation of sexual stimulation. It is achieved through a series of false mounts (allowing the bull to mount but not ejaculate) and restraint and ultimately results in an increase in the quantity and quality of sperm ejaculated. The type of preparation varies widely depending upon the libido and physical condition of the bull.

For all false mounts, the semen collector should be at the bull's side to hold the sheath aside so the penis does not come in contact with the rear quarters of the mount animal. This diminishes the chance of contaminating the penis and also serves to prevent possible injury. Due to physical and health conditions, especially rear limb and spinal disabilities, some bulls may need to be limited in the number of false mounts allowed. The seminal collection procedure for such bulls should be under the direction of a professional livestock person or a veterinarian.

## Collection of Semen by Artificial Vagina

The collector should work with the bull throughout the preparation procedure and determine the optimum time for seminal collection. Routinely the seminal collection is performed immediately after the false mounting regime is completed.

Semen is routinely collected through the use of an artificial vagina (AV). This device is made to simulate the natural breeding situation as much as possible. Intromission and ejaculation into the AV are performed by the bull in a manner nearly identical to natural mating. Since the final ejaculation cascade results from tactile stimuli to the bull's glans penis, the temperature, turgidity, and lubrication of the AV are important to successful sperm harvest.

The equipment used, assembly of the AV, collection with the AV, and proper care and cleaning of the equipment will be demonstrated by the instructor.

## Points to observe in using an artificial vagina:

1. Adequate facilities for handling bulls and mount animals during semen collection should be provided. It is recommended that the collection arena consist of an area large enough to accommodate the safe semen collection from one or more bulls (Figure 6.1). The size of the arena should be such that the individual bulls and mount animals can be led throughout the area without interfering with one another.

   It is important that the collection area provide good "footing" for bulls and mount animals to prevent slipping and subsequent injury. Concrete should be avoided unless surfaces are grooved.

   The passageway leading from the bull housing area to the collection arena should be equipped with a sturdy guard rail to allow the bull handlers to separate themselves from the

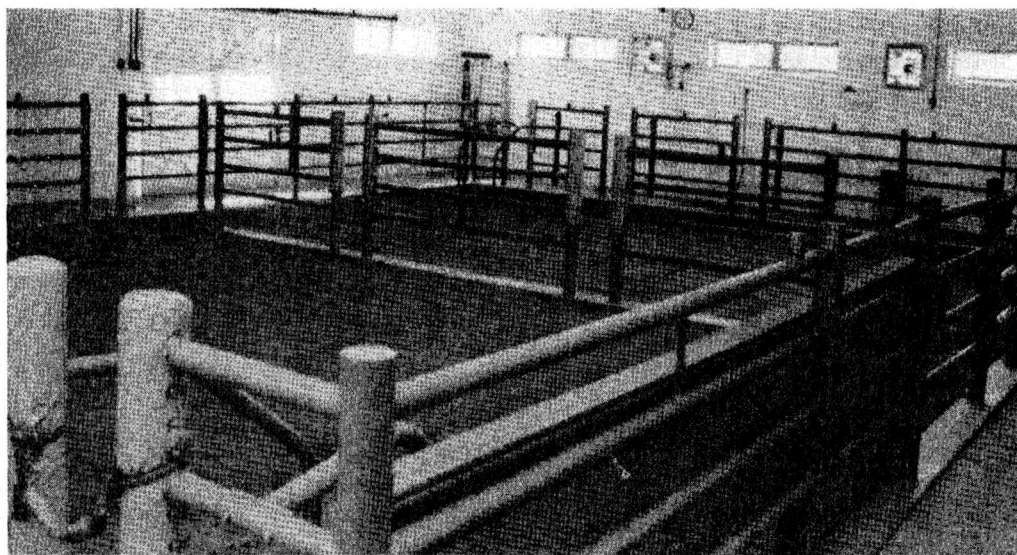

**Figure 6.1.** Collection arena facilities incorporate many features that provide for safety of bulls, mount animals, and personnel, as well as efficiency of semen collection. (Courtesy, the former Atlantic Breeders Cooperative, Lancaster, PA)

bulls. The railing is generally placed near the center of a walkway so that it allows a bull to be led on one side of the rail while the bull handler(s) walks on the opposite side of the rail. It is recommended that the railing be built in 7- to 14-foot lengths, with each length being separated by a gap, or safety pass, of approximately 14 inches. This safety pass provides the bull handler the opportunity to switch from one side of the railing to the other should the need arise. The 14-inch safety pass is of such size that the bull handler can easily pass through while a large bull cannot. It is also recommended that similar safety equipment and precautions be applied to the collection arena. The mount animal must be properly restrained. Because of health concerns, steers and, in some cases, other bulls are recommended as mount animals over females.

2. The bulls should be free of disease and kept clean and well groomed. Also, to prevent transmission of potential disease-producing agents during semen collection, the hindquarters of the mount animal need to be effectively and thoroughly disinfected between successively mounting bulls. The semen collector should use new disposable plastic gloves for each bull to avoid potential disease transmission. In addition, AV equipment is to be thoroughly cleansed and disinfected or sterilized prior to each use. A separate AV or AV liner must be used for each ejaculate to avoid unnecessary microbial contamination. (Care and management of bulls will be discussed in a later laboratory exercise.)

3. The AV used for the collection of semen from bulls consists of:
   a. An outer flexible rubber casing from 8 to 16 inches in length and from 2.25 to 3.50 inches in diameter.
   b. An inner liner of smooth or textured latex rubber, the ends of which are folded back over the ends of the casing to form a water jacket. The liner is usually held in place with large rubber bands. Care must be exercised to see that they do not slip off during collection. Severe penis injuries can result due to rubber bands slipping off the AV and becoming affixed to the penis during collection. Following collection it is important to check the AV equipment and make sure all bands are accounted for.
   c. A latex rubber director cone with air vent and with attached glass or plastic collection tube. The director cone is also secured with rubber bands. Alternatively, a one-piece or combination liner and cone may be used. In this case there are two inner liners— one that forms the water jacket, and the combination liner and cone that is inserted within the water jacket and secured only at the service end.

   The parts of a typical AV are shown in Figure 6.2, and a diagrammatic section is shown in Figure 6.3.

4. The water jacket of the AV is normally filled with water at 140° F (60° C) to within an inch or two of the top when held vertically. If a valve is not used, the inner liner can be loosened and the water introduced into the open end of the casing. The amount of wa-

ter used and the length and diameter of the AV are varied depending on penis development and thrusting characteristics of junk individual bulls. To save time when semen is to be collected from many bulls, some organizations maintain several AV's at collection temperature in an incubator. In this case, water is added to the AV's several hours before semen collection activity begins. Figure 6.4 shows AV's prepared for collection and ready to be placed in an incubator.

Smaller AV's are typically used for younger, immature bulls. Use of shorter AV's, even for mature bulls, is believed by some organizations to result in fewer penis injuries. A separate AV or AV liner should be used for each ejaculate. When the bull ejaculates into the AV, the semen should be deposited in the director cone portion of the AV. Ejaculation into the water-jacketed portion of the AV would result in thermal damage to sperm cells.

5. After the water jacket is filled, or, alternatively, after the AV is taken from an incubator, a thin coating of sterile, water-soluble lubricating jelly is applied by means of a sterile glass rod to the upper one-third of the open end of the vagina liner before use. The temperature of the AV should be checked before being used for collection. At the time of collection, the inside temperature of the

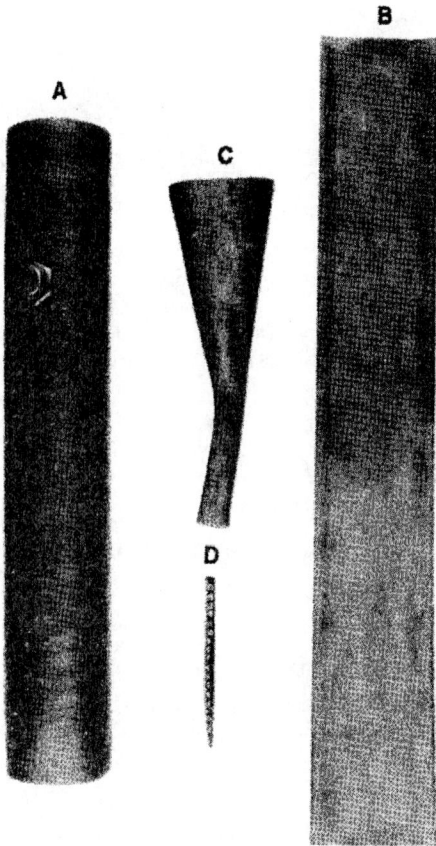

**Figure 6.2.** Component parts of an artificial vagina (AV). (A) outer flexible rubber casing, (B) latex rubber liner, (C) latex rubber director cone or funnel, (D) graduated collection tube.

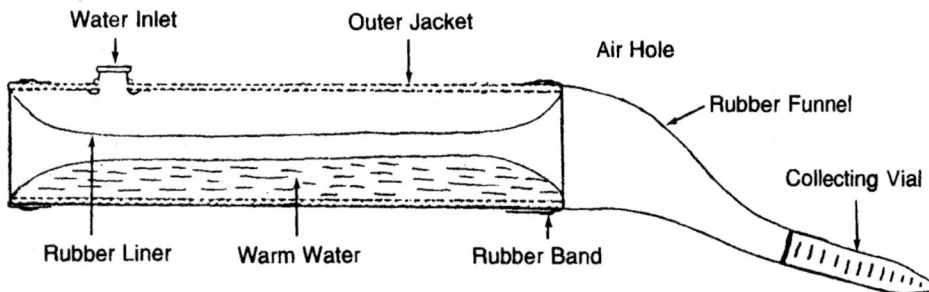

**Figure 6.3.** Cross-sectional view of an artificial vagina (AV), showing position of liner, director cone or funnel, and collection tube.

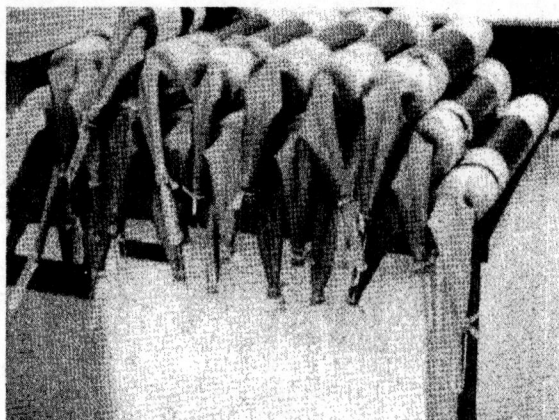

**Figure 6.4.** Artificial vaginas are assembled and then filled with water prior to placing them in a holding incubator several hours before collection. (Courtesy, Genex Cooperative, Shawano, WI)

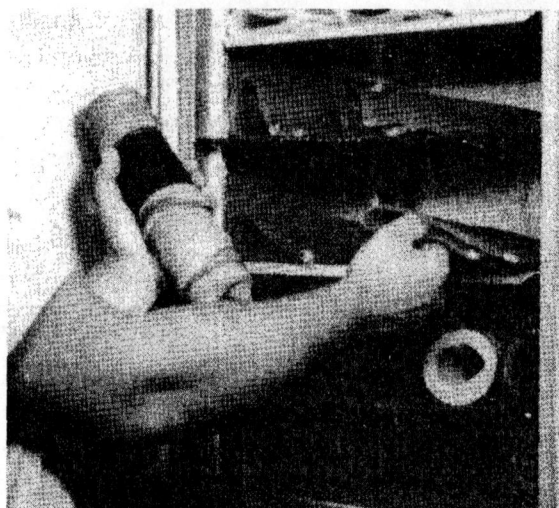

**Figure 6.5.** Prior to semen collection, an insulated protector is removed from the incubator and placed over the director cone and collection-tube portion of the AV. This will provide thermal protection for sperm cells during and after collection. (Courtesy, Select Sires, Inc., Plain City, OH)

AV should be between 113° and 131° F (45° and 55° C).

6. The semen should be protected against temperature shock (rapid changes in temperature) and strong light. Several AI organizations also use an insulated protector that fits over the director cone and collection-tube end of the AV (Figure 6.5). Also, an insulating sleeve or small water bath (containing 100° F [38° C] water) surrounding the collection tube can be used for thermal protection.

7. In order to obtain the maximum amount of good quality semen, the donor bull should be sexually stimulated and adequately prepared. Sexual preparation procedures recommended by Almquist[1] for dairy and beef bulls are as follows:

   a. **Dairy bulls**—One false mount plus two minutes of restraint plus two additional false mounts before each ejaculation.

   b. **Beef bulls**—Three false mounts (no restraint) before first ejaculation and no false mounts before second ejaculation.

   Figure 6.6 shows the semen collector holding the bull's sheath aside to avoid contact with the mount animal during sexual preparation prior to semen collection.

8. When the bull mounts for ejaculation following sexual preparation, the collector covers the extended penis with the AV, which is held at an angle of about 45 degrees. Contact of the penis with the warm, lubricated AV results in the ejaculation, which is instantaneous if all stimuli are adequate for the bull. Both hind feet of the bull leaving the ground during the ejaculatory thrust is an indication of proper stimulation and preparation. The extended penis should not be handled by the collector. Figure 6.7 depicts collection of semen from the bull. After ejaculation, the AV is held

[1] J. O. Almquist. 1978. Bull semen collection procedures to maximize output of semen. Proc. 7th Tech. Conf. on Artificial Insemination and Reproduction. NAAB. p. 33.

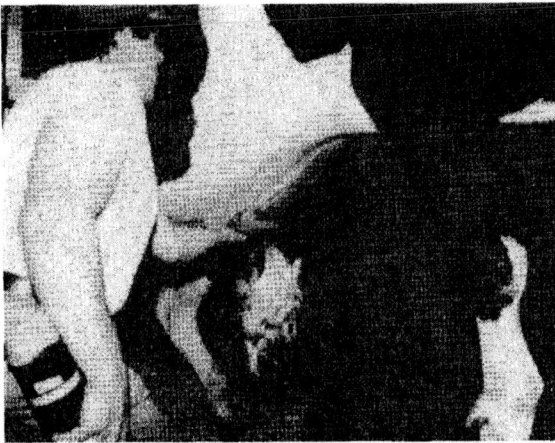

**Figure 6.6.** The collector grasps the bull's sheath posterior to the extended penis during a false mount. Gently pulling the sheath toward the collector during the false mount prevents contact of the penis with the rear quarters of the mount animal. Note that the collector wears a disposable plastic glove and does not directly handle the extended penis. (Courtesy, John O. Almquist Research Center, The Pennsylvania State University)

upright to permit the semen to drain from the director cone into the collection tube (Figure 6.8). The AV should not be squeezed or stripped, as this can introduce debris and contamination into the semen.

9. Proper identification of semen used in AI is critical. It is important that the bull's identity be verified before the semen is collected (Figure 6.9). Various systems used in the AI industry to insure proper identification have been described by Doak.[2] As soon as the semen has been collected, it should be labeled with at least the code number and the short name of the bull.

---

[2] G. A. Doak. 1978. Semen identification: Collection to sale. Proc. 7th Tech. Conf. on Artificial Insemination and Reproduction. NAAB. p. 16.

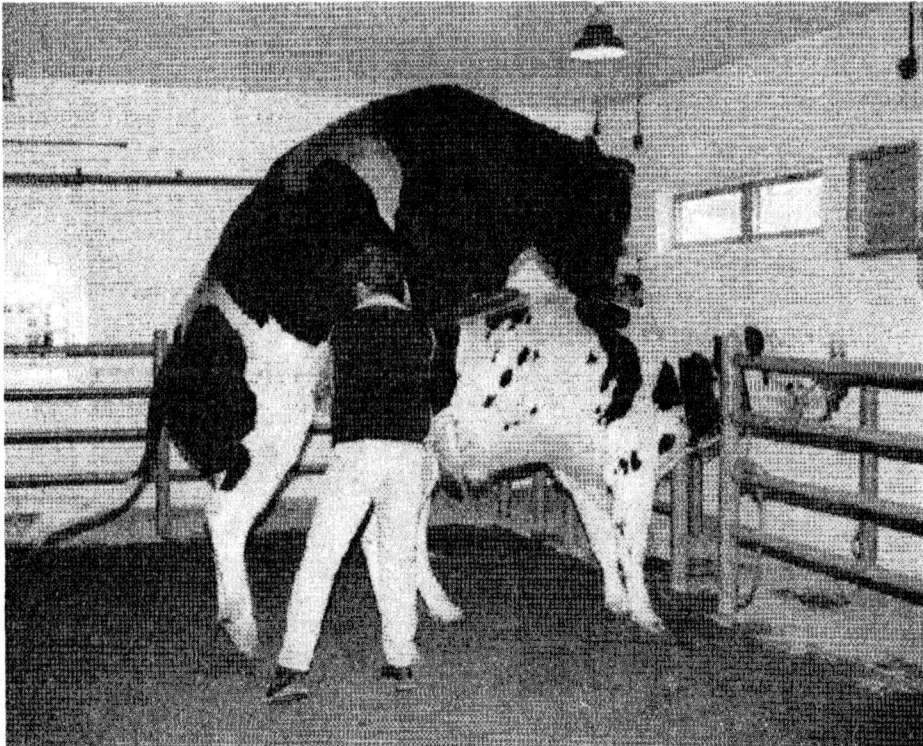

**Figure 6.7.** Semen collection from the bull, using an artificial vagina. Following false mounts and restraint, the mounting bull's penis is covered with the warm, lubricated AV, which elicits ejaculation. Note that both of the bull's hind feet are off the ground during the ejaculatory thrust. (Courtesy, the former Atlantic Breeders Cooperative, Lancaster, PA)

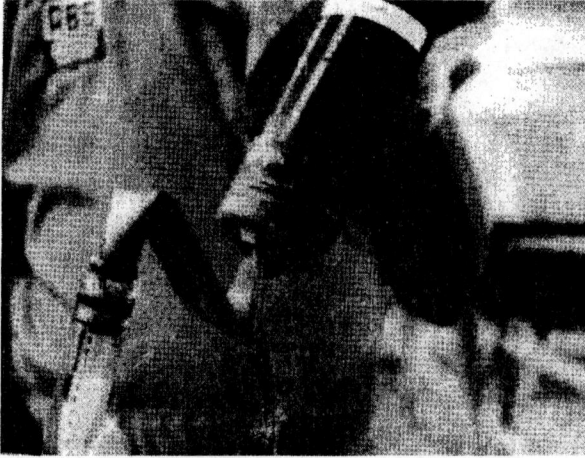

**Figure 6.8.** Following collection of semen from the bull, the semen is allowed to drain into the collection tube, which is thermally protected with a small water bath surrounding it. Note that an adhesive label with the bull's identification number and name has been affixed to the AV. (Courtesy, ABS Global, Inc., DeForest, WI)

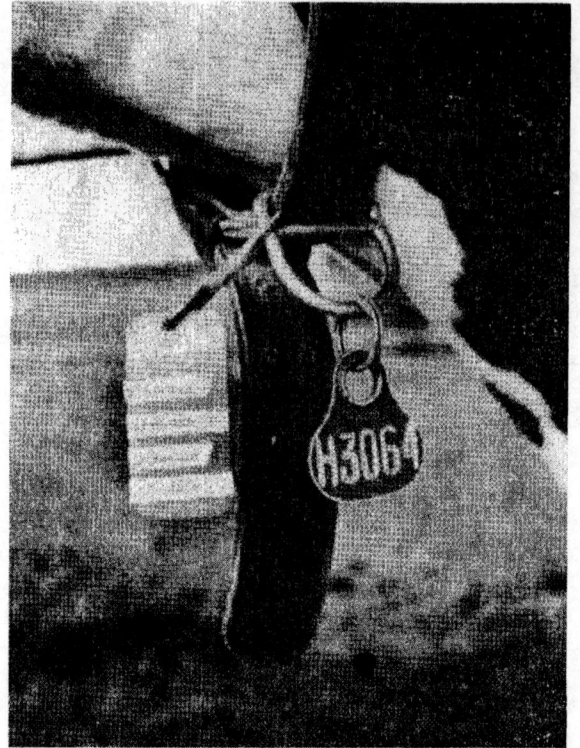

**Figure 6.9.** Proper identification of the sire and his semen is of critical importance in artificial insemination. Shown here is a plastic tag snapped onto the collar of a bull to be collected. A number of adhesive labels corresponding to ejaculates to be collected are affixed to the tag. These indicate the bull's identification code number and name. Identification of the bull is verified by collection personnel before semen is collected. Following collection of each ejaculate, the collector removes a label from the tag and places it on the AV. The AV, which is used for only one ejaculate, is taken to the lab area, and the label is then transferred to the collection tube to insure proper identification. Following collection, the plastic tag is removed from the bull's collar, cleaned, and labeled for next use. (Courtesy, ABS Global, Inc., DeForest, WI)

Typically this is accomplished by writing the information on a piece of tape that is applied to the collection tube. The semen collector routinely completes and initials a collection report that includes date, time, bull code, ejaculate number, volume of semen, and any comments pertinent to the collection. At some AI Centers the semen collector directly enters this information into a computer database (Figure 6.10) Processing begins when the semen enters the laboratory. This will be described in a later exercise.

10. Cleanliness and good hygiene should be followed in semen collection. The floor of the collection area should be throughly cleaned and periodically disinfected. The rear quarters of the mount animal should be cleansed and disinfected between collections from successive bulls. All collection equipment should be clean and sterile or disinfected.

All equipment used in collecting must be thoroughly cleaned after being used.

Suggested steps in cleaning include:

1. Rinse all equipment in cold water.

2. Wash all equipment in warm, soapy water (laboratory glassware detergent is preferred). Use various brushes for glassware, AV casings, AV liners, rubber bands, stoppers, and AV director cones. Liners and

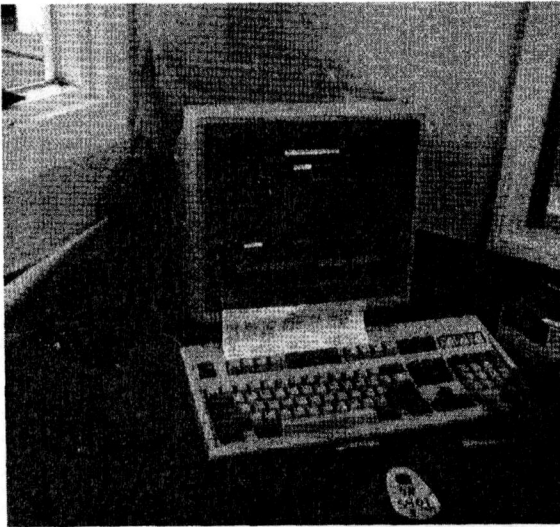

**Figure 6.10.** Semen collection information being entered into a computer database following collection of the bull. In addition to time of collection and identity of the ejaculate, other information may be recorded regarding: behavioral characteristics of the bull, the mount animal used, collection room location, etc. (Courtesy, Select Sires, Inc., Plain City, OH).

cones should be turned inside out so that all surfaces can be scrubbed.

3. Rinse all equipment in warm running tap water.

4. Air dry AV casings.

5. Rinse liners, director cones, rubber bands, rubber stoppers, and glassware in distilled water.

6. Dry-heat sterilize glassware in an oven (270° F [150° C] for 1.5 hours). After moisture has evaporated, cover openings with aluminum foil.

7. Immerse rubber goods in boiling distilled water for 15 minutes after water begins to boil or utilize appropriate steam sterilization methods.

8. Sterilize all rubber equipment by dipping it in 70 percent alcohol. Then allow drying in a dust-free environment.

9. Wrap liners and director cones individually in clean paper, or place in clean covered plastic containers for storage.

## Using Electrical Stimulation

Ejaculation may be brought about by electrical stimulation. In 1936, Gunn[3] and his co-workers first used this method for sheep. It has since been employed for many domestic and zoo animals. In 1950, two Brazilian workers, Mascarenhas and Gomes,[4] developed and used a bipolar type of electrode to obtain semen from bulls. Since 1950, the collection of semen by means of electro-ejaculation has been materially improved. Generally, semen collected by means of electro-ejaculation compares favorably to that collected by the AV. Although concentration may be lower and volume greater than AV collected semen, there are no apparent differences in freezability or fertility.[5]

The use of electro-ejaculation as an alternative seminal collection method should be limited to those circumstances when the temperament or physical condition of a bull renders collection of semen by AV unsafe or impossible. The electro-ejaculation method is convenient for obtaining semen from crippled bulls that are unable to serve the AV or for collecting semen from beef or range bulls unaccustomed to handling.

---

[3] R. M. C. Gunn. 1936. Fertility in sheep: Artificial production of seminal ejaculation and the characters of the spermatozoa contained therein. Res. Bull. 94. Australian Council for Science and Industry.

[4] H. Mascarenhas and W. V. Gomes. 1950. Contribuicao as estudo de electro ejaculacao em bovinos: Novo tipo de electrodo bipolar e technica de sua aplicacao. Publicacao N. 8. Instituto de Zootecnia, N.D.P.A.—Ministerio de Agricultura, Rio de Janeiro, Brasil.

[5] L. Ball. 1978. Semen collection by electro-ejaculation and massage of the pelvic organs. Proc. 7th Tech. Conf. on Artificial Insemination and Reproduction. NAAB. p. 37.

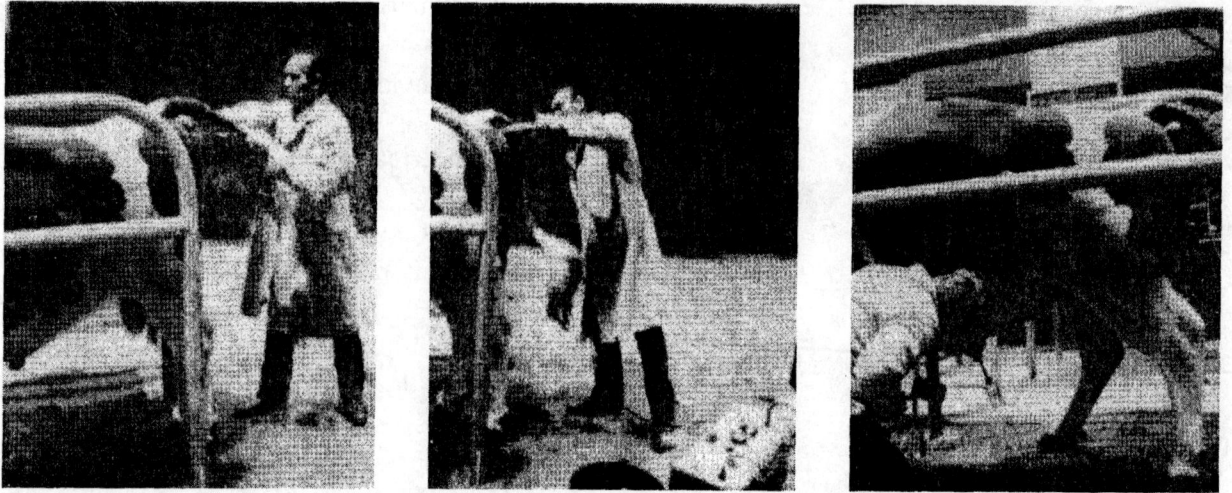

**Figure 6.11.** Semen collection by electrical stimulation of the reproductive tract (electro-ejaculation). *Left:* Removal of fecal material from bull's rectum. *Center:* Careful insertion of lubricated and sanitized probe. Ejaculation unit with power step and stimulator controls shown in foreground. *Right:* Thermally protected sanitary receptacle is used to collect semen emitted from bull's extended penis.

Briefly, the method involves the introduction of an electrode probe into the rectum. Excitation of the emission and ejaculatory nerve centers is produced by means of alternating current. Most ejaculators have a power step control and a stimulator control. The power step control limits the electrical potential and current to the bull by steps. The stimulator control allows variable application within the limits of each power step[6] (Figure 6.11).

Electro-ejaculators should be of the solid-state, low-amperage type with complete grounding of the electronics. Current output should not exceed 1 ampere at maximum power. Machines must be regularly maintained, with particular attention to possible short circuits. The use of rectal probes with ventrally oriented electrodes or finger electrodes is advocated to minimize extraneous skeletal muscle stimulation. The restraint chute selected for electro-ejaculation should provide lateral immobilization of the bull.

This technique may be of great value when bulls are unable to ejaculate into an AV. It has the disadvantage of requiring specialized equipment and skill. Proper training of machine operators must involve supervision by an experienced machine operator and/or veterinarian. An operator must be completely familiar with the instrument's controls, the restraint chute, and the bull.

The finger-electrode-massage method of electro-ejaculation of bulls described by Weidler[7] has been in use since 1971 as an alternative to the probe method. The advantages of this method are:

1. There is very little visible stress on the bull.

2. Since only selected areas are stimulated, the operator is in complete control of bull's erection and ejaculation.

### Massaging the Pelvic Accessory Genital Organs

Massaging the ampullae through the rectal wall is another method used to obtain se-

---

[6] Ibid.

[7] F. Weidler. 1978. Finger-electrode-massage method of electro-ejaculation of bulls. Proc. 7th Tech. Conf. on Artificial Insemination and Reproduction. NAAB. p. 39.

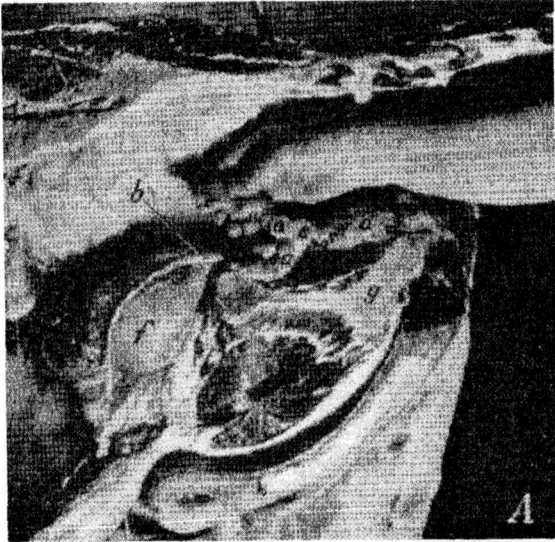

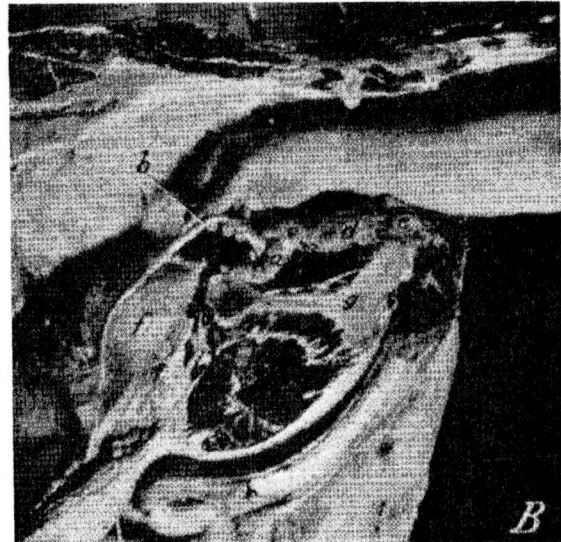

**Figure 6.12.** Semen collection by manual massage of pelvic genitalia of the bull. (A) Massaging the vesicular glands (seminal vesicles). (B) Massaging the ampullae of the ductuli deferentia (vas deferens).
(a) vesicular glands, (b) ampulla of ductus deferens, (c) body of prostate gland, (d) urethralis muscle surrounding pelvic urethra, (e) Cowper's gland, (f) urinary bladder, (g) pubis, (h) penis. (Adapted in part from Miller and Evans. 1934. USDA, Washington, DC)

men (Figure 6.12). This method of collection requires special training to be used successfully and is often less consistent in harvesting semen of acceptable quality. The advantages of this method are that collections can be made from bulls that are unable to mount and serve and less equipment is required for the collection.

## Collecting Semen from the Vagina of a Cow

This may be done with a sponge, pipet, spoon, or similar object. This method is *not* recommended because the semen is contaminated with mucus and urine, and there is an increased danger of spreading genital diseases.

## QUESTIONS

1. What are the methods available for the collection of bull semen? Which methods are preferable and why?

2. What is the general construction of the AV?

3. What is the proper temperature of the AV at the time of collection?

4. What precautions should be followed in handling bulls during semen collection?

5. What is the proper procedure for preparing and stimulating bulls prior to collection?

6. How should semen be handled immediately after it is collected? List steps and precautions.

7. What kind of a lubricant should be used for the AV?

8. What factors affect the quantity and quality of semen produced?

9. Under what conditions is it advisable to use the electro-ejaculation method?

10. How should semen be handled prior to processing?

## REFERENCES

Hafez, E. S. E. (Ed.). 1987. Reproduction in Farm Animals (5th Ed.). Lea & Febiger, Philadelphia. (Ch. 23.)

Sorenson, A. M., Jr. 1979. Animal Reproduction: Principles and Practices. McGraw-Hill, New York. (Ch. 4.)

# PART TWO

# Semen Evaluation; Extenders (Processing);

# Frozen Semen; Custom Collection

# EXERCISE 7

# Evaluation of Semen—General Considerations

## OBJECT

To understand the importance of evaluating semen quality in artificial insemination and to indicate certain evaluation limitations.

## DISCUSSION

Evaluations routinely conducted by the AI laboratory are used to determine whether the semen that is collected and processed is satisfactory for use. Immediately following collection, semen is screened for quality and number of spermatozoa in order to eliminate any substandard ejaculates. This initial screening also avoids wasting expensive supplies, antibiotics, semen extender, and so forth, because substandard samples are not processed. Semen that passes initial screening will be further extended, cooled, packaged into straws, and frozen. After freezing, a representative sample is normally thawed and evaluated using various laboratory tests. These post-thaw evaluations not only reflect the ability of the semen to withstand the processing conditions (process quality control) but also can give some indication of the potential fertility of the semen (fertility prediction). However, the best indication of the fertility of the bull is his actual breeding record, which may be estimated by non-return rate. Continual evaluation and interpretation of semen quality tests should always be followed up with a review of the fertility history of each bull, when available.

As pointed out by Saacke, et al.,[1] males differ in both fertility and the minimum number of sperm per inseminate needed to reach the maximum fertility of which they are capable. In this regard, two aspects of semen quality become important to the AI laboratory: those characteristics that are *compensable* and those that are *uncompensable*. Increasing sperm dosage to the female results in a response in fertility for compensable semen characteristics, whereas *differences in fertility among bulls cannot be removed by increasing sperm dosage for uncompensable semen characteristics*. Immotile or obviously malformed sperm would be compensable and have little effect on fertility if the female is inseminated with sufficient numbers of competent sperm. Viable abnormal ejaculates are believed to be uncompensable because they may not be able to maintain or sustain the fertilization process. Bulls with largely uncompensable semen characteristics would probably be subfertile at any dosage. Differences in these semen characteristics certainly need to be considered when making semen-processing decisions. Figure 7.1 illustrates this point for compensable and uncompensable semen deficiencies.

It should be recognized that the quality and quantity of frozen semen used to inseminate a cow or heifer are not the only factors influencing the opportunity for that female to become

---

[1] Saacke, R. G., et al. 1992. Semen: Its impact on fertility and embryo quality. Proc. 11th Ann. Conv., American Embryo Transfer Assoc. p. 1.

A
B

45%

U

55% | C | U | 15%

25% | C

30% | 30%

Compensable vs. Uncompensable
Semen Deficiencies

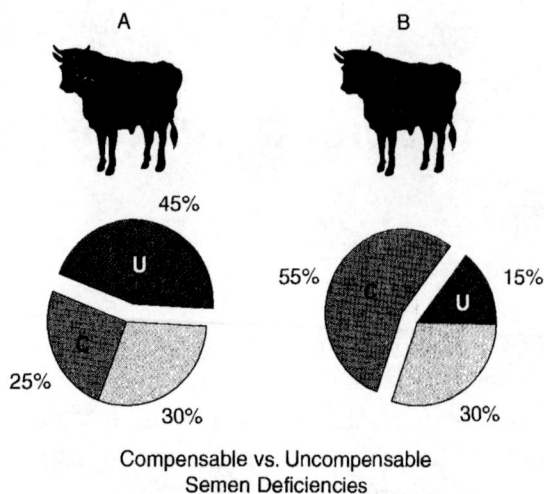

**Figure 7.1.** In the evaluation of semen, we would now consider the compensable (C) and uncompensable (U) deficiencies to comprise semen in any possible combination. In this scenario, a male such as Bull A should be recognized and eliminated from AI service since the larger portion of his deficiency is uncompensable and therefore cannot be overcome by increased dosage in the inseminate. On the contrary, Bull B may require higher than normal dosages to achieve pregnancy rates comparable to his peers with minimal compensable deficiencies. (Modified from R. G. Saacke. 2000. Fertility in the bovine male: current status and future prospects—An opinion. Proc. 18th Tech. Conf. Artificial Insemination and Reproduction. NAAB. p. 90)

pregnant. A myriad of other factors (e.g., heat detection accuracy, insemination skill, physiological stress from lactation, health and nutrition of the female, AI usage category, etc.) have also been shown to impact fertility. (See the references at the end of this exercise for further information.) These other factors are largely beyond the control of the AI laboratory but, nevertheless, must be dealt with by the AI technician or direct herd ("do-it-yourself") customer. Because herd fertility is the product of all these factors combined, it is very important that each factor be at an optimum level for a successful AI program.

Reputable AI organizations understand their responsibility for producing high-quality semen and therefore maintain complete quality control over all phases of their sire care, semen collection, processing, and distribution programs. Many different semen tests are used by the AI organizations to monitor changes that occur in their programs. Research has shown that these tests are not exact predictors of fertility, but they are effective quality control measures when used in an appropriate manner (by properly trained personnel using properly calibrated equipment). However, it is also known that results from these tests can be influenced by such things as the individual bulls, extenders, semen freezing and thawing rates, and so forth.

The Technical Committee of the National Association of Animal Breeders, Inc., published a position paper on laboratory tests for evaluating bovine semen[2] that lists evaluation techniques used in the AI industry with varied success. The position paper also points out that there can be considerable variation in test results when the same semen sample is evaluated by different personnel in the same laboratory or in another one. This is undoubtedly due to the subjective nature of various semen tests. It is important to note that evaluation of semen by other than the producing organization may result in incorrect conclusions, because semen evaluation methods are not exact and the fertility history of the bull is not usually known by others. Therefore, the reputation and the integrity of the semen-producing business continue to be the best indicator available to the customer of whether semen purchased directly from the organization is of high quality.

Although several valuable semen tests are being used in the AI industry today, there is no overwhelming evidence that conclusively demonstrates any one test or combination of tests to be an exact predictor of bull fertility. However, the AI industry continually conducts and supports research to identify improved tests for predicting fertility.

---

[2] NAAB Tech. Committee Position Paper. 1986. Laboratory tests for evaluating bovine semen. Proc. 11th Tech. Conf. on Artificial Insemination and Reproduction. NAAB. p. 102.

# QUESTIONS

1. When is semen routinely evaluated for quality in the AI laboratory?

2. How well do quality tests predict the fertility of a semen sample? List several factors that may influence fertility of an AI dose.

3. Do semen evaluation tests measure the inherent fertility of the bull? Explain.

4. Why do different lab technicians (in the same laboratory or in another one) sometimes obtain varying test results on the same semen freeze batch even though the same evaluation methods are employed? What factors can influence semen test results?

5. What are compensable and uncompensable semen characteristics?

6. Explain the concept of process quality control.

# REFERENCES

Foote, R. H. 1992. Collecting and processing semen with vision, decision and revision: Producing and maintaining a quality product. Proc. 14th Tech. Conf. on Artificial Insemination and Reproduction. NAAB. p. 68.

Rycroft, H., and B. Bean. 1992. Factors influencing non-return data. Proc. 14th Tech. Conf. on Artificial Insemination and Reproduction. NAAB. p. 43.

Saacke, R. G. 1982. Components of semen quality. J. Anim. Sci. 55 (Suppl. 2):1.

Saacke, R. G. 1998. AI fertility: Are we getting the job done? Proc. 17th Tech. Conf. on Artificial Insemination and Reproduction. NAAB. p. 6.

Saacke, R. G., et al. 2000. Relationship of seminal traits and insemination time to fertilization rate and embryo quality. Anim. Reprod. Sci. 60–61. p. 663.

# EXERCISE 8

# Evaluation of Semen—Appearance and Viability

## OBJECT

To become familiar with appearance and viability characteristics of semen.

## DISCUSSION

Monitoring of qualitative semen characteristics is an important function of the AI laboratory. Seasonal and even daily fluctuations in a bull's seminal characteristics are possible. Therefore, to maintain a quality AI program, constant vigilance is required. An integral part of this monitoring is an accurate system for keeping records of the bull's seminal quality. Such records document the bull's history of seminal quality and provide information on which to base production-related decisions.

## Appearance

The gross appearance of freshly collected bull semen is usually the first measure of quality made by the semen laboratory technician (Figure 8.1). Neat (unaltered) semen normally appears as a thick whitish to slightly yellowish fluid whose consistency is mainly determined by the number of spermatozoa it contains. Normal bull semen has very little odor.

Contamination of the semen can readily affect its appearance. Blood, urine, and feces are possible sources of contamination that can result in semen appearing off-color (pink to brownish). White clumps, flakes, or strands of material sometimes found in semen are due to the presence of pus, indicating a reproductive tract infection in the bull. Also, debris such as bedding material (straw, wood shavings) or

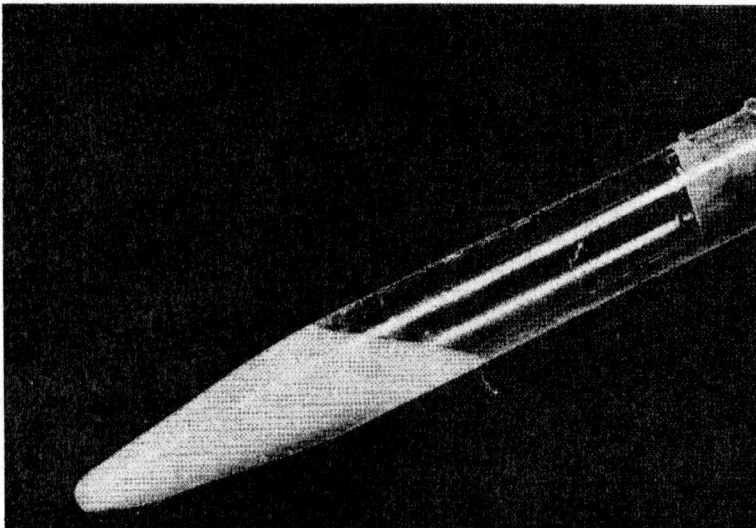

**Figure 8.1.** A freshly collected ejaculate of good quality bull semen. To the observer it appears creamy white in color, is thick, and is free from contamination.

other contamination is rare when responsible collection procedures are followed. Contamination from substances on the surface of the artificial vagina (AV) or from water that has leaked from the AV into the collection tube is also possible.

In the initial semen-screening process the laboratory technician will discard ejaculates that are abnormal in appearance or in initial quality or that are heavily contaminated. Often a low power microscopic examination will help determine the type of contamination that may be present. This is particularly useful in identifying the presence of blood cells in semen. When contamination of semen is discovered, it is important to follow up to determine its source and to correct the problem. Whether it is due to a change in the health status of the bull or to a human-made problem, contaminated semen should be avoided, since it could negatively affect the fertility or possibly the health of the females that are inseminated with it.

## Viability Measures

The viability characteristics of semen reflect important metabolic processes of the spermatozoa. Numerous aspects of sperm metabolic activity have been studied (Table 8.1), and various correlations with fertility have been demonstrated (see references). Although there are several measures available to monitor the viability characteristics of spermatozoa, this discussion will be limited to motility and acrosomal integrity, which are evaluations commonly used in the AI laboratory.

By virtue of their design, sperm are entirely dedicated to the fertilization process. They are mostly devoid of cytoplasm but contain a haploid DNA "payload," a complex propulsion mechanism, and a system of delicate membranes that mediate interactions between the sperm and their micro-environment.

Although relatively inactive during their storage in the extra-gonadal ducts of the male

**Table 8.1.** General Bases for Viability Measurements of Semen[a]

- Motility
- Velocity
- Penetration of cervical mucus
- Metabolic activity
- Cell content of:
  DNA
  Enzymes
  Lipids
- Structural integrity of:
  Cell membrane
  Acrosome
- Ability to agglutinate in presence of blood serum (head to head)
- Ability to pass through Sephadex—glass wool filter

[a]R. G. Saacke. 1984. Semen quality: Importance of and influencing factors. Proc. 10th Tech. Conf. on Artificial Insemination and Reproduction. NAAB. p. 30.

reproductive tract, sperm become committed to their mission and very vigorous upon mixing with accessory gland fluids during ejaculation. Sperm cells are generally at their peak in quality when ejaculated, and they decline in activity over a short period of time (usually within a few hours).

Quality and longevity are highly dependent upon the environments to which the sperm are exposed. In natural service, ejaculated sperm are sustained by conditions in the reproductive tract of the estrual female for a period that may span some 30 hours. However, when collected for use in artificial insemination, sperm cells are subjected to human-made conditions in which inherent quality could rapidly be compromised unless proper precautions are followed. Procedures and equipment used for seminal collection take this into account.

Thermal control of ejaculated semen is particularly important. The role of the AI laboratory is to preserve the viability of the ejaculated spermatozoa (through the addition of an extender and by a controlled cooling process) and to insure that the processed semen has the quality characteristics needed for acceptable fertility.

Assessing the progressive motility of the semen sample is probably the most common evaluation made. Motility characteristics of bull spermatozoa have been studied extensively (see references). Normal bull sperm move in a fairly straight to curvilinear path while rotating along their longitudinal axes. A three-dimensional tail wave that produces the cell rotation has been described.[1] Generally it is believed that motility is important for passage of sperm through the cervix (in the case

of natural service) and utero-tubal junction, and it likely facilitates penetration of the zona pellucida of the ovum during fertilization.

**Visual Motility**— Typically a small drop of neat semen or semen mixed with isotonic buffer is examined using, at low magnification ($100\times$ to $250\times$), a phase contrast microscope equipped with a heated stage (Figure 8.2). Since motility varies with temperature, it is important that the microscope stage, the microscope slides and cover glasses, and the buffer all be at a constant temperature (in the range of $95°$ to $99°$ F [$35°$ to $37°$ C]).

Some organizations prefer to use partially-extended semen for the initial motility evaluation. This acts to reduce the concentration for better viewing of individual spermatozoa and avoids the need to mix semen and buffer on the microscope slide.

Visual estimates of the percentage of motile sperm are quite subjective and can be influenced greatly by the evaluation technique and by technician bias. Consequently, it is important that standardized procedures be followed routinely. Overly-thick semen smears contribute to inaccurate estimates of motility, while very thin semen smears can dry out too rapidly. Use of a standard evaluation volume of semen (delivered by microliter pipet) and uniformly-sized cover glasses greatly improve accuracy and repeatability. Evaluation of multiple smears from the same semen sample usually result in a more representative estimation of the motility, since individual smears can vary. To avoid technician bias, samples should be evaluated "blindly" (i.e., sample identification is coded so that the evaluator will not know from which bull the semen was collected). Although this is not routinely done in initial semen screening, it is more practical for evaluations after freezing and thawing (post-thaw).

---

[1] R. Rikmenspoel. 1964. Measurements of motility and energy metabolism of bull spermatozoa. Transactions of NY Academy of Science II (Suppl. 8):1072.

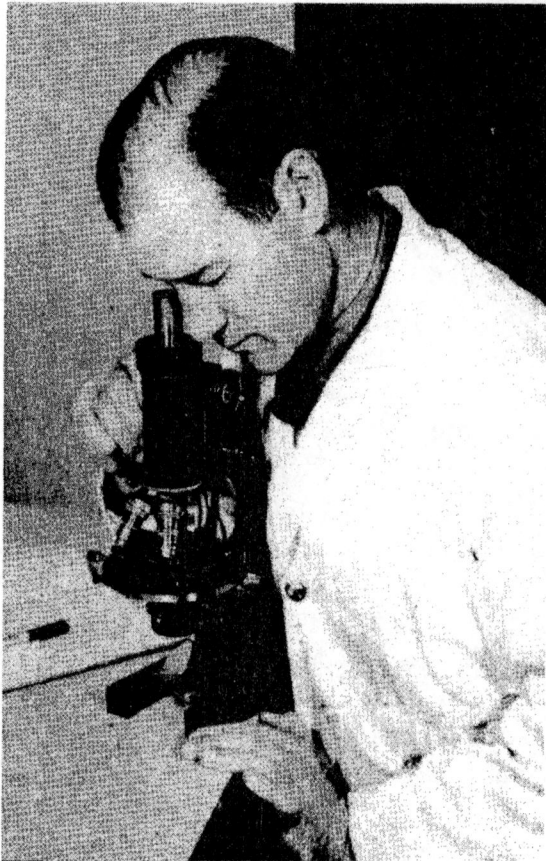

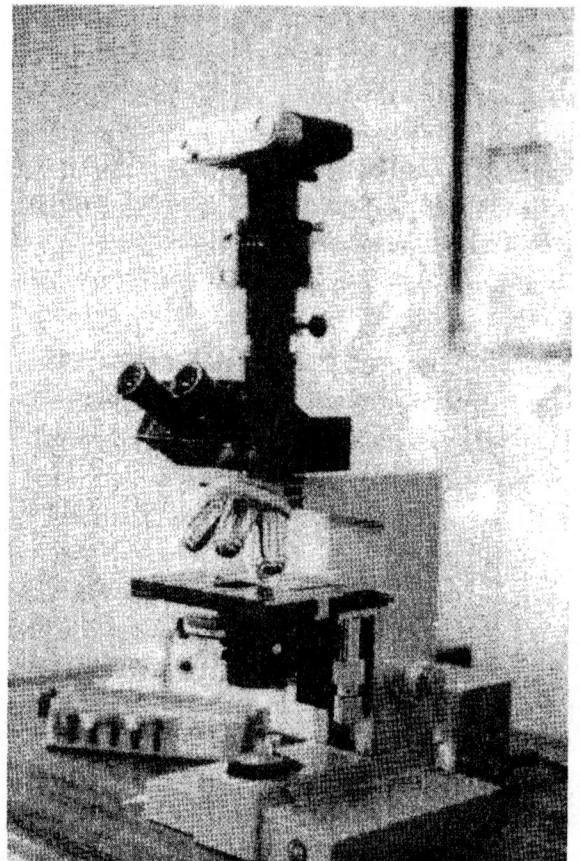

**Figure 8.2.** Former author Dr. H. Herman examining dairy semen for motility at Missouri Experiment Station in 1948 *(left)*. Although AI laboratory equipment and procedures are now much improved *(right)*, the same principles of evaluation apply today.

## PROCEDURE

Steps in examining semen for visual motility estimation include the following:

1. Be sure that all surfaces that come into contact with the semen are clean—preferably sterile—and free from spermicidal substances.

2. Maintain slides, cover glasses, sampling pipets, buffer, etc., on a slide warmer at an appropriate temperature (95° to 99° F [35° to 37° C]).

3. Mix the semen sample by gently inverting the vial several times. Remove the stopper, and place a small drop of the neat or extended semen on a prewarmed slide. A glass rod or sampling

pipet with disposable tip can be used. Gently place a cover glass over the sample. The cover glass makes a more uniform smear of the semen for better observation. Due to its high concentration, neat semen is frequently mixed with pre-warmed physiological saline or isotonic buffer to improve clarity. Normally a drop of saline or isotonic buffer is placed on the slide first, and a small amount of the semen added. The buffer and the semen are then mixed using the cover glass. Usually two semen smears from the same sample are placed on the slide for comparison.

4. Place the slide with the semen smears on the warm microscope stage, and examine the semen imme-

66

diately for motility, using low power objective(s) of the microscope.

5. Observe several fields of view on both semen smears for an approximation of the percentage of progressively motile sperm in the sample. Use the fine adjustment of the microscope to bring the sperm into sharp focus. At several loci try to determine the proportion of progressively motile sperm in the area being viewed (e.g., are four out of every six sperm progressively motile? etc.). Alternatively, the field diaphragm of the microscope can be closed down to restrict the view so that a smaller number of motile sperm are observed. An actual count of motile versus non-motile sperm cells could be made to determine percent motile. Areas along the edges of the smear where drying has occurred will give erroneous results. These areas should be avoided.

As stated above, to estimate the motility, several fields of view for each smear are examined to determine the percentage of progressively motile versus non-motile and/or aberrantly motile sperm. This is basically a rough estimate usually expressed to the nearest 10 percentage point. Good quality bull semen typically will range from 50 to over 90 percent initial (pre-freeze) progressive motility based on visual estimate (Figure 8.3).

The rate of progression (vigor) of the sperm cells in neat or extended semen is also observed and may be rated using the following numerical scale:

5 = Very rapid and vigorous forward motion. Swirls and eddies caused by movements of sperm are extremely rapid and changing constantly in neat semen preparations.

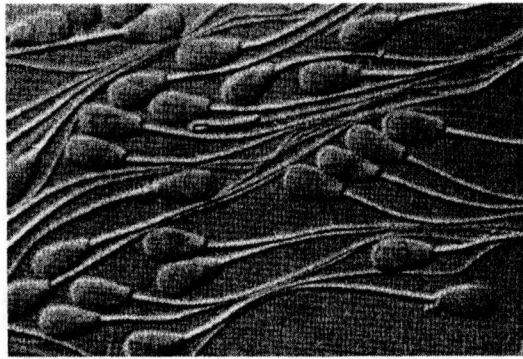

**Figure 8.3.** A stop-action view of motile bull spermatozoa (400×).

4 = Rapid progressive motion. Abruptly forming swirls and eddies are viewed in neat semen preparations.

3 = Steady progressive motion at a moderate speed. Swirls and eddies move more slowly across the field of view in neat semen preparations.

2 = Slow progression, including stop and start motion. No swirls or eddies are viewed in neat semen preparations.

1 = Weak undulation or oscillatory motion.

0 = No discernable motility.

**Photographic Motility**— Photographic or "track" motility evaluations have been shown to be more repeatable and objective than visual estimations. The method described by Van Dellen and Elliott[2] employs time-exposure darkfield photomicrography of thawed semen samples using a specially modified counting chamber. Several exposures are made for each semen sample. The film is developed, and the motility percentage is obtained by counting the number of

_____

[2] G. A. Van Dellen and F. I. Elliott. 1978. Procedure for time-exposure darkfield photomicrography to measure percentage progressively motile spermatozoa. Proc. 7th Tech. Conf. on Artificial Insemination and Reproduction. NAAB. p. 53.

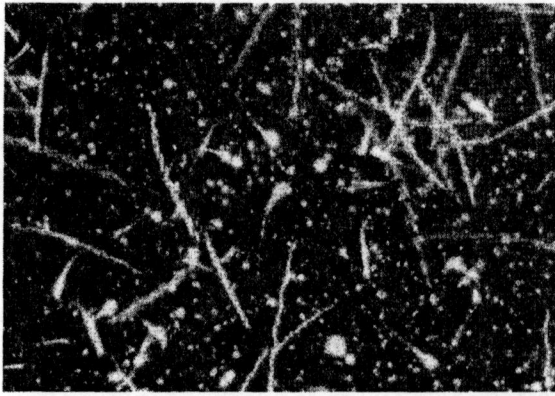

**Figure 8.4.** Time-exposure darkfield film of thawed bull semen. Live motile cells create "tracks" during the timed exposure while non-motile cells are recorded as stationary images. (Courtesy, ABS Global, Inc., DeForest, WI)

motility "tracks" in comparison to the number of single sperm cell images (those that did not exhibit motion and produce a photographic track during the time exposure). This method requires a considerable investment in photographic equipment and supplies and is more labor intensive. For optimum results, a non-opaque semen extender must be used. Figure 8.4 depicts an example of a photo-motility film.

**Computer-assisted Motility Analysis—** Computerized evaluations of sperm motion characteristics are available using technology found in various commercial semen analysis systems. These automated systems can generate detailed information on motion parameters of a semen sample, including curvilinear velocity, average path velocity, straight-line velocity, linearity, motile sperm, progressively motile sperm, lateral head displacement, and so forth. In addition, information on total sperm count and concentration can be obtained. Amann[3] has demonstrated that correlations between several computerized semen

analysis characteristics of sperm motion and competitive fertility index in cattle were found to be significant. Although computer-assisted motility analysis is not yet widely used in routine semen processing, it is likely to become more popular as research demonstrates these systems to be accurate, repeatable, and reliable for evaluating bovine semen. Correlations between various computerized sperm motion characteristics and field fertility need to be established.

In the initial semen screening process, samples that are found to be below a predetermined minimum motility level are suspect regarding their potential fertility and are usually discarded. Thus, pre-freeze motility evaluations are basically used to discriminate between ejaculates regarding eligibility for further processing. Some organizations, however, do not evaluate motility at all before freezing, since later quality checks will reveal any unacceptable semen that should be discarded.

Evaluations of semen after freezing and thawing (post-thaw) are more relevant to determining acceptability for field use. This is because post-thaw evaluations reflect the quality of the product that will actually be used for insemination and have been shown to correlate more highly with fertility. Additionally, bulls have been found to rank differently in fertility after freezing of the semen compared to their pre-freeze fertility ranking.[4]

**Acrosomal Integrity—** The acrosome of the sperm is a sac-like membranous structure that covers the anterior portion of the nucleus (Figure 8.5). Formed during the later stages of sperm development (spermiogenesis), the acrosomal cap is known to contain various enzymes believed essential for fertilization of the ovum. Although the process is not clearly un-

---

[3] R. P. Amann. 1988. Relationships between computerized evaluations of spermatozoal motion and competitive fertility index. Proc. 12th Tech. Conf. on Artificial Insemination and Reproduction. NAAB. p. 38.

[4] D. L. Stewart, et al. 1974. A second experiment with heterospermic insemination in cattle. J. Reprod. Fertil. 36:107.

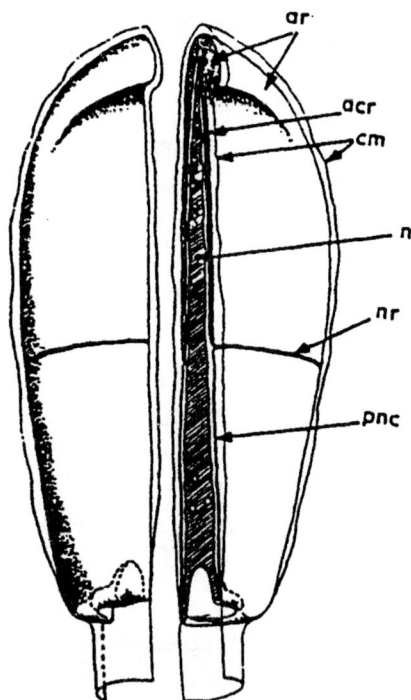

**Figure 8.5.** Graphic illustration of the bovine sperm head, cut to show the apical ridge (ar); acrosomal cap (acr); cell membrane (cm); nucleus (n); nuclear ring (nr); and post-nuclear cap (pnc). (R. G. Saacke. 1970. Morphology of the sperm and its relationship to fertility. Proc. 3rd Tech. Conf. on Artificial Insemination and Reproduction. NAAB. p. 17)

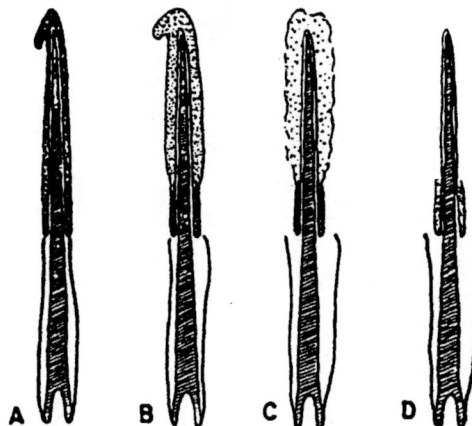

**Figure 8.6.** Schematic representation of sagittal section through the bovine sperm head as seen using an electron microscope. A through D show the sequential alterations of the acrosome due to sperm aging or injury. (R. G. Saacke and J. M. White. 1972. Semen quality tests and their relationship to fertility. Proc. 4th Tech. Conf. on Artificial Insemination and Reproduction. NAAB. p. 22)

derstood in mammals,[5] there is considerable evidence that the acrosomal cap plays a prominent role. This is underscored by the fact that males having elevated levels of sperm with acrosomal cap abnormalities have been shown to be subfertile or sterile.[6,7]

Saacke and Marshall[8] have described sequential alterations in the acrosome of bull sperm due to normal aging or as a result of cell

injury (Figure 8.6). The sequence of these acrosomal alterations was found to be constant and to be dependent upon semen handling techniques or the sperm environment.

Although classical staining techniques can be used to visualize the alterations in the acrosome, Saacke and Marshall demonstrated that differential interference contrast (DIC) microscopy of wet semen smears is a very effective and practical improvement for semen evaluation.

The most critical alteration of the bovine acrosomal cap is the loss of the apical ridge. Under DIC optics the apical ridge of the acrosome can be easily identified (Figure 8.7). In acrosomal deterioration there is an abrupt disappearance of the apical ridge, which is followed by swelling and by eventual loss of the anterior outer acrosomal membrane.

The rate of acrosomal change is a viability indicator that varies among bulls and among ejaculates of the same bull. It is influenced by conditions the sperm are exposed to during semen collection, processing, frozen storage, thawing, and post-thaw handling. Semen samples that are aged or that have sustained

[5] R. S. Prather and G. Schatten. 1988. Studies in fertilization. Proc. 12th Tech. Conf. on Artificial Insemination and Reproduction. NAAB. p. 94.

[6] J. L. Hancock. 1953. The spermatozoa of sterile bulls. J. Exptl. Biology 30:50.

[7] R. G. Saacke, R. P. Amann, and C. E. Marshall. 1968. Acrosomal cap abnormalities of sperm from subfertile bulls. J. Anim. Sci. 27:1391.

[8] R. G. Saacke and C. E. Marshall. 1968. Observations on the acrosomal cap of fixed and unfixed bovine spermatozoa. J. Reprod. Fertil. 16:511.

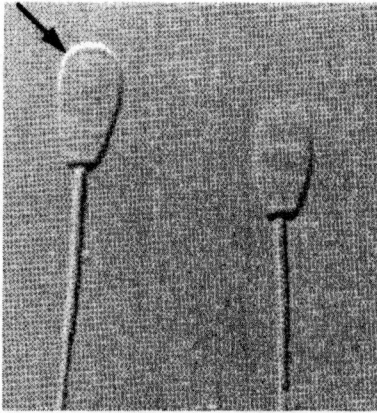

**Figure 8.7.** Comparison of bovine sperm heads as observed in an unfixed wet smear using a differential interference contrast microscope. Sperm on left exhibits intact acrosome characterized by distinct apical ridge (arrow); sperm on right has altered acrosomal cap due to aging or injury (1,000×).

injurious conditions typically exhibit lower acrosomal integrity.

Quantitative measurements of acrosomal integrity (i.e., presence of the apical ridge expressed as percent intact acrosomes) during incubation of bovine semen at 99° F (37° C) post-thaw have been shown to correlate highly with non-return rate and competitive fertility index.[9,10]

Many AI laboratories have incorporated acrosomal integrity into their quality control programs. This requires investment in one or more differential interference contrast microscopes and in related equipment for incubation of semen samples.

For routine semen evaluation, samples are thawed and then incubated at 99° F (37° C). Percent intact acrosomes (PIA) is determined by direct count, usually after two, three, or four hours of incubation. The post-thaw incu-

bation time chosen is largely a matter of convenience as long as it is within limits of the original research. A standard incubation time should be followed for all routine evaluations.

Saacke, et al. (see references at end of exercise), have discussed the rationale for incubation of post-thaw semen at or near body temperature. Incubation post-thaw is consistent with the fact that sperm, when deposited in the cow's genital tract, must survive for several hours before ovulation and a subsequent opportunity for fertilization. It is recognized, however, that conditions in the cow are probably much different from those in the incubation tube. More importantly, incubation is believed to reveal injury that may have been sustained by sperm cells but is expressed latently (latent injury) after cells are aged under incubation conditions.

## POST-THAW VIABILITY PROCEDURES

1. Two or three straws per collection code are thawed, and the contents emptied into stoppered 5-ml disposable culture tubes. These tubes are placed in a water bath or dry block warmer at 99 F (37° C). Following a five-minute thermal equilibration period, the pooled sample is mixed thoroughly, and two thin wet smears are made and examined for 0-hour motility using procedures described previously. Alternatively, straws of semen can be incubated after thawing for the appropriate period of time, and the contents pooled into a sample tube just prior to evaluation.

   To avoid bias, a technician other than the one evaluating the semen should thaw and code the samples so that the evaluator does not know which bull is being evaluated. After all

[9] R. G. Saacke and J. M. White. 1972. Semen quality tests and their relationship to fertility. Proc. 4th Tech. Conf. on Artificial Insemination and Reproduction. NAAB. p. 22.
[10] R. G. Saacke, et al. 1980. Semen quality and heterospermic insemination in cattle. Proc. 9th International Congr. Animal Reproduction and Artificial Insemination (Madrid) 5:75.

evaluations are completed, the samples are then decoded and the evaluation results recorded.

2. After the semen has been incubated for the appropriate period of time (e.g., two hours, three hours, four hours, etc.), a second motility estimate is made and recorded. The same slide used for the second motility estimate is then examined under DIC optics at $1,000\times$ magnification. Presence of an apical ridge is used to differentiate between sperm having intact acrosomes and sperm that have aged or been damaged. Two random DIC counts of 100 sperm each are made using a differential counter. The counts are averaged together in order to objectively quantitate percent of sperm with intact versus altered acrosomes. If variation in the two counts is greater than 7 percent, a recount is made, and either all three counts or the two closest counts are averaged.

As indicated previously, use of standardized evaluation volume and uniformly sized cover glasses greatly improves accuracy and repeatability.

Semen in whole milk extender is more difficult to evaluate for acrosomal integrity because the high concentration of milk fat globules present reduces optical clarity. Dilution with a suitable buffer may improve this situation.

3. Samples may also be fixed for acrosomal evaluation. A solution of 0.2 percent buffered glutaraldehyde has been shown to be effective.[11] Typi-

cally a subsample of the semen is mixed with an equal volume of fixative solution. Chief advantages of fixation are that motility is arrested and samples can be stored for later evaluation at a convenient time. However, fixation artifacts and clumping of cells have been experienced.

Acrosomal integrity may also be assessed using Giemsa, Wells-Awa, and Spermac staining under brightfield microscope optics.[12] Staining procedures, however, may introduce artifacts and cause damage to the acrosome, thereby giving unreliable results.

Good quality bull semen normally ranges from 30 to 70 percent estimated motility and from 45 to 80 percent intact acrosomes post-thaw. Values for percent motility and percent intact acrosomes are typically highest at 0-hour post-thaw and usually decline over the incubation period. The actual percentages per se are not critically important to fertility. Rather, it is the number of viable sperm per inseminate, as emphasized in Exercise 7, that influences the attainment of maximum fertility for a particular bull. Depending upon the semen extension rate used, the post-thaw percentages determine whether the acceptable number of viable sperm are available in the breeding unit. Obviously, AI organizations want to minimize any losses in seminal quality during processing and maintain inherent bull fertility. Each organization, therefore, establishes quality standards for viability and other characteristics to meet these needs. Since individual bulls may vary in their inherent fertility, it is important to integrate bull fertility history information into quality control decisions. Semen that is found to be substandard is routinely discarded.

[11] L. Johnson, et al. 1976. An improved method for evaluating acrosomes of bovine spermatozoa. J. Anim. Sci. 42:951.

[12] A. D. Barth and R. J. Oko (Eds.). 1989. Abnormal Morphology of Bovine Spermatozoa. Iowa State Univ. Press, Ames. (Ch. 2.)

# QUESTIONS

1. Why is it important to maintain a record of each bull's semen quality?

2. Is semen that appears thick to the naked eye always good-quality semen? Explain.

3. List several types of contaminants that may be found in bull semen. What course of action would you follow if you discovered blood in a bull's ejaculate?

4. Of what significance are sperm viability characteristics? What is their correlation with fertility?

5. Is it possible for sperm cells to improve in viability characteristics following collection? Explain.

6. Why is thermal control of ejaculated semen important?

7. What is the advantage of evaluating multiple smears for visual motility?

8. What effect on motility percentage would evaluating cold semen have? What would be the result of having the microscope slide too hot?

9. Why is a thin smear preparation important?

10. Explain motility "tracks."

11. Are pre-freeze or post-thaw evaluations of semen more important to the AI organization? Explain.

12. What type of optical system is needed for evaluations of acrosomal integrity?

13. For post-thaw semen evaluations, why are samples incubated for specified periods of time?

14. What is the minimum number of viable sperm needed to achieve fertility?

# REFERENCES

Foote, R. H. 1992. Collecting and processing semen with vision, decision and revision: Producing and monitoring a quality product. Proc. 14th Tech. Conf. on Artificial Insemination and Reproduction. NAAB. p. 68.

Graham, E. F. 1984. Research 1984–2004. Proc. 10th Tech. Conf. on Artificial Insemination and Reproduction. NAAB. p. 24.

Graham, E. F., M. K. L. Schmehl, and R. C. M. Deyo. 1984. Cryopreservation and fertility of fish, poultry and mammalian spermatozoa. Proc. 10th Tech. Conf. on Artificial Insemination and Reproduction. NAAB. p. 4.

Graham, E. F., M. K. L. Schmehl, and D. S. Nelson. 1980. Problems with laboratory assays. Proc. 8th Tech. Conf. on Artificial Insemination and Reproduction. NAAB. p. 59.

Hafez, E. S. E. (Ed.). 1987. Reproduction in Farm Animals (5th Ed.). Lea & Febiger, Philadelphia. (Ch. 22.)

Marshall, C. E., et al. 1988. The relationship of semen quality and fertility: A heterospermic study II (A sequel). Proc. 12th Tech. Conf. on Artificial Insemination and Reproduction. NAAB. p. 35.

Saacke, R. G. 1984. Procedures for identifying source and solution to a low quality ejaculate. Proc. 10th Tech. Conf. on Artificial Insemination and Reproduction. NAAB. p. 81.

Saacke, R. G. 1984. Semen quality: Importance of and influencing factors. Proc. 10th Tech. Conf. on Artificial Insemination and Reproduction. NAAB. p. 30.

Saacke, R. G. 1992. Considerations in the laboratory evaluation of semen. Proc. 11th Ann. Conv., American Embryo Transfer Assoc. p. 21.

Saacke, R. G., et al. 1991. Assessing bull fertility. Proc. Ann. Mtg., Soc. Theriogenology. p. 56.

Saacke, R. G., et al. 1992. Semen: Its impact on fertility and embryo quality. Proc. 11th Ann. Conv., American Embryo Transfer Assoc. p. 1.

Salisbury, G. W., N. L. Van Demark, and J. R. Lodge (Eds.). 1978. Physiology of Reproduction and Artificial Insemination of Cattle (2nd Ed.). W. H. Freeman, San Francisco. (Chs. 14, 15.)

# EXERCISE 9

# Evaluation of Semen-Enumeration of Spermatozoa

## OBJECT

To become familiar with the technique of enumerating spermatozoa in semen by use of the hemacytometer and to understand the principles of other rapid methods of estimating sperm numbers.

## DISCUSSION

Accurate determination of the number of spermatozoa per unit volume of semen harvested from the bull is of utmost importance to the AI laboratory. It is necessary to know the concentration of the neat (unaltered) semen that is collected from the bull in order to adequately ensure numbers of sperm for optimum fertility in the extended semen (breeding unit). Accurate determination of sperm concentration is also important for carefully monitoring the sperm output or reproductive capacity of the sire over a period of time.

There can be a wide variation in the sperm concentration of semen ejaculated by different bulls as well as in the sperm concentration of ejaculates collected from the same bull over a period of several weeks. Individual differences in sperm production among healthy bulls are due largely to the size (weight) of the testes and the efficiency of their production (spermatozoa produced per gram of testis per day). Differences observed in the same bull over a period of time can be due to age of the bull, collection frequency, and intensity of the sexual stimulation employed. Table 9.1 demonstrates the de-

velopment of sperm production capability in Holstein bulls over time. It is obvious that the daily number of sperm produced increases as the size of testes and the efficiency of production increase with age. Sperm concentration is also influenced to some extent by the volume of semen ejaculated at one time. The volume of semen in bulls can vary with age, weight, health, nutrition, breed, frequency of collection, and temperament. Young bulls may produce from 2 to 5 ml of semen per ejaculate, which may be somewhat thin and watery if masturbation is excessive, and older mature bulls may produce from 6 to 15 ml per ejaculate, with an average of about 8 ml.

The number of spermatozoa per milliliter of fresh bull semen ranges from a few hundred thousand to well over 2 billion, with an average of about 1 billion. It is necessary to determine the concentration of sperm to guide the rate of semen extension. The concentration of a semen sample can be determined accurately by making a direct count of spermatozoa using the hemacytometer method. This method is also employed for calibrating instruments, such as the spectrophotometer, which is used for rapid determination of sperm concentration.

## PROCEDURE

### Hemacytometer Method

The hemacytometer is a specialized microscope slide usually containing two ruled counting fields (Figure 9.1). The depth of each

**Table 9.1.** Development of Sperm Production in Holstein Bulls[a]

| Age | Testis Wt. | Daily Sperm Production | |
|-----|-----------|---------|----------|
| | | $10^6$/g | $10^6$/Bull |
| | (g) | | |
| 5-7 mo. | 97 | (1) | (104) |
| 8-10 mo. | 284 | 7 | 1750 |
| 11-12mo. | 370 | 10 | 3300 |
| 17 mo. | 480 | 10 | 4480 |
| 3 yr. | 586 | 11 | 6040 |
| 4-5 yr. | 647 | 11 | 6530 |
| ≥7 yr. | 806 | 11 | 8000 |

[a]R. P. Amann. 1990. Management of bulls to maximize sperm output. Proc. 13th Tech. Conf. on Artificial Insemination and Reproduction. NAAB. p. 84.

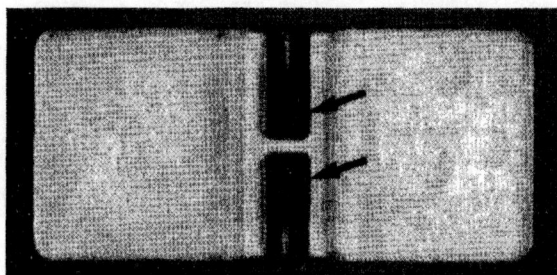

**Figure 9.1.** The improved Neubauer hemacytometer. Each counting field (arrows) contains a volume of 0.1 cu mm in which sperm are counted under the microscope.

counting field is 0.1 mm, and the ruled counting area is 1.0 sq mm. This results in a known volume of 0.1 cu mm in which sperm are counted. The improved Neubauer hemacytometer is recommended. A reduced-thickness version of this hemacytometer is also available, allowing use under phase contrast objective lenses. Each ruled counting area includes 25 large double-ruled squares, each containing 16 small squares, for a total of 400 small squares in the entire counting field. It is preferable to obtain a sperm count from each field and then determine the average value. To improve accuracy, some workers use two different hemacytometers and average the sperm counts from all four of the counting fields. Although sperm may be counted over the entire counting field (400 small squares), this can be very tedious if the sperm concentration is high. Routinely, accurate estimates are obtained when sperm are counted over at least 5 of the double-ruled squares (80 small squares). The number of squares counted depends upon the concentration of the sample and uniform distribution of spermatozoa over the counting field. Typically, the 5 double-ruled squares chosen for counting are located diagonally from an upper to lower corner of the counting field or at the 4 corners and center of the counting field. The steps in making the sperm count are as follows:

1. Mix the semen thoroughly by gently inverting the vial several times. Do not shake the vial.

2. Draw the neat semen into a standard red cell dilution pipet (to the appropriate mark in the capillary portion below the bulb).

3. Draw a small bubble of air into the pipet, and wipe the end of the pipet clean. The air prevents the capillary

removal of semen when inserting the pipet into the diluting fluid.

4. Fill the pipet to the mark (above the bulb) with diluting fluid. Depending on the manufacturer, this should result in a 1:200 dilution.

Note: As an alternative to using the standard red cell dilution pipet, accurate dilutions can also be made using fixed- or variable-volume mechanical pipets. The pipeted semen is dispensed into accurately measured volumetric or weighed volumes of dilution fluid. Following thorough mixing, a sample of the diluted semen can be loaded into the counting chamber by using a capillary tube or pipet tip. To minimize variation and improve accuracy, it is important to use the same standardized mixing and sampling procedures for each semen sample prepared for counting.

5. Agitate the pipet by bumping it against the heel of your hand for about three minutes to insure thorough mixing.

6. Discard the first four or five drops (to get properly diluted semen from the bulb).

7. Place the cover glass over the ruled field of the cytometer slide, and load the counting fields by letting a drop run under the hemacytometer cover glass.

8. Wait about five minutes before starting to count to allow the spermatozoa to settle. Counting is done at room temperature. Figure 9.2 illustrates the hemacytometer counting field.

9. Make the count under low magnification (approximately 200×).

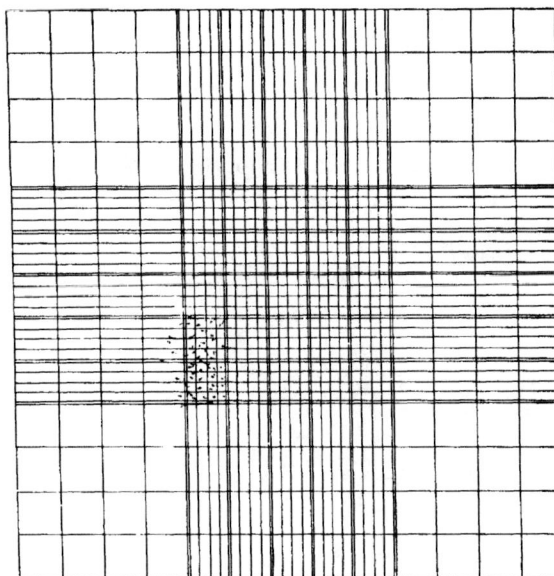

**Figure 9.2.** Improved Neubauer ruling on hemacytometer slide showing spermatozoa within two of the double-ruled squares.

10. Count only sperm nuclei (heads) that have settled over at least 80 small squares (5 large double-ruled squares). Do not count sperm tails. Use a hand tally counter to record the counts.

Note: To avoid counting twice any sperm that are at the boundary of adjacent double-ruled squares, routinely count only those boundary sperm on or within the top and left edges of each double-ruled square.

The number of sperm per milliliter (cubic centimeter) is equivalent to the number of sperm counted over 80 small squares × 5 (because only one-fifth of the total of 400 small squares were counted) × 10,000 (to convert the number of sperm counted in the 0.1 cu mm volume to a milliliter or cubic centimeter basis) × the dilution factor.

Examples:

1. A bull ejaculate having a volume of 5.5 ml was taken to the laboratory

for a determination of its sperm concentration by hemacytometer. A sample of the neat semen was diluted 1:200 in diluting fluid, and sperm were counted over 80 small squares in each of the two counting fields of the hemacytometer. 200 sperm were counted in one field, and 224 in the other. Therefore, the average count was 212.

The calculated sperm concentration for this semen sample is $212 \times 5 \times 10,000 \times 200 = 2,120,000,000$ sperm per milliliter.

At this concentration the entire ejaculate would contain 11.66 billion spermatozoa ($2,120,000,000 \times 5.5$ ml).

2. A routine evaluation of a breeding unit of semen (0.5-ml medium-straw) for sperm concentration was made using the hemacytometer method. A sample of the semen was diluted 1:50 in diluting fluid, and sperm were counted over 80 small squares in each of the two counting fields of the hemacytometer. 24 sperm were counted in one field, and 18 in the other. The average count was 21.

The calculated sperm concentration for this sample is $21 \times 5 \times 10,000 \times 50 = 52,500,000$ sperm per milliliter.

Since the straw volume is 0.5 ml, it would contain approximately 26.25 million spermatozoa.

A satisfactory dilution fluid for counting spermatozoa in the hemacytometer consists of a weak eosin solution made up of 50 ml of distilled $H_2O$ (to dilute for counting purposes), 1 ml of 2 percent eosin (to provide a background and facilitate counting), and 1 ml of 3 percent sodium chloride solution (to kill sperm and prevent movement).

The hemacytometer has been explained first because it is basic in determining the number of sperm.

## Spectrophotometer Method

The sperm concentration may be measured by an instrument called a spectrophotometer. This measurement is based upon the amount of light (550-nanometer wavelength) transmitted through a standard dilution of semen (generally a 1:100 dilution of semen using 2.9 percent sodium citrate dihydrate solution). The spectrophotometer or photoelectric colorimeter is commonly used throughout the AI industry for rapidly determining the sperm concentration of the collected semen (Figure 9.3). The spectrophotometer is accurate, relatively inexpensive, and reliable. Spectrophotometers can be calibrated for AI laboratory work by using direct sperm counts made on the hemacytometer chamber. Spectrophotometer calibration involves constructing a linear relationship between the hemacytometer sperm counts and the converted spectrophotometer readings (optical density) for several semen samples that represent a "normal" range of sperm concentration for the bull. A regression equation is then used to determine a sperm concentration value for each division on the spectrophotometer scale. After the "standard curve" has been constructed, sperm concentration values can be determined readily from the instrument reading.

## Other Methods of Sperm Enumeration

Other methods of rapidly determining sperm concentration include the use of electronic particle counters, flow cytometry, the DNA assay method, and computer-assisted semen analyzers.

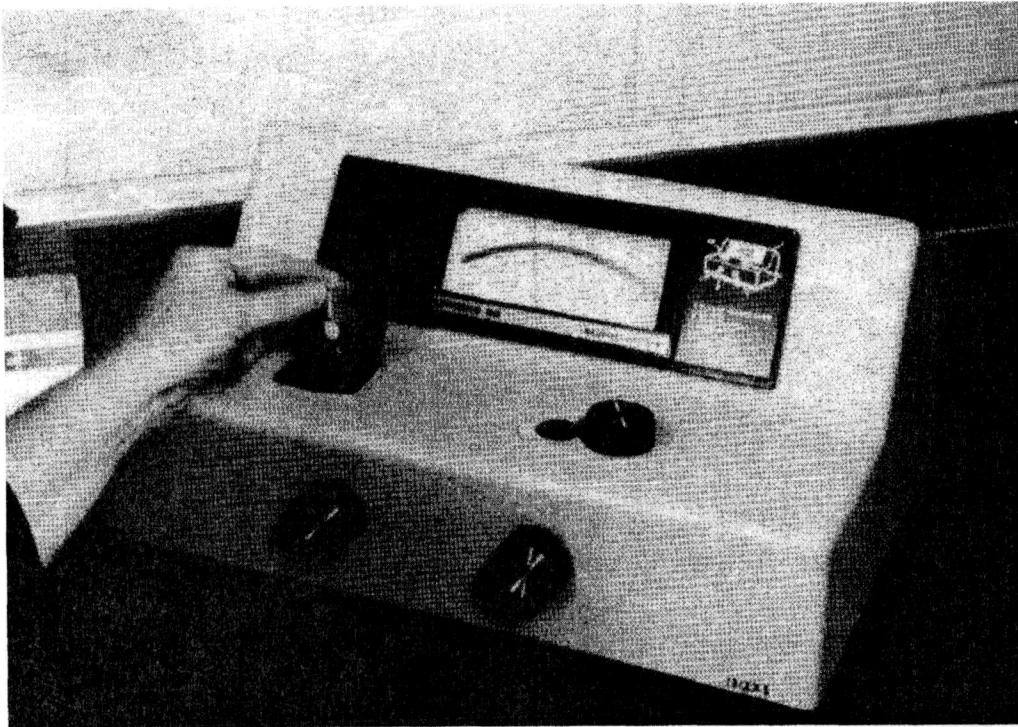

**Figure 9.3.** A sample of neat semen is checked in a spectrophotometer to determine sperm concentration. The sperm concentration is read directly from a chart based on the optical density of the sample (meter reading). The chart, or "standard curve," is constructed by comparing a scale of hemacytometer sperm counts with optical density readings. (Courtesy, Select Sires, Inc., Plain City, OH)

**Electronic Particle Counters—** In an electronic particle counter, a capillary aperture is located between two electrodes across which a current is applied. Particles to be counted (i.e., blood cells, sperm cells, etc.) are suspended in physiological electrolyte solution that is free of other particles. When a particle (sperm) passes through the aperture, it displaces its own volume of electrolyte, causing an abrupt change in current flow between the electrodes. The electrical pulse generated is proportional to the volume of the particle and will be amplified by the electronic circuitry. A multichannel analyzer allows for upper and lower threshold discrimination of pulses to be counted. The electronic particle counter registers the number of particles in a specific quantity of electrolyte that passes through the aperture.

Electronic particle counters have not been widely used in the AI processing laboratory due to their cost. Also, the time required to process individual semen samples with this method has not been conducive to the processing work flow. However, they have gained popularity for quality control applications after semen freezing and thawing. Enumeration of sperm in randomly selected breeding units (straws) and enumeration of sperm following filtration through a Sephadex column are examples. Figure 9.4 shows an electronic particle counter used for quality control in an AI laboratory.

**Flow Cytometry—** Flow cytometry is an analytical technique used for studying individual cells. Cells of interest (i.e., the sperm sample) are stained with fluorescent dye(s) and then subjected to a laminar flowing liquid stream, which is intersected with a laser beam. The laser excites the dye, resulting in the

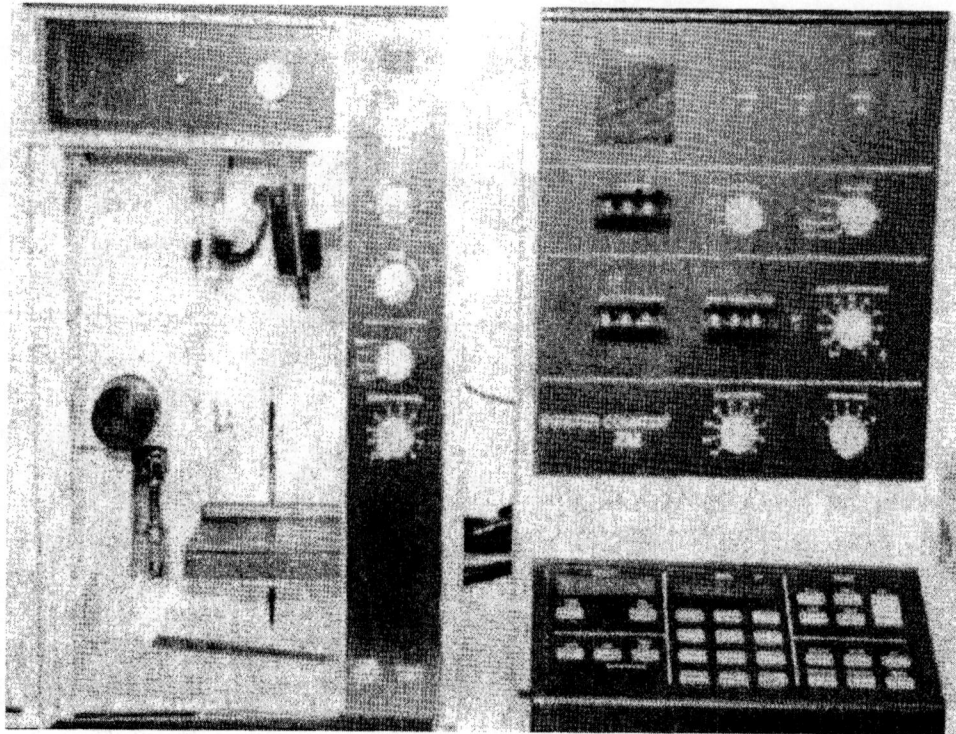

**Figure 9.4.** The Coulter Model ZM particle counter adapted to electronically count sperm cells. (Courtesy, Alta Genetics, Watertown, WI)

emission of fluorescence. The fluorescence is subsequently converted to electrical signals that are processed through a multichannel analyzer to determine the amount of specific fluorescence per cell. Flow cytometry is a very rapid method of single-cell analysis, and numerous fluorescent probes are available that allow various cellular components to be analyzed. Flow cytometry is well suited for determining the concentration of extended semen, because there is little interference from the extender particulate matter, which has often been a limiting factor encountered when using other methods of enumeration. Parks[1] has demonstrated that flow cytometric analysis of sperm concentration in whole-milk-extended semen compares favorably with hemacytome-

ter and electronic cell counter methods. One AI organization has used this method to determine sperm concentration in semen processed, packaged, and frozen in 0.5-ml straws as a quality control measure.

**The DNA Assay Method**—The DNA assay method of sperm enumeration is based on the concept that each bovine sperm cell contains the same known quantity of DNA (3.3 pg). By measuring the amount of DNA in a semen sample, the concentration of sperm can then be accurately calculated. This procedure can be used to compare a semen sample diluted in saline that would be read in a spectrophotometer, or it can determine how many sperm are in a breeding unit (straw). The procedure requires a DNA assay buffer, a dye reagent (Hoescht 33258), and use of a fluorometer. The fluorometer measures the fluorescence emitted when the dye reagent binds to DNA that is released from sperm cells in the

---

[1] J. E. Parks. 1992. Applications of flow cytometry in semen processing and handling. Proc. 14th Tech. Conf. on Artificial Insemination and Reproduction. NAAB. p. 12.

**Table 9.2.** Total Sperm in 0.5-ml Straw $(10^6/Straw)^a$

| | Volume Assayed (Dilution Rate) | |
|---|---|---|
| μg DNA | 20μl (1/25) | 50μl (1/10) |
| | (million sperm/straw) | |
| 1.0 | 7.57 | 3.03 |
| 2.0 | 15.14 | 6.06 |
| 3.0 | 22.71 | 9.09 |
| 4.0 | 30.28 | 12.12 |
| 5.0 | 37.85 | 15.15 |
| 6.0 | 45.42 | 18.18 |
| 7.0 | 52.99 | 21.21 |
| 8.0 | 60.56 | 24.24 |
| 9.0 | 68.13 | 27.27 |
| 10.0 | 75.70 | 30.30 |

[a]R. L. Ax, et al. 1988. How many sperm are in a straw? Proc. 12th Tech. Conf. on Artificial Insemination and Reproduction. NAAB. p. 32.

semen sample. Known DNA standards are used to calibrate the fluorometer, and a blank sample (a sample containing no sperm cells) of the saline or semen extender is used to zero the fluorometer, thus accounting for any "background" fluorescence. Table 9.2 demonstrates corresponding sperm concentration values per breeding unit for amount of DNA assayed in two different sample volumes of extended semen using this method. The DNA assay method is likely to see more use by AI centers in the future.

**Computer-assisted Semen Analyzers—**
Various computer-assisted semen analyzers are on the market that, among other features, provide a determination of sperm concentration and/or total sperm count in the semen sample. Independent research by Anzar, et al.,[2] has demonstrated that these types of in-

strumentation can be accurate for AI laboratory use when adjustments are made for species-specific sperm characteristics and semen extender background.

Visual estimates of sperm concentration based on the opacity of the collected semen were often used in the early years of AI. However, since such estimates of concentration tend to be highly inaccurate, they should be avoided in the modern AI laboratory.

Because accurate determination of sperm numbers in the bull ejaculate is vital to the AI organization, sources of error in sperm enumeration must be accounted for. Measurement errors that underestimate sperm concentration in the semen sample can result in significant losses in a superior sire's semen production over a period of time. On the other hand, measurement errors that tend to overestimate sperm concentration in a semen sample might result in the extension of semen into breeding units that contain fewer than the desired numbers of sperm.

[2] M. Anzar, et al. 1991. Efficacy of the Hamilton Thorn Motility Analyzer (HTM-2030) for the evaluation of bovine semen. Theriogenology 36:307.

## QUESTIONS

1. What factors may influence the volume of semen and the concentration of spermatozoa in any given collection of bull semen?

2. What is the most important reason for determining the concentration of spermatozoa?

3. Does the concentration of spermatozoa influence the fertility of the semen? Does it influence the storage capacity of the semen? Explain.

4. Can concentration be roughly estimated by visual inspection of the semen at the time of collection? If so, is this method reliable?

5. What accounts for the great variation in the number of sperm in different ejaculates from the same bull?

6. What are some of the causes of a low sperm concentration in semen?

7. What are the potential sources of error in determining sperm concentration?

8. What are some of the advantages and disadvantages of using the spectrophotometer, electronic particle counter, flow cytometer, DNA assay, and computer-assisted semen analyzers for sperm enumeration?

## REFERENCES

Amann, R. P. 1990. Management of bulls to maximize sperm output. Proc. 13th Tech. Conf. on Artificial Insemination and Reproduction. NAAB. p. 84.

Ax, R. L., et al. 1988. How many sperm are in a straw? Proc. 12th Tech. Conf. on Artificial Insemination and Reproduction. NAAB. p. 32.

Deibel, F. C., et al. 1978. Technique and application of electronic counting and sizing of spermatozoa. Proc. 7th Tech. Conf. on Artificial Insemination and Reproduction. NAAB. p. 45.

Evenson, D. P., and B. E. Ballachey. 1988. Flow cytometry evaluation of bull sperm chromatin structure. Proc. 12th Tech. Conf. on Artificial Insemination and Reproduction. NAAB. p. 45.

Foote, R. H., et al. 1978. Principles and procedures for photometric measurement of sperm cell concentration. Proc. 7th Tech. Conf. on Artificial Insemination and Reproduction. NAAB. p. 55.

Perry, E. J. (Ed.). 1968. Artificial Insemination of Farm Animals (4th Ed.). Rutgers Univ. Press, New Brunswick, NJ.

Salisbury, G. W., N. L. Van Demark, and J. R. Lodge (Eds.). 1978. Physiology of Reproduction and Artificial Insemination of Cattle (2nd Ed.). W. H. Freeman, San Francisco. (Chs. 8, 9, 10.)

Sorenson, A. M., Jr. 1979. Animal Reproduction: Principles and Practices. McGraw-Hill, New York.

# EXERCISE 10

# Evaluation of Semen–Live–Dead (Vital) Staining

## OBJECT

To become familiar with the differential staining technique used to determine the percentage of live sperm in semen.

## DISCUSSION

In addition to viability measures of semen, which have already been discussed, the percentage of live sperm can also be determined by means of a differential vital stain. The measure of the live–dead sperm ratio may be useful in conjunction with the motility examination for a more complete analysis. A certain percentage of dead sperm may not be apparent in initial microscopic motility examinations, since these inactive sperm might be moved about merely by action of the live motile sperm. Also, a proportion of sperm estimated to be motile may be weak and show only slow oscillatory movements. Differential live–dead staining, although not widely used today, may help reveal these differences, thus supplementing initial motility estimations and providing more conclusive results.

The staining procedures can also be used for general morphological examination of neat semen. However, as with all staining procedures, smear preparation can cause mechanical damage to sperm cells, and artifacts may be introduced that contribute to unreliable results. Care must be taken to standardize all procedures to obtain repeatable results.

## PROCEDURE

The live–dead stain is based upon differences between live and dead sperm cells in absorbing certain dyes. Sperm that are presumed to be dead become stained, while sperm that are presumed to be alive (motile) do not become stained. Undoubtedly, the characteristic of a cell absorbing certain dyes reflects the quality (integrity) of the cell membranes. Cells having damaged membranes apparently react with or absorb the dyes more readily than cells having undamaged membranes. In this evaluation method, the sperm that are dead at the time the slide is made will react with or absorb the eosin stain and appear pink to red; those that are alive will remain unstained, appearing white (Figure 10.1). The background stain provides contrast for easier observation of the sperm cells.

A satisfactory vital stain is the eosin-aniline blue mixture reported by Shaffer and Almquist.[1] Preparation of this staining solution, preparation of slides, and the procedure for examining slides have been described by Saacke[2] as follows:

I. Preparation of staining solution

    A. Dissolve 1.0 g of certified eosin bluish (alcohol and water soluble, 88 percent

---

[1] H. E. Shaffer and J. O. Almquist. 1948. Vital staining of bovine spermatozoa with an eosin-aniline blue staining mixture. J. Dairy Sci. 31:677.

[2] R. G. Saacke. 1970. Morphology of sperm and its relationship to fertility. Proc. 3rd Tech. Conf. on Artificial Insemination and Reproduction. NAAB. p. 17.

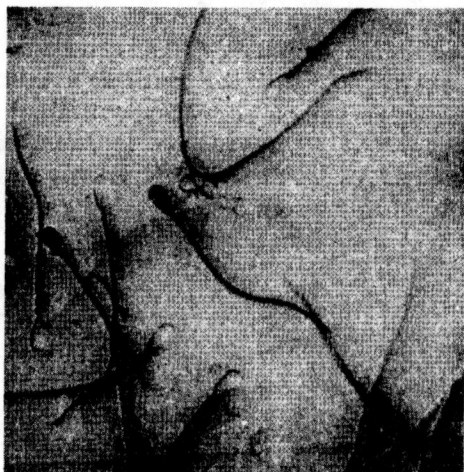

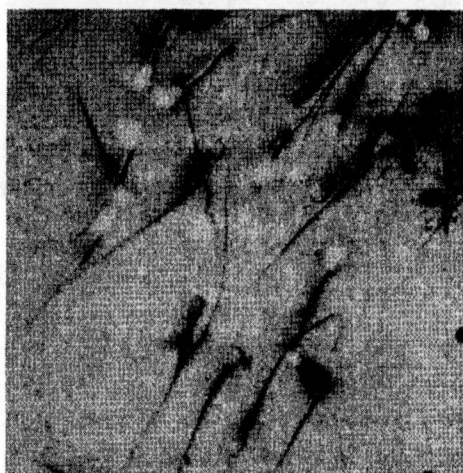

**Figure 10.1.** Photomicrograph of differentially stained sperm cells. Live sperm do not become stained, while damaged or dead sperm absorb the stain.

dye content) and 4.0 g of certified aniline blue (water soluble) in 100 ml of M/8 phosphate buffer prepared as follows:

1. Dissolve 1.702 g $KH_2PO_4$ in 100 ml of distilled water.

2. Dissolve 1.776 g anhydrous $Na_2HPO_4$ in 100 ml of distilled water.

3. Mix 28.5 ml of the $KH_2PO_4$ solution and 71.5 ml of the $Na_2HPO_4$ solution. The pH of this buffer so-

lution should be approximately 7.2. (The buffer solution should be prepared fresh as needed, but does not require sterilization.)

B. Warm the staining mixture for 10 minutes in a water bath at 185° F (85° C). Since the dyes dissolve readily, it is not necessary to filter the solution.

C. The final pH of the staining solution should be approximately 6.6.

D. Store the solution in a refrigerator at 41° F (5° C) when not in use.

II. Preparation of slides

A. The 1-inch × 3-inch microscope slides should be carefully cleaned and should be free from scratches. Immediately prior to use, each slide should be wiped with a lint-free cloth to remove particles of ground glass. In addition, the slides should then be flamed to remove traces of dust or lint.

B. Place 0.03 ml of the staining mixture, previously warmed to room temperature, near the center of the slide by means of a 0.1-ml pipet (graduated in 0.01-ml subdivisions).

C. Add a small amount of undiluted semen to the drop of staining solution, and mix gently. This step can be accomplished best with an O-shaped platinum or nichrome wire loop approximately 1 to 3 mm in diameter. The loop should be rinsed in distilled water and flamed before it is used. Be sure the loop has cooled after flaming.

D. Immediately place a second slide flatly upon the first so that about 1/2 inch of the slide remains free of contact. Allow the liquid to spread evenly between the slides.

E. Hold the slides so that their long axes are vertical, and pull them apart with a gentle, even motion.

F. Immediately place both slides (stained surface up) on an electric hot plate adjusted to maintain a temperature of 113° to 131° F (45° to 55° C), with an electric fan directing a current of air across the surface of the heated hot plate.

   Rapid drying and careful attention to details of the technique described are essential to achieve uniform differentiation between stained and unstained cells. The slides should be placed on the hot plate within 15 seconds after the semen and the dye are mixed. Also, it should take no more than 30 seconds to dry the slides after they are placed on the hot plate.

III. Examination of slides

A. The slides should be examined under an oil-immersion objective at a total magnification of approximately 1,000×.

B. Stained spermatozoa (presumed to be dead) appear pink or red against a blue background, while those that are not stained appear white. Cells that stain only in the posterior portion of the head are classified as stained.

C. To obtain an accurate estimation of the percent of unstained spermatozoa (presumed to be living) in a semen sample, a minimum of 100 sperm cells should be counted per slide.

For further reading on staining methods and formulas for semen evaluation, see references.

# QUESTIONS

1. How does percentage of live spermatozoa influence the motility of semen?

2. What is the correlation between the percentage of live sperm and the conception rate of semen?

3. What are some of the disadvantages of the live–dead staining technique?

# REFERENCES

Barth, A. D., and R. J. Oko (Eds.). 1989. Abnormal Morphology of Bovine Spermatozoa. Iowa State Univ. Press, Ames. (Ch. 2.)

Salisbury, G. W., N. L. Van Demark, and J. R. Lodge (Eds.). 1978. Physiology of Reproduction and Artificial Insemination of Cattle (2nd Ed.). W. H. Freeman, San Francisco. (Ch. 14.)

# EXERCISE 11

# Evaluation of Semen—Morphology

## OBJECT

To gain an understanding of the morphological assessment of sperm cells and obtain practice in preparing smears for examination.

## DISCUSSION

The structure, or morphology, of sperm cells has been studied extensively using light and electron microscopy techniques. It is quite apparent that sperm are amazingly complex cells (see references for detailed information). The head of a sperm, which varies in shape by species, contains the nucleus, where chromosomes carrying genes that determine individual traits are located. Also, as discussed in Exercise 8, the acrosomal cap that covers the anterior portion of the sperm head is intimately involved in the initiation of the fertilization process. The tail of the sperm produces the motion of the cell. It contains a highly-organized bundle of contractile elements that runs longitudinally through its center and is responsible for the helical tail wave. The tail is often described as having three regions: (1) the middle piece adjacent to the head of the sperm, containing the mitochondrial sheath that supplies energy to the tail; (2) the principal piece; and (3) the end or terminal piece. It is important to recognize that a plasma or cell membrane envelopes the entire sperm cell. Figure 11.1 shows diagrammatic representations of the structure of a typical bull sperm.

The relationship of sperm abnormalities to fertility is of prime importance to the AI lab-

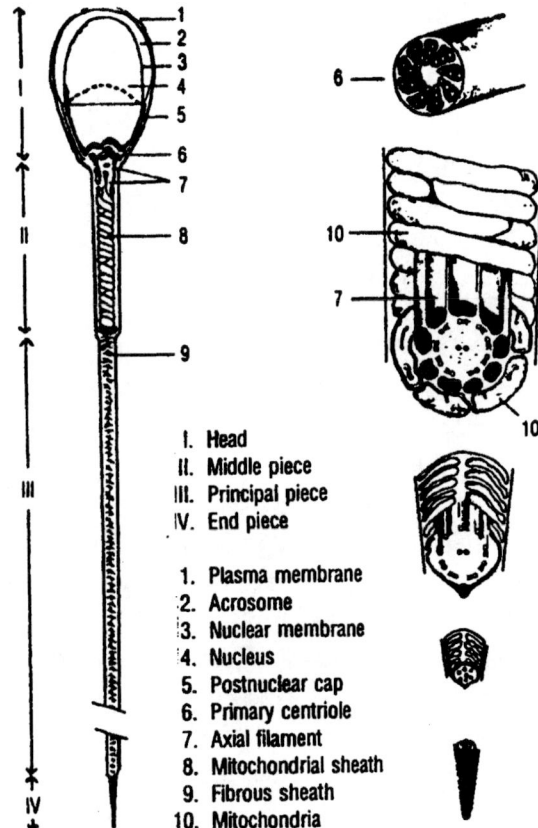

I. Head
II. Middle piece
III. Principal piece
IV. End piece

1. Plasma membrane
2. Acrosome
3. Nuclear membrane
4. Nucleus
5. Postnuclear cap
6. Primary centriole
7. Axial filament
8. Mitochondrial sheath
9. Fibrous sheath
10. Mitochondria

**Figure 11.1.** Diagrammatic representations of the fine structure of a bovine spermatazoon. (A. S. H. Wu. Microstructure of mammalian spermatozoa. June 1966. The A.I. Digest 14:7)

oratory. Early investigations[1,2] demonstrated that semen from subfertile and sterile bulls contained elevated levels of certain types of morphologically abnormal sperm. Over the

[1] W. W. Williams and A. Savage. 1925. Observations of the seminal micropathology of bulls. Cornell Vet. 15:353.
[2] W. W. Williams. 1927. Methods of determining the reproductive health and fertility of bulls: A review with additional notes. Cornell Vet. 17:374.

years, other studies have shown correlations between elevated levels of abnormal sperm in the inseminate and lowered fertility.[3,4,5,6] Apparently, fertility is reduced because certain morphological defects interfere with the sperm's abilities (1) to gain access to the site of fertilization, resulting in fewer sperm than are required by the female, or (2) to successfully fertilize the ovum or sustain the embryo should they reach the site of fertilization. Generally, abnormalities of the sperm head have been considered to be more detrimental to fertility than those of the tail.

Numerous morphological deviations of sperm cells have been identified. As shown in Figures 11.2a, b, and c, abnormalities can occur in the head, middle piece of the tail, or tail proper of the sperm. It is important to note here that individual bulls may vary in certain morphological characteristics of their sperm and still achieve "normal" fertility. For example, one bull's sperm may have slightly longer heads than those of another bull. A key consideration, however, is that the morphological characteristics are uniform for a bull's sperm. On the contrary, there is also evidence that sperm with normal-appearing morphology may contain defective chromatin, resulting in subfertility.[7] Consequently, a thorough examination of the semen and a knowledge of the field fertility of the bull are essential.

From a research standpoint it has been difficult to determine the effect of each specific type of misshapen sperm on fertility. This is because ejaculates seldom contain only one type of abnormality, and the viability of the normal cells in the ejaculate may compensate for the level of abnormalities present.

In one series of experiments, Barth[8] was able to evaluate the effect on fertility of inseminating heifers with frozen-thawed semen from bulls that contained high levels of a single specific type of abnormality (i.e., 65 to 95 percent narrow sperm heads). He concluded that a moderate degree of sperm head narrowness, in the absence of other signs of disturbed spermatogenesis, was not detrimental to fertility.

It is known that sites in the female reproductive tract can act as selective barriers to the transport of types of abnormal sperm (see Saacke, 1990, for review). These barriers are believed to exclude those sperm cells with abnormalities of the tail or head that cause a distortion in motility characteristics.

In order to assess the morphological characteristics of sperm that actually reach the site of fertilization, Saacke, et al.,[9] compared sperm head abnormalities in the cattle inseminate with abnormalities recovered as accessory sperm in the zona pellucida of the ovum. This work demonstrated a significant improvement in the proportion of sperm with normal heads that become accessory sperm (i.e., sperm able to pass through barriers in the female tract and reach the ovum) (Table 11.1). It was apparent that only those sperm with subtle abnormalities were found as accessory sperm.

[3] R. A. Beatty, et al. 1969. An experiment with heterospermic insemination in cattle. J. Reprod. Fertil. 19:491.

[4] R. G. Saacke and J. M. White. 1972. Semen quality tests and their relationship to fertility. Proc. 4th Tech. Conf. on Artificial Insemination and Reproduction. NAAB. p. 22.

[5] E. Linford, et al. 1976. The relationship between semen evaluation methods and fertility in the bull. J. Reprod. Fertil. 47:283.

[6] R. G. Saacke, et al. 1980. Semen quality and heterospermic insemination in cattle. 9th International Congr. Animal Reproduction and Artificial Insemination (Madrid) 5:75.

[7] B. L. Gledhill. 1983. Cytometry of deoxyribonucleic acid content and morphology of mammalian sperm. J. Dairy Sci. 66:2623.

[8] A. D. Barth. 1992. The relationship between sperm abnormalities and fertility. Proc. 14th Tech. Conf. on Artificial Insemination and Reproduction. NAAB. p. 47.

[9] R. G. Saacke, et al. 1988. Transport of abnormal spermatozoa in the artificially-inseminated cow based upon accessory sperm in the zona pellucida. 11th International Congr. Animal Reproduction and Artificial Insemination (Dublin) 3:292.

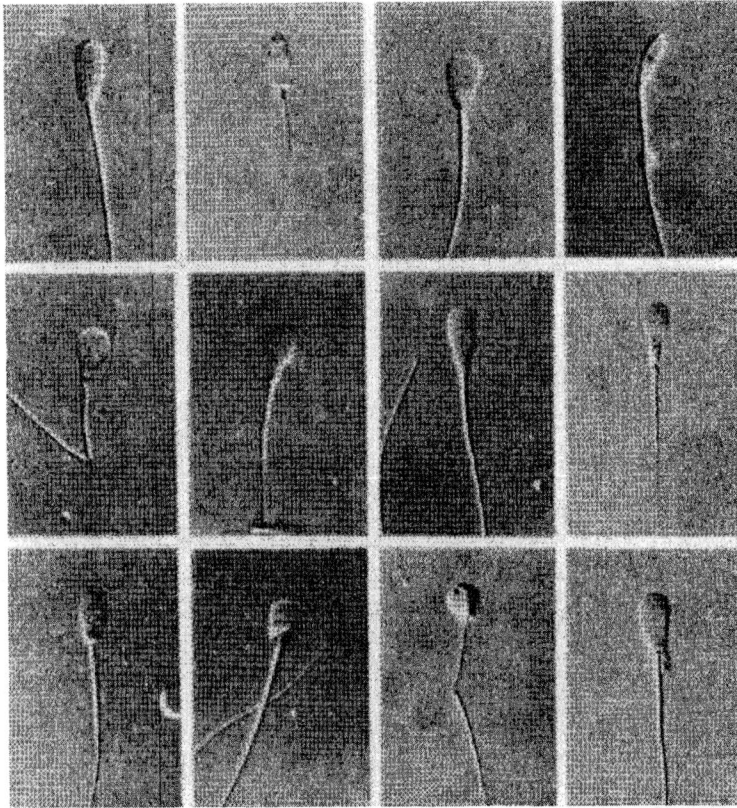

**Figure 11.2a.** Primary (1°) abnormalities of bovine spermatozoa observed at 1,000× magnification under DIC optics.

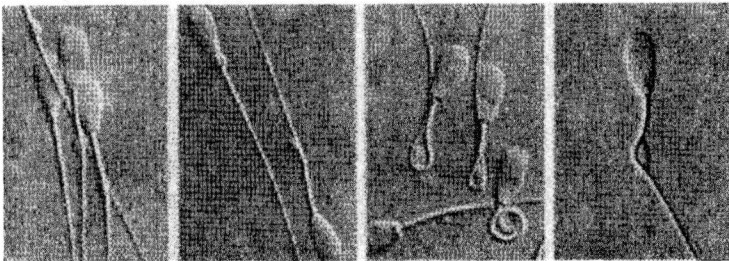

**Figure 11.2b.** Secondary (2°) abnormalities of bovine spermatozoa observed at 1,000× magnification under DIC optics.

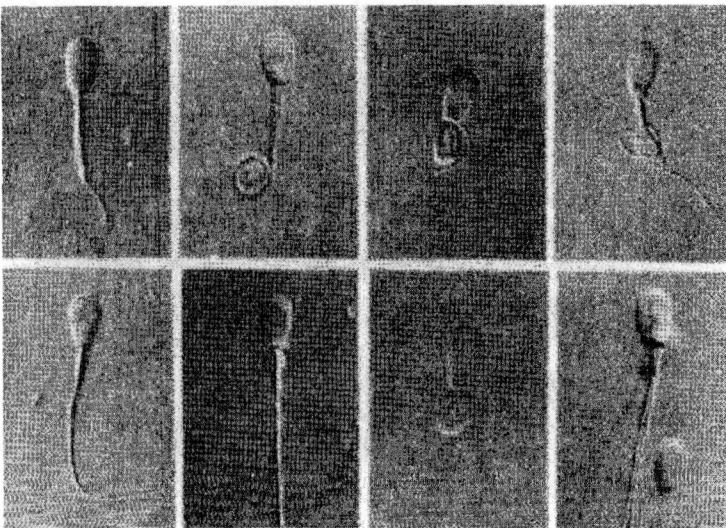

**Figure 11.2c.** Tertiary (3°) abnormalities of bovine spermatozoa observed at 1,000×H magnification under DIC optics.

**Table 11.1.** Morphological Characteristics of Accessory Sperm Heads Compared to Those of the Inseminated Sperm[a,b]

| Characteristic | Inseminate | Accessory |
|---|---|---|
| | (%) | (%) |
| Normal sperm heads | 61.8 | 75.5[c] |
| Cratered/diadem, but normal shape | 17.3 | 19.9[d] |
| Tapered | 13.6 | 1.6 |
| Pyriform | 4.6 | 1.5 |
| Asymmetrical | 1.5 | 1.5 |
| Short, giant, double, or flat | 1.0 | 0 |

[a]R. G. Saacke. 1990. What is abnormal? And is abnormal dependent upon the animal? Proc. 13th Tech. Conf. on Artificial Insemination and Reproduction. NAAB. p. 67.

[b]Weighted average of inseminates of four bulls based upon numbers of accessory sperm recovered per inseminate.

[c]Significant P<.05.

[d]Non-significant.

Interestingly, bull ejaculates that contain severe forms of abnormalities also have proportionate populations of sperm with subtle abnormalities. Thus, even though severe forms of abnormalities might be excluded from the female tract, more subtle abnormal sperm in the inseminate that are viable may reach the ovum and initiate fertilization but not be able to complete it successfully. The result would be degeneration and early embryonic death.

Although a great deal of information has been learned in recent years, it is evident that much more research needs to be done to gain a complete understanding of the relationship between sperm morphology and fertility.

In the bull, elevated levels of abnormal sperm can be manifested as a persistent condition reflecting a chronic dysfunction in the genital tract or a more transient condition related to age or numerous environmental factors (e.g., season of the year, disease, shipping, etc.). There can be wide variations in the percentages of abnormal sperm among bulls and in different ejaculates from the same bull. In one study, Mitchell[10] observed that there were episodic patterns in the incidence of abnormal sperm in ejaculates of Holstein bulls with histories of normal and elevated levels of abnormalities. These bulls were on a routine semen collection schedule of four ejaculates per week. Absolute fluctuations in percentage of abnormal sperm from one ejaculate to the next were greatest in bulls with high levels of abnormalities (Figure 11.3).

Obviously it is important for the AI laboratory to monitor morphological characteristics of semen in order to identify any changes that may occur in a bull's production. Typically, every collection from new bulls entering production or from bulls with a history of seminal problems is evaluated for morphology. However, bulls that have established a normal pattern of morphology may be evaluated less frequently, although on a routine basis.

In appraising morphologically abnormal sperm, attention should always be directed to

[10] J. R. Mitchell. 1984. Distribution of abnormal sperm in the bull genital tract. Proc. 10th Tech. Conf. on Artificial Insemination and Reproduction. NAAB. p. 99.

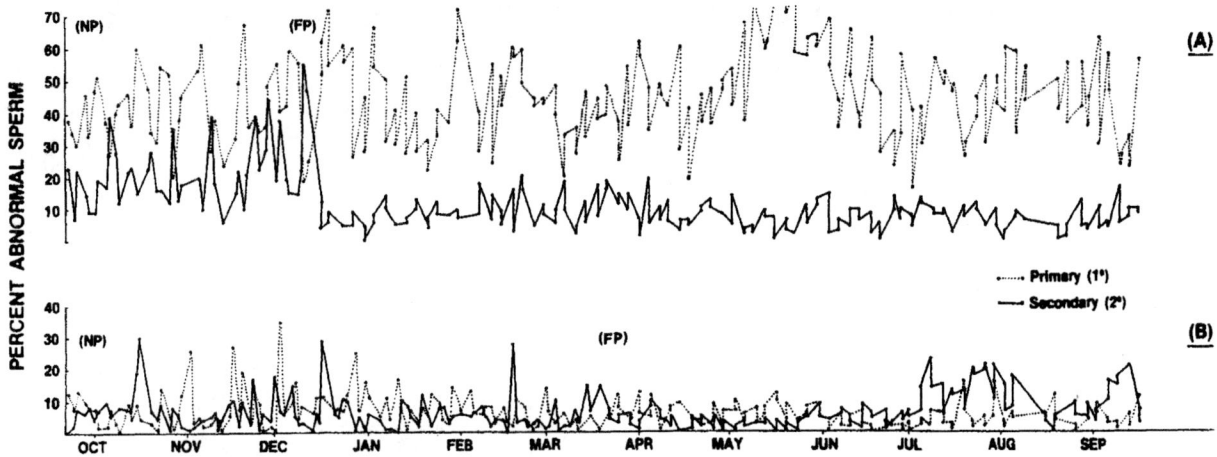

**Figure 11.3.** Typical one-year collection histories for bulls with (A) high levels and (B) normal levels of abnormal sperm. Only primary (sperm head) and secondary (protoplasmic droplets) abnormalities are included. 4×/week collection regimen (NP = no sexual preparation, FP = full sexual preparation).

conditions of environment and management of the sire. Although in certain cases, impaired spermatogenesis may appear to be genetically transmitted, studies have demonstrated that heritability estimates for types of sperm abnormalities are relatively low.[11, 12]

Several classification systems for morphological characteristics have been developed. (For discussion, see the work edited by Barth and Oko cited in the references at the end of this exercise.) One system classifies abnormalities that originate in the testis during spermatogenesis as "primary" and those that originate in the epididymis as "secondary." Another system classifies abnormal sperm as either "major" or "minor" based on whether or not they have been associated with infertility. Possible drawbacks to these systems are that it may not always be clear at what level in the genital tract an abnormality originates and that there may be conflicting reports in the literature about the effects on fertility of specific abnormalities.

A practical system commonly used by many laboratories in the AI industry classifies sperm abnormalities as primary (1°), secondary (2°), or tertiary (3°), based on structural components of the cell involved. Primary abnormalities are associated with the sperm head and acrosome, secondary abnormalities refer to the presence of protoplasmic droplets enveloping the middle piece of the tail, and tertiary abnormalities are other tail-related defects. This system emphasizes a description of the morphological defects of the sperm in the sample, rather than a classification based on presumptions of reproductive tract origin or fertility. Nevertheless, this descriptive classification can easily be related to the reproductive health and fertility of the bull. An example of morphological data collected from a commercial AI center using this classification system is shown in Table 11.2.

Regardless of what system is employed, the laboratory must establish strict rules and procedures defining what to include in each category and how to classify sperm cells with multiple defects that do not easily fall into one category or another. Such procedures will improve repeatability.

Recently researchers have reported on a new approach for evaluating the head (nuclear)

---

[11] R. E. Pearson, et al. 1984. Heritability and repeatability. Proc. 10th Tech. Conf. on Artificial Insemination and Reproduction. NAAB. p. 41.

[12] M. D. Dentine. 1988. Puberty and seminal quality. Proc. 12th Tech. Conf. on Artificial Insemination and Reproduction. NAAB. p. 26.

**Table 11.2.** Summary of Spermatozoan Abnormalities in Dairy Bulls over a Six-Month Period[a]

| Category | No. of Bulls | No. of Counts | Mean Percent | | | |
|---|---|---|---|---|---|---|
| | | | 1° | 2° | 3° | Total |
| Young Holsteins < 2 yrs. | 60 | 1,190 | 2.5 ± 2.9 | 3.1 ± 2.1 | 5.0 ± 2.4 | 10.6 ± 5.9 |
| Aged Holsteins > 4 yrs. | 64 | 2,354 | 1.8 ± 1.5 | 2.7 ± 1.8 | 3.3 ± 1.7 | 7.8 ± 3.6 |
| Colored dairy | 13 | 377 | 1.7 ± 1.5 | 3.1 ± 2.2 | 5.1 ± 4.0 | 9.9 ± 5.9 |
| Overall dairy | 137 | 3,921 | 2.1 ± 2.3 | 2.9 ± 1.9 | 4.2 ± 2.5 | 9.2 ± 5.1 |

[a]J. R. Mitchell, R. D. Hanson, and W. N. Fleming. 1978. Using differential interference contrast microscopy for evaluating abnormal spermatozoa. Proc. 7th Tech. Conf. on Artificial Insemination and Reproduction. NAAB. p. 64.

shape of bovine sperm cells using the analysis of Fourier harmonic amplitudes.[13] This method has been shown statistically to identify previously described sperm head abnormalities and has potential to more objectively characterize differences in sperm head shape; particularly from the live cells in a sample. With this method, computerized image analysis of the stained sperm (nuclear perimeter data) and mathematical manipulation are used to create the Fourier harmonic data. Figure 11.4 shows how sperm head (nuclear) shapes in Cartesian coordinates convert to polar coordinates with this procedure. Additional research is needed to determine whether Fourier harmonic analysis can improve the ability to evaluate noncompensable sperm defects. Further information can be found in the references listed at the end of this exercise.

## PROCEDURE

Evaluation of semen samples for levels and types of morphological abnormalities must be performed using high-resolution microscopy.

Wet mounts using differential interference contrast (DIC) microscopy or conventional staining techniques using brightfield microscopy are frequently used, as follows:

1. **Wet mounts**—To critically evaluate sperm abnormalities, the motility of the sample must be stopped. This is accomplished by extending the semen sample 1:1 with a stock solution of 40.0 mM sodium fluoride or 0.35 M potassium chloride made up in 2.9 percent sodium citrate buffer. A thin wet smear is made from this preparation and examined under oil at 1,000× magnification. A total of 100 cells are differentially counted per sample.

   Morphological evaluations can be made at any time prior to or after freezing. Several AI organizations prefer a post-thaw evaluation, since this more closely reflects the quality of the inseminate. The DIC microscope provides an excellent method of directly examining sperm samples for abnormalities with a high degree of precision. Specimen preparation is simple, requires little time expenditure, and reduces mechanical injury of sperm associated with smear preparation for staining.

[13] J. J. Parrish, et al. 1998. Fourier harmonic analysis of sperm morphology. Proc. 17th Tech. Conf. on Artificial Insemination and Reproduction. NAAB. p. 25.

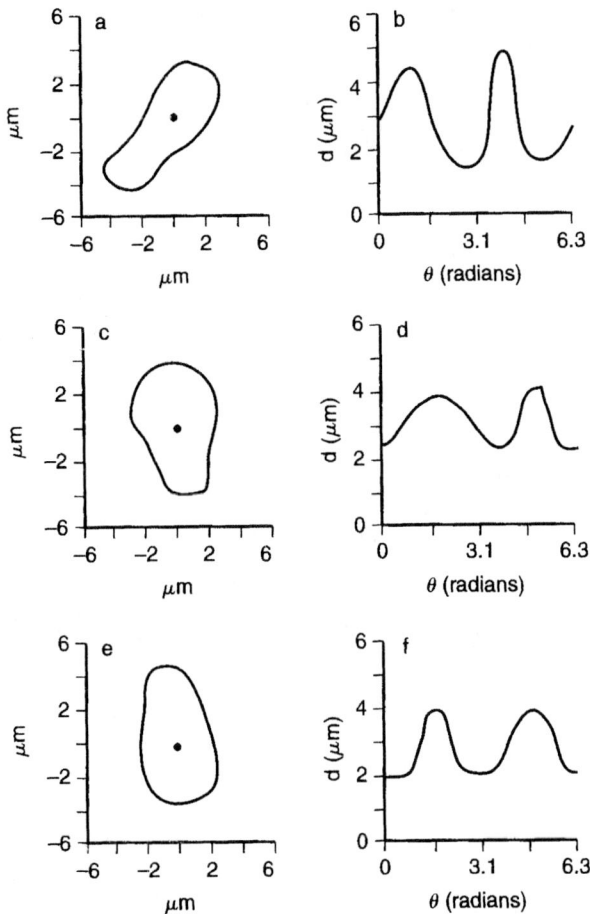

**Figure 11.4.** Conversion of Cartesian coordinates to polar coordinates. The nuclear perimeters for three different bovine sperm are shown in Cartesian coordinates (X, Y) in a, c, and e while the same data is presented in polar coordinates (d, θ) in b, d, and f, respectively. The centroid for each sperm is shown as the dot in the center of the sperm nucleus in a, c, and e. The d in polar coordinates represents the radius from the centroid at specific angles, θ. (From J. J. Parrish et al. 1998. Fourier harmonic analysis of sperm morphology. Proc. 17th Tech. Conf. on Artificial Insemination and Reproduction. NAAB. p. 25)

2. **Staining techniques**—The procedure outlined in Exercise 10 using the eosin–aniline blue vital staining mixture should be followed. Alternatively, an eosin-nigrosin stain, which is similar, may be substituted. The amount of semen used for the smear preparation varies with the sperm cell concentration. If neat se-men is used, a smaller amount should be added to the stain compared to the amount added for ex-tended semen. The Feulgen staining technique, which is specific for DNA, may also be used to examine nuclear defects. The Feulgen proce-dure does not stain the acrosome or tail of the sperm (see Barth and Oko in references).

Another procedure utilizes the Rose-Bengal stain, as follows:

a. Place two or three drops of any physiological buffer (such as phos-phate buffer) on a clear slide.
b. Add one drop of semen, and mix.
c. Spread by covering with a second slide, but do not exert excess pres-sure on the second slide, as this may damage the sperm.
d. Air dry the smear thoroughly.
e. Flood the dry smear with a Rose-Bengal stain.
f. Dry for 5 to 10 minutes; then care-fully rinse off excess stain by dip-ping slide in distilled water.
g. Dry and evaluate for morphology. Count 100 cells under the oil im-mersion objective of the micro-scope (1,000×).

A Rose-Bengal stain is made up as follows:

3 g powdered Rose-Bengal
99 ml distilled water
1 ml 40 percent Formalin

In studying morphology, care must be taken not to shock or alter the spermatozoa in any way before examination. Diluting fluids that are not of equal osmolality to the semen may produce abnormalities of the sperm re-lated to osmotic shock. Also, lack of thermal control during collection or in cooling the se-men may cause an increase in tail abnormali-ties related to thermal shock.

Although most ejaculates possess some abnormal spermatozoa, good quality bull semen generally contains a relatively low percentage of these cells. For many bulls, when total abnormalities in the ejaculate exceed the 20 to 30 percent range, fertility becomes adversely affected. Obviously the types of abnormalities involved would determine the magnitude of any problem encountered.

## QUESTIONS

1. Explain some of the differences between normal and abnormal sperm morphology.

2. How do abnormalities of sperm interfere with fertility?

3. Explain the interrelationships between viability and morphological characteristics of spermatozoa.

4. What factors may be responsible for the production of abnormal spermatozoa in the bull? Explain.

5. Indicate why it is important to follow a standard classification system when evaluating abnormal sperm. Give examples of various classification systems.

6. What are the advantages and disadvantages of using wet mounts and DIC microscopy for evaluating sperm morphology?

7. What precautions should be followed when utilizing staining techniques for evaluating sperm morphology?

8. Are sperm abnormalities heritable? Are sperm abnormalities caused by environmental factors? Explain.

## REFERENCES

Barth, A. D., and R. J. Oko (Eds.). 1989. Abnormal Morphology of Bovine Spermatozoa. Iowa State Univ. Press, Ames. (Chs. 2, 8.)

Mitchell, J. R., R. D. Hanson, and W. N. Fleming. 1978. Using differential interference contrast microscopy for evaluating abnormal spermatozoa. Proc. 7th Tech. Conf. on Artificial Insemination and Reproduction. NAAB. p. 64.

Ostermeier, G.C. 2001. The measurement of bovine sperm nuclear shape using Fourier harmonic amplitudes. J. Androl. 22(4). p. 584.

Saacke, R. G. 1970. Morphology of sperm and its relationship to fertility. Proc. 3rd Tech. Conf. on Artificial Insemination and Reproduction. NAAB. p. 17.

Saacke, R. G., 1990. What is abnormal? And is abnormal dependent upon the animal? 13th Tech. Conf. on Artificial Insemination and Reproduction. NAAB. p. 67.

Saacke, R. G. 2001. What is a BSE-SFT standards—The relative importance of sperm morphology: an opinion. Proc. Ann. Conf. Soc. Theriogenology. p. 81.

Sullivan, J. J. 1978. Morphology and motility of spermatozoa. In: G. L. Salisbury, N. L. Van Demark, and J. R. Lodge (Eds.). Physiology of Reproduction and Artificial Insemination of Cattle (2nd Ed.). W. H. Freeman, San Francisco. (Ch. 10.)

# EXERCISE 12

# Evaluation of Semen—Other Measurements and Methods

## OBJECT

To recognize other measures used to evaluate semen.

## DISCUSSION

The more commonly applied tests for evaluating bull semen are discussed in Exercises 7 through 11. However, investigators and some laboratory workers have also utilized the methods described in this exercise with varied success.

### Metabolic Reaction Rates

Important biological reactions of spermatozoa include glycolysis and respiration. By laboratory measurement of the rates of glycolysis and respiration over a defined period of time, the relative number of live, active spermatozoa in the semen is demonstrated. Good quality semen contains a high percentage of vigorous, active spermatozoa and normally exhibits higher glycolytic and respiratory rates than does semen containing a preponderance of weak or immotile sperm. Thus, the measurement of these reaction rates may serve as a direct indicator of activity and vigor reflecting the combined effects of sperm cell motility and concentration.

**Glycolysis—** Glycolysis by spermatozoa is generally the reduction of glucose (and other

simple sugars) to acids (lactic and others) by action of the cell enzymes and other reducing substances that may be in the seminal plasma. Some investigators suggest the glycolytic reaction as the source of energy for spermatozoan activity. Temperature, motility of sperm, sugar concentration, hydrogen ion concentration, and acid level are important factors that may influence the glycolytic rate.

In measuring the rate of glycolysis for sperm, a chemical analysis of glucose content and lactic acid level is made before and after a definite time interval. This is generally done by the micromodification of the Shaffer-Hartman-Somogyi method as described by Moore and Mayer.[1] The increase in acid level and the decrease in glucose content of the medium can be determined. These changes are proportional to the concentration and activity of the spermatozoa.

**Respiration—** The respiration rate, or oxygen uptake and conversion to carbon dioxide by spermatozoa, is closely related to the glycolytic rate. Such factors as diluting medium, extension rate, hydrogen ion concentration, temperature, various gases, certain chemicals, and age of the semen affect the respiration rate of sperm. Different investigators (see references) disagree concerning the respiratory activities of sperm and the degree of correlation of this process with sperm quality.

---

[1] B. H. Moore and D. T. Mayer. 1941. The concentration and metabolism of sugar in ram semen. Mo. Agr. Exp. Sta. Res. Bull. No. 338.

*Respiration rate* may be measured with a modified Barcroft-Warburg respirometer (as described by Walton and Edwards[2]), other modifications of the respirometer, or an oxygen electrode. In all cases, the concentration of spermatozoa should be controlled so that this variable will not influence the measurements, since the rate is determined in terms of microliters of oxygen consumed per number of sperm per unit of time. The percentage of live sperm should be determined before and after the test is made. The oxygen uptake of the medium must be determined, since this element is variable within a limited range. There is evidence indicating that oxygen consumption in extended semen is greater in the presence of evolved carbon dioxide than in its absence.[3]

The *methylene blue reduction test* is a laboratory exercise that enables students to observe and learn firsthand about some of the metabolic characteristics of bull semen. In semen that contains a high concentration of active sperm, the oxygen is used at a more rapid rate than in poor quality semen. This causes an excess of hydrogen, which combines with the methylene blue (chloride) to form leuco–methylene blue. The relative length of time required for this bleaching out or reduction of blue color serves as an indication of the number and activity of the spermatozoa in the semen.

Methylene blue is a quinoid dye that may be hydrogenated to the colorless leuco–methylene blue form. Certain reducing enzymes are necessary to activate the hydrogen, since molecular hydrogen alone does not cause the color reduction. Biological substances such as semen may contain these enzymes, or the methylene blue may act as a catalyst to activate the

hydrogen. Semen contains free and loosely combined oxygen, which, due to bacteria or enzymes, is used to change the material from a mildly oxidizing to a mildly reducing substance. The rate of this reduction in semen depends largely upon the concentration and activity of the spermatozoa; however, it can be influenced to some degree by such factors as presence of microflora, enzymes, light, and temperature, which may vary the hydrogen reduction.

## PROCEDURE

A recommended procedure for the methylene blue reduction test is:

1. Prepare a methylene blue solution by dissolving 50 mg of methylene blue in 100 ml of 3.6 percent sodium citrate buffer ($Na_3C_6H_5O_7 \cdot 2H_2O$).

2. Dilute 0.2 ml of semen with 0.8 ml of egg yolk–citrate extender in a 10-ml vial and thoroughly mix (extended 1:4).

3. Add 0.1 ml of methylene blue solution (as prepared in step 1) and mix.

4. Seal tube with ½-inch layer of mineral oil.

5. Place in water bath at 110° to 115° F (43° to 46° C).

6. Observe time required for sample to lose its blue color.

The blue color will be lost (by reduction) within three to six minutes in good quality semen. Any semen that retains the color for nine minutes or longer would not be useful for insemination purposes, because in such a sample, there would be very few live sperm. Some of the color reduction may be caused by reducing substances other than the spermato-

[2] A. Walton and J. Edwards. 1938. Criteria of fertility in the bull: I. The exhaustion test. Proc. American Soc. of Animal Production 31:254.

[3] J. R. Lodge and G. W. Salisbury. 1963. Factors influencing metabolic activity of bull spermatozoa: VI. Metabolic $CO_2$ and fructose. J. Dairy Sci. 45:140.

zoa; thus, there are no definite standards for the various reduction times.

## Hydrogen Ion Concentration (pH)

The acidity or alkalinity of a solution is determined by the hydrogen ion concentration. When there is an excess of hydrogen ions, the solution is acidic, and when there is an excess of basic salts, the solution is alkaline. This measurement is generally referred to in terms of pH. The pH is a figure representing the negative logarithm of the free hydrogen ion concentration. This characteristic of semen is important because a shift in pH may reflect pathological or inflammatory conditions in the reproductive tract. Also, any semen extender used should be approximately the same pH as the semen or should act as a buffer against excessive acidity or alkalinity.

Freshly collected bull semen is slightly acidic, typically ranging from about pH 6.5 to 6.9 (average pH 6.75). However, pH can vary considerably. For example, in studies by Swanson and Herman,[4] 295 samples of semen had a pH range from 5.8 to 7.4, with an average of 6.3.

The pH of semen is determined mainly by the proportions of various seminal plasma constituents (i.e., rete testis fluid, epididymal fluid, and vesicular, prostate, and bulbo-urethral gland secretions). It has been shown that the method of collecting semen affects its pH. Davis[5] and Kuhne[6] reported that bull semen collected by the massage method was ordinarily alkaline, while that collected with an artificial vagina was usually acidic.

Changes in pH of bull semen during storage at 40° F (~5° C) have been attributed to the production of lactic acid from glycolysis. The formation of lactic acid and the decrease in pH may be considered as an approximate measure of sperm metabolic activity. Bernstein and Slovohotov[7] reported that fresh ejaculates of bull and human semen contained about 40 to 50 mg percent of lactic acid and that the content of lactic acid increased as the semen was kept outside the body. The motility of the spermatozoa decreased, but complete cessation of motility occurred at different levels; hence, it was not thought to be due to lactic acid alone. Another study[8] found lactic acid level in fresh bull semen to range from 0 to 88 mg percent, with an average of 25 ± 18.2 mg percent for 75 samples.

There are many different types of test solutions and papers that may be used as acid-base indicators. These materials change color based on different pH ranges. Some of these indicators are more specific than others, being suitable only for a definite pH or for a very limited range of pH values. Other indicators are suitable for a wider range of pH values but are much less accurate or may change color to indicate only an acid (pH less than 7) or a base (pH greater than 7). Examples of various acid-base indicators include nitrazine paper (pH 4.5 to 7.5), Hydrion paper (pH 0 to 14 in various ranges), litmus paper, bromphenol blue, methyl red, bromcresol purple, phenol red, cresol red, and phenolphthalein. The pH is determined by

[4] E. W. Swanson and H. A. Herman. 1944. The correlation between some characteristics of dairy bull semen and conception rate. J. Dairy Sci. 17:297.

[5] H. P. Davis. 1938. Some factors affecting artificial insemination in cattle. Proc. American Soc. of Animal Production 32:232.

[6] W. Kuhne. 1936. Untersuchengen von Bullensperma auf Beschaffenheit und Eignung für die künstliche Besamung. Dissertation. University Giessen.

[7] A. Bernstein and I. Slovohotov. 1931. Glucose metabolism in semen. Orenburg Vet Inst.—Studies of Physiol. of Spermatozoa 9 (Abstr.). In: Physiol. Abstr. 26:331.

[8] C. N. Graves. Semen and its components. 1978. In: G. L. Salisbury, N. L. Van Demark, and J. R. Lodge (Eds.). Physiology of Reproduction and Artificial Insemination of Cattle (2nd Ed.). W. H. Freeman, San Francisco. (Ch. 9.)

matching the reacted test paper or indicator solution to a standard color chart. For the most part, these indicators are only a rough measure of pH and must be properly stored to remain effective. For AI laboratory and research purposes, the pH is determined more accurately using a pH meter equipped with an appropriate combination electrode.

## Binding of Glycosaminoglycans

Glycosaminoglycans (GAG's) are high-molecular-weight polysaccharides found in seminal plasma and in the female reproductive tract. GAG's have been shown to be effective in capacitating bull sperm and increasing the incidence of acrosome reactions in vitro. In the female reproductive tract (in vivo), the acrosome reaction must occur before a sperm can fertilize an oocyte. Heparin has been found to be one of the most potent GAG's for enhancing the occurrence of acrosome reactions, and it appears to attach to specific binding sites on sperm cells.[9] The ability of sperm to respond to GAG's and undergo an acrosome reaction in vitro has been shown to correspond with the bull's non-return rate. Binding affinity that sperm possess for the GAG heparin appears to increase with increasing fertility[10] and decrease with decreasing seminal quality (e.g., as a result of summer heat stress) (Table 12.1). As reported by Ax and Lenz,[11] binding of GAG's may prove to be a valuable method to monitor cellular changes of sperm in vitro that reflect bull fertility.

## Flow Cytometry

Flow cytometry has become an important research tool for evaluating sperm cells. In addition to applications for determining sperm concentration (refer to Exercise 9), flow cytometry has also been utilized to correlate sperm chromatin structure with fertility (see below), to measure intracellular calcium changes in the acrosome, and to assess sperm cell viability. A simultaneous analysis of sperm cell viability, acrosomal integrity, and mitochondrial

[9] R. L. Ax and R. W. Lenz. 1986. Laboratory procedures to assess fertility of bulls. Proc. 11th Tech. Conf. on Artificial Insemination and Reproduction. NAAB. p. 80.

[10] Ibid.
[11] R. L. Ax and R. W. Lenz. 1987. Glycosaminoglycans as probes to monitor differences in fertility of bulls. J. Dairy Sci. 70:1477.

**Table 12.1.** Seminal Characteristics and Binding Parameters for $^3$H-Heparin in Sperm Collected from Bulls Prior to, During, and Following a Period of Heat Stress[a]

| Trait Examined | Collection Relative to Heat Stress | | |
| --- | --- | --- | --- |
| | Prior to | During | After |
| Concentration ($\times 10^9$) | 1.95 | 1.48 | 2.02 |
| Motility (%) | 65.0 | 50.0 | 66.7 |
| Abnormal sperm (%) | 25.0 | 50.7 | 19.0 |
| Dissociation constant (nmolar) | 30.4 | 151.3 | 18.1 |
| Binding sites per sperm ($\times 10^6$) | 1.5 | 1.1 | 1.4 |

[a]Data from R. L. Ax and G. R. Gilbert. 1986. Binding of $^3$H-heparin to bull sperm corresponds to semen quality. 81st Ann. Mtg. American Dairy Science Assoc. (Abstr.).

function using this technique has been reported by Graham.[12] Flow cytometry/cell sorter techniques have also made it possible to identify and separate X- and Y- bearing sperm in semen sexing applications (refer to Exercise 21).

## Sperm Chromatin Structure

Sperm nuclear material consists of DNA molecules and a unique basic protein called "protamine." This complex, called "chromatin," is highly condensed due to the presence of disulfide bonds and, as such, may protect the genetic material from environmental damage. Denaturation of the DNA results in a separation of the normal double-stranded material into single-stranded molecules. DNA in sperm with normal chromatin is very resistant and does not denature at low pH or high heat, while DNA in sperm with abnormal chromatin exhibits greater susceptibility to denaturation. As indicated previously (Exercise 11), morphologically abnormal sperm from subfertile bulls have been shown to contain abnormal sperm chromatin, which may be responsible for early embryonic death after fertilization.

Evenson and Ballachey[13] developed an assay that assesses the chromatin structure of sperm cells by using flow cytometry techniques to measure relative amounts of double- to single-stranded DNA in individual sperm cells subjected to denaturation. (A brief description of the flow cytometry can be found in Exercise 9.) In this assay, fresh or frozen-thawed semen is diluted, subjected to denatu-

$$\text{ALPHA } (\alpha) \text{ T} = \frac{\text{RED FLUORESCENCE}}{\text{RED + GREEN (TOTAL) FLUORESCENCE}}$$

PURPOSE: TO DETERMINE THE SUSCEPTIBILITY OF DNA IN SITU TO ACID OR HEAT DENATURATION

MEASURE: SHIFT FROM GREEN TO RED FLUORESCENCE NATIVE DNA VALUE OF 0 SHIFTS TO DENATURED DNA VALUE OF 1.0

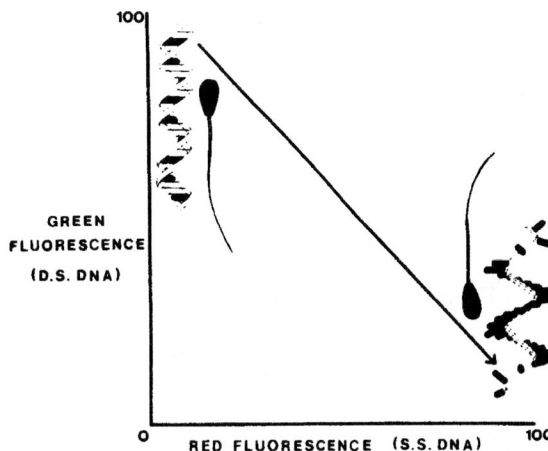

**Figure 12.1.** Outline of the principles of the sperm chromatin structure assay. A color photograph would show the left-hand sperm cell with a green nucleus and green fluorescing accretion orange molecules intercalated into the DNA helix (D.S. DNA); the right-hand sperm cell would show a red fluorescing nucleus with red fluorescing accretion orange molecules attached to the single-stranded DNA molecules (S.S. DNA). The amount of single- and double-stranded DNA is quantitated by the expression $\alpha_t$, which is the ratio of single-stranded DNA to total DNA measured. (D. P. Evenson and B. E. Ballachey. 1988. Flow cytometry evaluation of bull sperm chromatin structure. Proc. 12th Tech. Conf. on Artificial Insemination and Reproduction. NAAB. p. 45)

ration, stained, and then analyzed by flow cytometry, all in a relatively short period of time. In sperm stained with a metachromatic dye (e.g., acridine orange) and then excited by a laser beam, the double-stranded DNA produces green fluorescence and the single-stranded DNA produces red fluorescence. The flow cytometry precisely measures the red and green fluorescence in each cell, and a ratio ($\alpha_t$) is determined (Figure 12.1). Typically, 5,000 individual sperm per sample are evaluated. Theoretically, a normal sperm with all-green fluorescence would have an $\alpha_t$ of 0

---

[12] J. K. Graham. 1994. In vitro assays of bull fertility. Proc. 15th Tech. Conf. on Artificial Insemination and Reproduction. NAAB. p. 74.

[13] D. P. Evenson and B. E. Ballachey. 1988. Flow cytometry evaluation of bull sperm chromatin structure. Proc. 12th Tech. Conf. on Artificial Insemination and Reproduction. NAAB. p. 45.

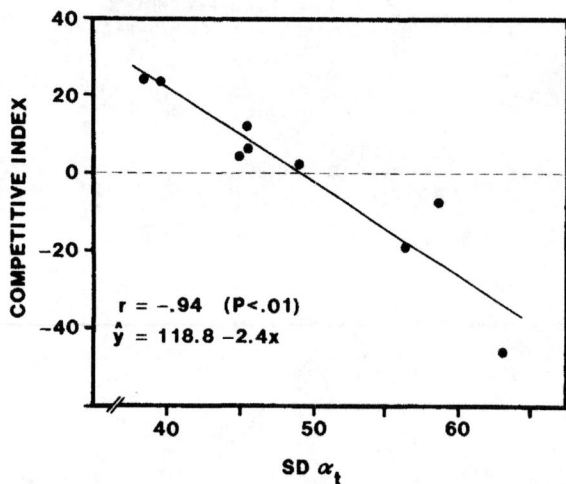

**Figure 12.2.** Correlation between competitive index of nine bulls and the standard deviation (SD) of $\alpha_t$. (D. P. Evenson and B. E. Ballachey. 1988. Flow cytometry evaluation of bull sperm chromatin structure. Proc. 12th Tech. Conf. on Artificial Insemination and Reproduction. NAAB. p. 45)

while a sperm that was entirely denatured would have an $\alpha_t$ of 1.0. The standard deviation (SD) of $\alpha_t$ is a useful determinant of the chromatin structure abnormalities and has been shown to have a highly negative correlation with the competitive fertility index (Figure 12.2). A modification of the sperm chromatin structure assay (SCSA) using an epifluoresence/DIC microscope has been developed by Acevedo, et al.[14] This procedure allows for the observation of chromatin structure and morphology of the same sperm cells with equipment that is less costly than a flow cytometer. Initial research has demonstrated that chromatin aberrations due to experimentally induced heat stress of the bull's scrotum was accompanied by the appearance of classical sperm abnormalities. A significant finding of this work was that chromatin aberrations were also found in many normally shaped sperm. Thus, conventional morphology evaluations alone may not be revealing the full extent of problems that can exist in an ejaculate. Additional research will be needed to further evaluate this new assay.

## Penetration of Hamster Ova

Penetration of hamster ova has been used as a test system to evaluate the fertilizing ability of sperm from humans and other species (see references). Hamster ova are obtained by superovulation and recovery from the oviducts. The zona pellucida of the hamster ova must first be removed enzymatically before sperm of species other than the hamster can penetrate and have an opportunity for their chromatin to decondense. Before bull sperm are capable of penetrating the hamster ova, it is necessary to remove the semen extender by washing the sample in buffer and to induce capacitation/the acrosome reaction. A controlled number of test sperm and hamster ova are then incubated together for a few hours under appropriate culture conditions. Ideally, 20 to 30 hamster ova per semen sample are used. This is followed by the ova being fixed, stained, and observed microscopically to determine the number that are penetrated by sperm having a decondensed/swollen nucleus and an associated tail. A semen sample from a bull of known fertility may be tested concurrently as a control. The correlations between ova penetration and the competitive fertility index for a group of bulls have been demonstrated.[15] A possible drawback to this assay is an apparent lack of uniformity between

---

[14] N. J. Acevedo, J. H. Bame, L. A. Kuehn, W. D. Hohenboken, D. P. Evenson, R. G. Saacke. 2001. Effects of elevated testicular temperature on spermatozoal morphology and chromatin stability to acid denaturation. Biol. Reprod. 64: p. 217. (Suppl 1).

[15] R. H. Foote, S. Hough, and C. Blanpain-Tobback. 1988. Heterospermic field trials: Hamster egg penetration. Proc. 12th Tech. Conf. on Artificial Insemination and Reproduction. NAAB. p. 49.

batches of hamster ova, which could vary the results.

## Filtration

The filtration of extended semen through a column of Sephadex gel/glass wool and the electronic counting of the filtered cells has been shown to correlate well with bull fertility.[16, 17] In this assay, Sephadex gel is prepared and layered over a glass wool plug placed in the bottom of a plastic syringe barrel, creating a filtration column. The column is flushed with buffer, and a small volume of the semen sample is added. More buffer is used to flush the system, and the filtrate is recovered for enumeration of sperm. Dead or damaged sperm cells and certain types of abnormal sperm are retained in the filtration column, and the more normal, viable cells pass through. The factors responsible for the entrapment of certain sperm cells in the Sephadex gel/glass wool have not been completely determined; however, the integrity of the cell membranes and sperm surface structure is believed to be important. Semen samples that exhibit a higher proportion of cells passing through the filter would presumably have a higher number of viable cells eligible and available for fertilization upon insemination.

Details of column preparation and procedures have been described by Graham, et al.[18] This assay requires use of an electronic particle counter, which may be quite expensive for general AI laboratory purposes.

## Additional Tests

Several other assays and tests for evaluating quality of semen have been applied to the bull. For example, release of the enzyme glutamic oxaloacetic transaminase (Pace and Graham, 1970), acrosin activity (Johnson, et al., 1976; Garner and Palencia, 1996), serum-induced head-to-head agglutination (Senger and Saacke, 1976), and hypo-osmotic swelling (Smith and Graham, 1976; Jeyendran, et al., 1985) represent various approaches that have been used to measure sperm quality. For further reading, see the indicated references.

In reviewing numerous laboratory tests pertaining to bull semen quality, Graham[19] emphasized the importance of these tests being:

1. **Objective**—Not easily affected by human judgment/bias.

2. **Repeatable**—Able to be repeated with the same result.

3. **Reliable**—Faithfully measuring specific quality trait(s) (reflecting any processing damage and relating to fertility).

4. **Economically feasible**—Worth the time and expense to the laboratory.

Generally laboratory tests and assays used in the AI industry encompass these characteristics. However, since all methods have some limitations and there are no single semen tests that are complete indicators of quality, combinations of viability, morphology, and sometimes additional tests are employed.

---

[16] E. F. Graham, et al. 1978. Viability assays for frozen semen. Cryobiology 15:242.

[17] R. G. Saacke, et al. 1980. The relationship of semen quality and fertility: A heterospermic study. Proc. 8th Tech. Conf. on Artificial Insemination and Reproduction. NAAB. p. 71.

[18] E. F. Graham, et al. 1978. An overview of column separation of spermatozoa. Proc. 7th Tech. Conf. on Artificial Insemination and Reproduction. NAAB. p. 69.

---

[19] E. F. Graham, M. K. L. Schmehl, and D. S. Nelson. 1980. Problems with laboratory assays. Proc. 8th Tech. Conf. on Artificial Insemination and Reproduction. NAAB. p. 59.

# QUESTIONS

1. Is there a correlation between the glycolytic rate and the fertility of the semen? Between the respiratory rate and the fertility? Explain.

2. What factors, other than the concentration and motility of sperm, may cause variations in metabolic reaction rates?

3. In general terms, what are the important changes that occur during glycolysis and respiration of spermatozoa?

4. What are the main advantages and disadvantages of the methylene blue reduction test?

5. What is the optimum pH of semen?

6. How does the pH of neat semen and extended semen change during storage?

7. Is there any correlation between pH of semen and fertility or storage time? Explain.

8. Does the pH of semen vary between bulls and/or between different collections from one bull? Explain.

9. Explain how GAG binding may be used to assess sperm cell quality.

10. How does the sperm chromatin structure assay relate to fertility? What is the significance of condensed and decondensed chromatin?

11. Why must the zona pellucida of hamster ova be enzymatically removed to accommodate penetration by sperm of other species?

12. Explain how a sperm's ability to pass through a Sephadex gel column reflects its quality. Would it be useful or practical to filter an entire bull ejaculate and use only filtered sperm cells for artificial insemination?

13. List the important characteristics of quality tests and assays. Indicate which tests you would use to evaluate semen for artificial insemination. Briefly support your choices.

# REFERENCES

Ax, R. L., and G. R. Gilbert. 1986. Binding of $^3$H-heparin to bull sperm corresponds to semen quality. 81st Ann. Mtg. American Dairy Science Assoc. (Abstr.).

Beck, G. H., and G. W. Salisbury. 1953. Rapid methods for estimating the quality of bull semen. J. Dairy Sci. 26:483.

Garner, D. L. and D. D. Palencia. 1996. Relationship of activable proacrosin to bull sperm fertility. Proc. 16th Tech. Conf. on Artificial Insemination and Reproduction. NAAB. p. 81.

Hafez, E. S. E. (Ed.). 1987. Reproduction in Farm Animals (5th Ed.). Lea & Febiger, Philadelphia. (Ch. 22.)

Jeyendran, R. S., et al. 1985. The hypo-osmotic swelling (HOS) test as an indicator of the fertilizing capacity of human spermatozoa. Current Clinical and Basic Investigations. 33rd Clinical Mtg., ACOG. p. 24.

Johnson, L. A., et al. 1976. Comparison of several extraction procedures for boar Spermatozoan acrosin. Biol. Reprod. 15:79.

Mann, T. 1975. Biochemistry of semen. In: R. O. Greep and E. Astwood (Eds.). Handbook of Physiology. American Physiological Soc., Washington, DC. Vol. 5, Sec. 7.

Pace, M. M., and E. F. Graham. 1970. Release of glutamic oxaloacetic transaminase from bovine spermatozoa as a test method of assessing semen quality and fertility. Biol. Reprod. 3:140.

Salisbury, G. W., N. L. Van Demark, and J. R. Lodge (Eds.). 1978. Physiology of Reproduction and Artificial Insemination of Cattle (2nd Ed.). W. H. Freeman, San Francisco. (Ch. 11.)

Senger, P. L., and R. G. Saacke. 1976. Serum-inducted head to head agglutination of bovine spermatozoa. J. Reprod. Fertil. 47:215.

Smith, J. E., and E. F. Graham. 1976. High resolution size distributions of bull spermatozoa. Proc. 8th International Congr. Animal Reproduction and Artificial Insemination (Krakow, Poland). p. 943.

Van Demark, N. L., E. Mercier, and G. W. Salisbury. 1945. The methylene blue reduction test and its relation to other measures of quality in bull semen. J. Dairy Sci. 28:121.

Weeth, H. J., and H. A. Herman. 1949. The relationship between semen quality and conception rate in artificial insemination of cattle. Mo. Agr. Exp. Sta. Res. Bull. No. 447.

# EXERCISE 13

# Extenders and Extension of Semen

## OBJECT

To study the preparation of extenders and the extension of semen.

## DISCUSSION

The object of extending semen is to increase the volume of the ejaculate and aid in preserving the viability of sperm so that a large number of females may be successfully inseminated to a single collection. A satisfactory extender should not only increase the volume of the semen but also should aid in the preservation and longevity of the spermatozoa. Semen may be extended many fold, depending upon sperm numbers present in the ejaculate, its quality, and the fertility history of the sire in question.

Extension of semen is one of the advantages of artificial insemination. In natural service, one ejaculate might settle one cow, but in artificial insemination, with the use of extenders, one collection may be used for from 300 to more than 1,000 cows and heifers.

Since spermatozoa do not survive in neat semen for long periods of time, even at cool temperatures, it is necessary that extenders be utilized to improve or maintain the media surrounding the sperm by furnishing a supply of energy and providing protection against by-products of metabolism and against temperature changes. A desirable extender should (1) furnish energy and nutrients for the stored sperm, (2) provide buffering action to compensate for shifts in pH due to lactic acid for-

mation, (3) provide protection against rapid cooling and temperature shock, (4) maintain the optimum osmotic pressure and balance of electrolytes for the media, (5) inhibit the growth of microorganisms, including those that are pathological, and (6) increase the volume of the original semen so that its use can be extended to many animals.

The extender should be economical and relatively simple to prepare under routine conditions, and the ingredients should be readily available through the usual laboratory supply or chemical firms.

Materials used for semen extenders are quite varied and may differ from one semen processing laboratory to another or from one country to another. In regard to semen quality or fertility, there is no one best semen extender. However, egg yolk–citrate, milk, and egg yolk–tris extenders are commonly used throughout the U.S. AI industry, having stood the test of time. It is important to recognize that no extender can make good-quality, highly-fertile semen from that which was inferior when collected. From a health standpoint, the interaction of the type of extender or its components with the added antibiotics is an important consideration. Certified Semen Services, Inc., requires its participating organizations to use semen extenders that have been tested and approved for use, in order to insure efficacy of the CSS combination of antibiotics (see Exercise 24).

Despite the intrinsic ability of spermatozoa to withstand processing, freezing, and storage, conditions can vary between individual bulls and occasionally between ejaculates of the same bull over extended periods of time. Bulls that maintain above-average fertility or non-return rates are normally found in every AI organization. There are also those sires making up the bulk of the population that are average in fertility, as well as those that may be below average. It is important that the semen extender help preserve the inherent quality of the semen so that each sire's genetic contributions are realized.

Bull semen extenders usually contain (1) a buffer, such as sodium citrate dihydrate or tris (hydroxymethyl) aminomethane; (2) egg yolk or milk, which contains macromolecules that provide protection against cold shock; (3) simple sugars, such as glucose and fructose, that serve as a source of energy for sperm; (4) glycerol, which is added as a cryoprotectant to reduce the intercellular formation of ice crystals and solute effects during the freeze–thaw process; and (5) antibiotics, such as gentamicin, tylosin, and Linco-Spectin (GTLS), which inhibit a variety of microorganisms found in semen.

Semen is isotonic with body fluids such as blood plasma, milk, and other secretions (approximately 300 milliosmols). Semen extenders should be isotonic, or iso-osmotic. The pH should be near neutral to slightly acidic in the range of 6.5 to 6.9. For routine quality control, each batch of buffer that is prepared, as well as the final semen extender, should be checked for osmolality and pH. These measurements will detect possible errors in preparations. If values are outside normal tolerances, the buffer or extender should be discarded and a new batch prepared.

The preparation of semen extenders is not difficult; however, it requires attention to detail. It is also important that the laboratory be clean, properly equipped, and adequately supplied and that personnel be thoroughly trained to insure accuracy. Typical equipment and supplies may include a water purification system (e.g., distillation unit, reverse-osmosis unit, ion exchange unit), an electronic top-loading balance, a pH meter, an osmometer, a magnetic stirrer unit, a sterilization oven and/or autoclave, cold sterilization equipment (filtration), a vacuum pump, temperature monitoring equipment (thermometers, thermocouples, recording instrumentation), a large assortment of laboratory glassware (e.g., volumetric flasks, graduated cylinders, reagent bottles, Erlenmeyer flasks, beakers), reagent grade chemicals (buffer salts, sugars, glycerol), fresh disease-free components, such as eggs or milk, and appropriate antibiotics approved for drug use.

All equipment and glassware used in the preparation of extenders must be cleaned and sterilized before use. Strict control of microbial contamination and toxic substances is a must. Glassware and equipment are normally washed in warm soapy water (e.g., water with anionic laboratory detergent), rinsed in tap water, then rinsed repeatedly in distilled water. These materials are allowed to air dry in a dust-free environment. The openings are covered with aluminum foil, and glassware is dry-heat sterilized in an oven at 365°F (185°C) for two to three hours. Materials that cannot withstand dry-heat temperatures (e.g., rubber goods, stoppers, some types of plastic) can be autoclaved for 20 to 30 minutes (250°F [121°C] at 15 psi). Various sterility indicators can be used to monitor the sterilization process and insure that the equipment or materials have actually reached sterilization conditions.

Figure 13.1 depicts the preparation of semen extender at a large commercial AI organization.

Probably no phase of artificial insemination has been more heavily studied than the formulation of semen extenders. The literature is voluminous, and numerous semen extender recipes have been developed, many of them in the early AI years (1940's, 1950's, 1960's). Over the decades extenders have been continually investigated and improved. A few of the

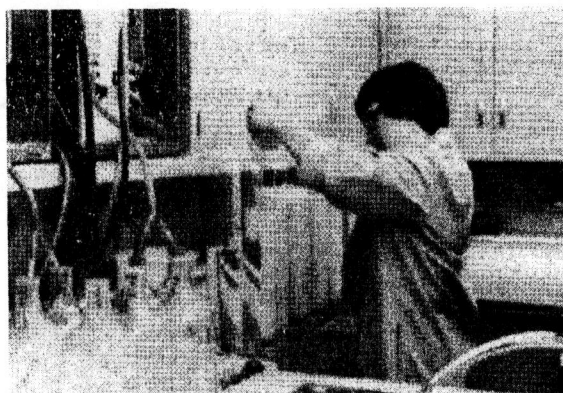

**Figure 13.1.** Semen extender is prepared daily under strict quality control procedures. It contains the necessary ingredients to protect sperm cells during cooling, freezing, and thawing and allows many females to be inseminated to a single collection. (Courtesy, ABS Global, Inc., DeForest, WI)

dependable extenders for frozen semen are explained here. In addition, other extenders used for liquid semen, frozen semen, ambient temperature storage, and so forth, are included to demonstrate a wide spectrum of semen extender applications. For a more comprehensive review of semen extenders, consult the references at the end of this exercise.

In this exercise, all semen extenders will apply to cattle. Extenders for other species will be included with the discussion of artificial insemination of those species.

# PROCEDURE

## Egg Yolk–Citrate Extender

Citrate as a buffer for semen diluting fluids was proposed by Schersten[1] in 1936. Phillips,[2] in 1939, also reported the value of hen's yolk in a semen extender. In 1941, Salisbury and his co-workers[3] developed an egg yolk–citrate extender that is widely used today.

**2.9 Percent Sodium Citrate Buffer**—To prepare 1 liter of a 2.9 percent solution of sodium citrate dihydrate ($Na_3C_6H_5O_7 \cdot 2H_2O$), weigh exactly 29 g of reagent grade (AR) crystalline sodium citrate on the analytical or top-loading balance. Add the salt to an appropriate sized volumetric flask (1 liter) and bring to one-half volume (about 500 ml) with distilled/ultrapure water.

Swirling the solution in the flask will cause most of the sodium citrate crystals to dissolve. After the salts are initially dissolved, bring to volume with distilled/ultrapure water, add a stir bar, and thoroughly mix using a magnetic stirrer. When the stir bar is removed, make sure that the solution is up to the volume mark on the flask. The sodium citrate buffer is then transferred to a storage bottle and sterilized in an autoclave or cold sterilized by vacuum filtration through a 0.45μ filter membrane into a sterile reagent bottle. A sample of the buffer is then checked for osmolality and perhaps pH.

If acceptable, the buffer is labeled, dated, and stored in the coldroom or refrigerator (41°F [5° C]) until use. Typically a one- to two-week supply of buffer is prepared at a time.

An advantage of this buffer solution is that the sodium citrate effectively binds calcium and other heavy metals. It also disperses the fat globules in the egg yolk, thus making it possible to observe individual sperm cells on microscopic examination.

**Yolk Preparation**— Eggs used to provide yolk must come from disease-free flocks and must be fresh—preferably not over one day old. To remove possible contamination, the

---

[1] B. Schersten. 1936. Studies on the occurrence and biological importance of citrate in the sexual gland secretions of man and various animals. (Trans. title.) Scand. Arch. Physiol. 74:3.

[2] P. H. Phillips. 1939. Preservation of bull semen. J. Biol. Chem. 130:415.

[3] G. W. Salisbury, H. K. Fuller, and E. L. Willett. 1941. Preservation of bovine spermatozoa in yolk-citrate diluent and field results from its use. J. Dairy Sci. 24:905.

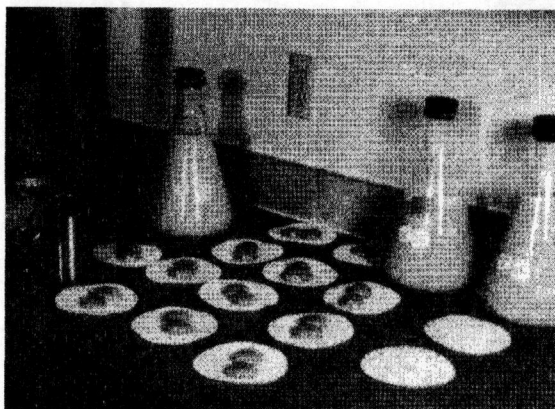

**Figure 13.2.** Filter paper method of processing egg yolks for preparation of yolk-based extender. (Courtesy, Select Sires, Inc., Plain City, OH)

eggs are washed in warm water with mild detergent and then rinsed in warm tap water followed by distilled water. The egg shells are wiped or sprayed with isopropyl or 70 percent ethyl alcohol and are then allowed to dry.

A clean and sterilized metal egg separator is used to separate each yolk from the egg white. Break an egg midway on a clean beaker, and transfer its contents to the egg separator. By gravity, most of the egg white falls through the openings in the separator. The white is then discarded. The yolk is transferred to a sterile filter paper and is rolled to absorb any remaining egg white (Figure 13.2). The paper is folded over the yolk, and the yolk membrane is ruptured by pressure or by puncturing it with a sterile probe. The egg yolk is then collected in a sterile receptacle (graduated cylinder or reagent bottle). Frequently, sterile gauze is placed over the mouth of the receptacle to filter out any egg yolk membranes. Another method is to place the yolk on a card that has a ½-inch hole in it, so that the yolk is centered over the hole. When the card is tapped on the mouth of the container, the yolk membrane breaks and the yolk drains into the receptacle. After the desired volume is obtained, the combined yolks can be thoroughly mixed or homogenized using a sterile mixer or blender. Yolks that are off-color or have blood spots are not used.

**Extender Preparation—** Most extenders for frozen semen are prepared in two fractions. A non-glycerol portion (A fraction) is used for the initial extension and cooling of semen, and a portion containing twice the desired concentration of glycerol (B fraction) is added after the semen is cooled to 41°F (5°C). The final ratio of A fraction plus semen to B fraction is 1:1. The glycerol fraction is added after initial cooling to 41°F (5°C) to avoid any potential damage to sperm cells and interference with efficacy of antibiotics.

### For 500 ml of A and B Fraction Egg Yolk–Citrate Extender

| Component | Non-glycerol Fraction A | Glycerol Fraction B | Final % of 1:1 Mixture |
|---|---|---|---|
| 2.9% sodium citrate buffer | 400 ml | 330 ml | 73 |
| Fresh hen's yolk (20%) | 100 ml | 100 ml | 20 |
| Glycerol | — | 70 ml | 7 |
| | 500 ml | 500 ml | |

Antibiotics (as per Appendix 1 of CSS Minimum Requirements—Exercise 24)

Some laboratories use a higher proportion of egg yolk (i.e., up to 28 percent) with good results. Also fructose or glucose is frequently included in either one or both fractions of the extender (final extender concentration from 1.0 to 1.25 percent). Depending upon the final components used, egg yolk–citrate extender normally has the following characteristics:

pH: 6.8 to 6.9
Osmolality: 285 to 300 mOsms

## Whole Milk Extender

The use of milk as an extender for frozen semen is popular, particularly since it obtains good results and requires fewer steps to prepare than egg yolk extenders. It is estimated that in 2001 about one-fifth of the semen marketed in the United States by NAAB members was processed in whole milk. One possible disadvantage of this extender is that it is optically opaque due to the presence of lipid globules. This makes it difficult to observe individual sperm cells microscopically for quality evaluations.

Fresh or pasteurized milk is harmful to sperm because of adverse enzymes that it contains; however, if the milk is heated for about 10 minutes at 198° to 203°F (92° to 95°C), the deleterious enzymes are destroyed.

**Milk Preparation**— Following is the recommended procedure:

1. Use fresh, pasteurized, homogenized whole milk (approximately 3.5 percent fat).

2. Heat the milk in a covered double boiler (Pyrex glass preferred) at 198° to 203°F (92° to 95°C) for 10 minutes.

3. Remove the milk from the heat, and allow it to cool to room temperature.

4. Pour the cooled milk into a sterile container, leaving the scum in the boiler. If necessary, strain the milk through sterile gauze or filter to remove scum.

**Extender Preparation**— The milk extender is prepared in two fractions as follows:

**For 500 ml of A and B Fraction Whole Milk Extender**

| Component | Non-glycerol Fraction A | Glycerol Fraction B | Final % of 1:1 Mixture |
|---|---|---|---|
| Heated milk | 500 ml | 430 ml | 93 |
| Glycerol | — | 70 ml | 7 |
| | 500 ml | 500 ml | |

---

Antibiotics (as per Appendix 1 of CSS Minimum Requirements—Exercise 24)

Normal characteristics of milk extender:

pH: 6.5 to 6.6
Osmolality: 260–290 mOsms

## Egg Yolk–Tris Extender

Tris-buffered semen extenders have gained in commercial application in recent years. When combined with egg yolk and other components, tris is a buffer that has proven to be as effective as other common semen extenders.

**Tris Buffer**— To prepare 1 liter of 0.2 M tris buffer, weigh 30.28 g tris hydroxymethyl aminomethane ($C_4H_{11}NO_3$) and 17.30 g citric acid monohydrate [$HOC(COOH)(CH_2COOH)_2$] on a top-loading or analytical balance. Add the salts to an appropriate sized volumetric flask (1 liter), and bring to volume with distilled/ultrapure water following the procedures outlined for sodium citrate buffer. Sterilize the buffer by filtration or autoclaving, and store at 41°F (5°C) until use.

**Yolk Preparation**— Egg yolk is prepared according to procedures described for egg yolk–citrate extender.

**Extender Preparation**— The egg yolk–tris extender is prepared as follows:

**For 500 ml of A and B Fraction Egg Yolk–Tris Extender**

| Component | Non-glycerol Fraction A | Glycerol Fraction B | Final % of 1:1 Mixture |
|---|---|---|---|
| 0.2 M tris buffer | 400 ml | 330 ml | 73 |
| Fresh hen's yolk | 100 ml | 100 ml | 20 |
| Glycerol | — | 70 ml | 7 |
| | 500 ml | 500 ml | |

---

Antibiotics (as per Appendix 1 of CSS Minimum Requirements—Exercise 24)

As with egg yolk–citrate extender, egg yolk–tris may incorporate a higher proportion of egg yolk and/or inclusion of fructose or glucose in either one or both fractions of extender (e.g., 1.0 to 1.25 percent, final concentration). Depending upon the final components used, egg yolk–tris extender normally has the following characteristics:

pH: 6.5–6.75
Osmolality: 275 to 290 mOsms

The egg yolk–citrate, milk, and egg yolk–tris extenders are considered fairly basic in the AI industry. However, modifications of these basic extenders are used by certain laboratories. Amounts of egg yolk, sugars, glycerol, citric acid, enzymes, etc., may be added or modified by some laboratories. The intent here in suggesting semen extenders in common use is to emphasize the basic formulas that have demonstrated their dependability. When a semen-producing business adopts a semen extender and finds it doing the job from the standpoint of cows in calf under field conditions, it generally stays with it. Changes are made only when research clearly demonstrates the superiority of new extenders or of modifications of those in use.

## Minnesota GO Extender

### Formula and Preparations

1. Basic Minnesota GO buffer:

   | | |
   |---|---|
   | Adonitol | 1.0 g |
   | Sorbitol | 1.0 g |
   | Mannitol | 1.0 g |
   | Erythritol | 1.0 g |
   | Inositol | 1.0 g |
   | Dulcitol | 1.0 g |
   | Dextrose | 3.0 g |
   | Fructose | 5.0 g |
   | Sodium citrate | 21.0 g |
   | Citrate acid | 0.4 g |

   Dissolve in 1,000 ml distilled water.

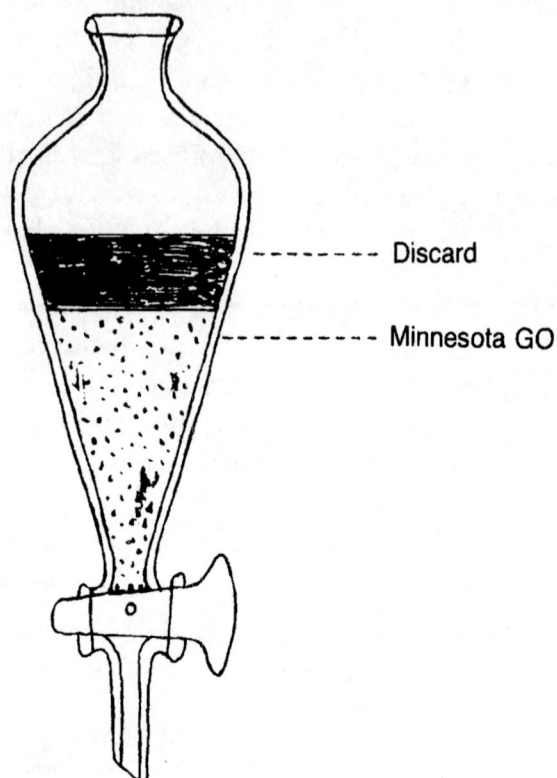

**Figure 13.3.** Minnesota GO extender in separatory funnel.

2. Dried egg yolk:

   Dispense 50 g of spray-dried egg yolk solids in 1,000 ml pre-cooled (41° F [5° C]) Minnesota GO buffer, and allow to separate in a separatory funnel in a cool room for two hours (Figure 13.3).

3. Final steps:

   a. Discard the colloidal packed upper fraction.

   b. Collect the lower clear fraction. This constitutes the Minnesota GO extender. Add antibiotics in usual amounts. Add 7 percent glycerol when using extender as freezing extender.

Following are comparisons of the Minnesota GO extender with egg yolk–citrate and with milk-glycerol extenders:

| Extender | First Service No. | 30- to 60-Day Non-return | Percent Non-return |
|---|---|---|---|
| Yolk-citrate | 7,438 | 5,266 | 70.79 |
| Minnesota GO | 6,821 | 5,422 | 79.48 |

### Preliminary Results—Milk Glycerol vs. Minnesota GO

| | | | |
|---|---|---|---|
| Milk-glycerol | 270 | 191* | 80.9 |
| Minnesota GO | 236 | 208* | 77.0 |

---

*90-day non-returns.

## Other Extenders

**Egg Yolk–Phosphate Extender—** Egg yolk–phosphate extender was developed by Phillips[4] and modified by Phillips and Lardy.[5] It is also known as the Phillips buffer or the Wisconsin buffer.

Following is the formula for the solution of phosphate buffer:

> 0.2 g $KH_2PO_4$
> 2.0 g $Na_2HPO_4 \cdot 12H_2O$
> 100 ml $H_2O$ distilled over glass (pH of 6.7 to 6.8)

Mix with boiling hot water to aid in dissolving crystalline material. Store in a cool (59°F [15°C]) place. Prepare fresh egg yolk by aseptically removing all white from the yolk, mechanically removing the yolk membrane, and allowing the freed yolk to run into a sterile container. When using, mix equal volumes of fresh egg yolk and phosphate buffer, and mix thoroughly.

### CUE (Cornell University Extender)

For liquid (unfrozen) bull semen:

a. Buffer:

> Sodium citrate dihydrate . . . .14.5 g
> Sodium bicarbonate . . . . . . . .2.1 g
> Potassium chloride . . . . . . . . .0.4 g
> Glucose . . . . . . . . . . . . . . .3.0 g
> Glycine . . . . . . . . . . . . . . .9.4 g
> Citric acid . . . . . . . . . . . . . .0.9 g
> Sulfanilamide . . . . . . . . . . . .3.0 g
> Distilled water,
>      final volume . . . . . . . .1,000 ml

b. Extender in which spermatozoa are stored:

> Buffer (above solution)
>      . . . . . . .80 percent by volume
> Egg yolk . . . .20 percent by volume
> Penicillin (units per ml) . . . . .1,000
> Streptomycin (Fg/ml) . . . . . .1,000

### Raffinose Extender

For frozen bull semen:

a. Buffer:

> Raffinose . . . . . . . . . . . . . .185 g
> Distilled water,
>      final volume . . . . . . . .1,000 ml

b. Extender:

> Buffer (above solution)
>      . . . . . . .75.3 percent by volume
> Glycerol . . . .4.7 percent by volume
> Egg yolk . . .20.0 percent by volume
> Penicillin (units per ml) . . . . .1,000
> Streptomycin (µ g/ml) . . . . . .1,000

**Milk-Glycerol Extender—** Milk-glycerol extender was developed in 1962 by Almquist and co-workers[6] and is particularly well adapted to packaging and shipping liquid (unfrozen) semen.

---

[4] Phillips, op. cit.

[5] P. H. Phillips and H. A. Lardy. 1940. A yolk buffer pablum for the preservation of bull semen. J. Dairy Sci. 23:399.

[6] J. O. Almquist. 1962. Diluents for bovine semen: XI. Effect of glycerol on fertility and motility of spermatozoa in homogenized milk and skim milk. J. Dairy Sci. 45:911.

1. Extend the fresh semen to about one-half the final desired sperm concentration with fresh, previously heated and cooled homogenized or skim milk containing the recommended antibiotics.

2. Slowly cool the partially extended semen to 41°F (5°C) over a period of about four hours.

3. Add an equal volume of cooled milk extender (41°F [5°C]) containing 20 percent glycerol by volume. For best junk sperm survival, the milk-glycerol fraction should be added gradually. To accomplish this:

   a. Add, in stepwise fashion, 20, 30, and 50 percent of the milk-glycerol solution at 10-minute intervals, or

   b. Add three equal amounts at 10-minute intervals, or

   c. Add one drop at a time from a reservoir equipped with a stopcock or flow control device continuously over a 30-minute period.

4. The final concentration of glycerol is now 10 percent, and the diluted semen is ready for packaging and shipping. Storage and shipping are at 41°F (5°C).

**Commercial Extenders—** Several commercial extenders are on the market that are easy to prepare and may be suitable for the small laboratory. These extenders may require the addition of distilled/ultrapure water, egg yolk, and/or glycerol, based on the directions of the supplier.

Examples are Plus-X Extender, available from Edwards Agri-Supply; Biladyl Extender, available from Minitube of America; Europhos Diluter, available from IMV International Corporation; Continental Concentrated Two-Step Extender, available from Continental Plastic Corporation; and Two-Step Extender available from Viam Pac, Inc.

Recent international biosecurity concerns raised by animal health regulators have prompted interest in developing semen extenders that are devoid of components containing animal proteins (e.g., milk, egg yolk, etc.). It is likely that non-animal protein extenders will be utilized to a greater extent in the future.

*Note:* It should be recognized that not all semen extenders have been approved by Certified Semen Services (CSS), regarding efficacy of the CSS combination of antibiotics. Therefore, it is important to refer to the CSS Minimum Requirements or contact CSS directly before using an unknown semen extender.

## Some Early Extenders Not in General Use

**Saline Solution Extender—** A 0.9 g saline solution (0.9 g NaCl per 100 cc distilled water), used as a physiological solution for short-time dilutions, has not been satisfactory for storage and has actually been harmful to the spermatozoa.

**Lipid Glucose Buffer (LGB) Gum—** Phillips and his co-workers[7] developed a pablum for semen storage, as follows:

Glucose . . . . . . . . . . . . . . . . . . . . .0.6%
Galactose . . . . . . . . . . . . . . . . . . . .0.2%
$KH_2PO_4$ . . . . . . . . . . . . . . . . . . . .0.2%
$Na_2HPO_4 \cdot 2H_2O$ . . . . . . . . . . . . .2.0%
Lipositol, or purified lecithin . . . . .1.0–2.0%
Gum acacia . . . . . . . . . . . . . . . . . . .3.0%
Distilled $H_2O$ to volume of 100 ml . . . . . . . .
Sulfathalidine, sulfasuxidine,
    or streptomycin . . . . . . . . . . . . . .0.03%

---

[7] P. H. Phillips and R. R. Spitzer. 1946. A synthetic pablum for the preservation of bull semen. J. Dairy Sci. 29:407.

In this formula, glucose can be used as the only sugar, but frequently the results are improved by the addition of traces of galactose. Lipositol (made after the method of Wooley[8]) or highly purified soybean lecithin can be used as the source of the lipid. Such preparation should be freshly made or have been stored under conditions that prevent deterioration. An initial pH of 6.9 with this mixture seems to be optimum.

Field tests with similarly compounded extenders that contained glucose-galactose, lipid, gum acacia, and buffer gave results comparable to yolk-buffered semen.

## PROCEDURE

### Extension and Cooling of Semen

Following collection, semen is properly identified, labeled, and placed in the laboratory for initial evaluation and subsequent extension and cooling. Typically, the collection tube of semen is held in a dry-block or water bath at 90° to 95°F (32° to 35°C). Quantitative and qualitative measurements are made, and appropriate quantities of antibiotics are added to the semen. Then, after allowing the necessary time for antibiotics to be in contact with the neat semen (three to five minutes), the sample can be initially extended and cooling begun.

Individual or combined ejaculates can be partially extended and gradually cooled to 41°F (5°C) over a period of time (two to three hours). Generally, a 1:1 up to a 1:4 extension of the semen is made with the non-glycerol fraction of extender (containing appropriate antibiotics) at the same temperature as the semen. The ratio used is often determined by the sperm concentration of neat semen. Alternatively, a standardized volume of extender can be used for each ejaculate or collection.

---

[8] D. W. Wooley. 1943. Isolation and partial determination of structure of soybean lipositol, a new inositol-containing phospholipid. J. Biol. Chem. 147:581.

Semen must be held in contact with the non-glycerol extender for a minimum of two hours prior to the addition of any glycerol-containing extender (see Appendix 1 of CSS Minimum Requirements—Exercise 24). The tube, flask, or plastic bag of partially extended semen is placed in an individual water bath (e.g., beaker) containing a standard volume of 90° to 95°F (32° to 35°C) water and then set in the coldroom or refrigerator (41°F [5°C]). Controlled cooling can also be achieved in an air flow cabinet. The purpose of only partially extending the semen initially is to avoid having to cool down large volumes that would require longer cooling times.

Following cooling of the partially extended semen, the remainder of the non-glycerol fraction of extender is added, followed by the glycerol-containing fraction. If individual ejaculates were cooled, they will be combined before the addition of the glycerol fraction extender. The glycerol fraction is added to the non-glycerol fraction of extender plus semen at a 1:1 ratio. These fractions of extender are added in the coldroom at a temperature of about 41°F (5°C). The glycerol fraction is usually added in incremental steps or by slow dripping to avoid osmotic shock. After the semen is fully extended it is packaged into straws for subsequent freezing and distribution.

*Note*: One-step semen extenders are not fractionated into non-glycerol and glycerol components. Rather, the complete extender contains the total percentage of glycerol (e.g., 7%) [See Appendix 1 of CSS Minimum Requirements—Exercise 24 for information on a one-step extender acceptable to CSS].

Generally, semen is collected from the bulls in the morning hours (6:00 AM to noon), and it is frozen by the end of the work day (late afternoon). However, some organizations do not begin freezing until late evening or the next morning.

During extension and cooling, great care is exercised to insure that any semen misidentification is avoided. Each container of

## SEMEN EXTENSION WORKSHEET

Date_____

Collection Code_____

| BULL CODE | EJACULATE VOLUME | INITIAL EXTENSION VOLUME | TIME IN RACK | COOL DOWN TO 41°F (5°C) COMPLETED (TIME) | REMAINING A FRACTION | INCREMENTS OF B FRACTION | | | | CALCULATED STRAWS | ACTUAL STRAWS | REMARKS |
|---|---|---|---|---|---|---|---|---|---|---|---|---|
| | | | | | | 20% | 30% | 50% | TOTAL | | | |
| | 1. | | | | | | | | | | | |
| | 2. | | | | | | | | | | | |
| | 3. | | | | | | | | | | | |
| | 1. | | | | | | | | | | | |
| | 2. | | | | | | | | | | | |
| | 3. | | | | | | | | | | | |
| | 1. | | | | | | | | | | | |
| | 2. | | | | | | | | | | | |
| | 3. | | | | | | | | | | | |
| | 1. | | | | | | | | | | | |
| | 2. | | | | | | | | | | | |
| | 3. | | | | | | | | | | | |
| | 1. | | | | | | | | | | | |
| | 2. | | | | | | | | | | | |
| | 3. | | | | | | | | | | | |
| | 1. | | | | | | | | | | | |
| | 2. | | | | | | | | | | | |
| | 3. | | | | | | | | | | | |
| | 1. | | | | | | | | | | | |
| | 2. | | | | | | | | | | | |
| | 3. | | | | | | | | | | | |
| | 1. | | | | | | | | | | | |
| | 2. | | | | | | | | | | | |
| | 3. | | | | | | | | | | | |

**Figure 13.4.** Worksheet used in AI laboratory coldroom for monitoring semen extension procedures.

semen is accurately labeled and must match the appropriate volume(s) or weight(s) according to the semen-processing calculations. A coldroom worksheet is used to record and monitor the semen extension operations (Figure 13.4).

## Determination of Extension Rate

The object of extending semen is to maximize the number of females that can be in-seminated to a collection of semen while maintaining satisfactory fertility. Obviously, the number of viable sperm per milliliter collected and the inherent fertility of the semen are important factors influencing the semen extension rate. It has also been postulated that individual bulls differ in the threshold number of sperm needed to reach their maximum fertility. In other words, their fertility level apparently cannot be improved by increasing sperm number above their optimal threshold number.

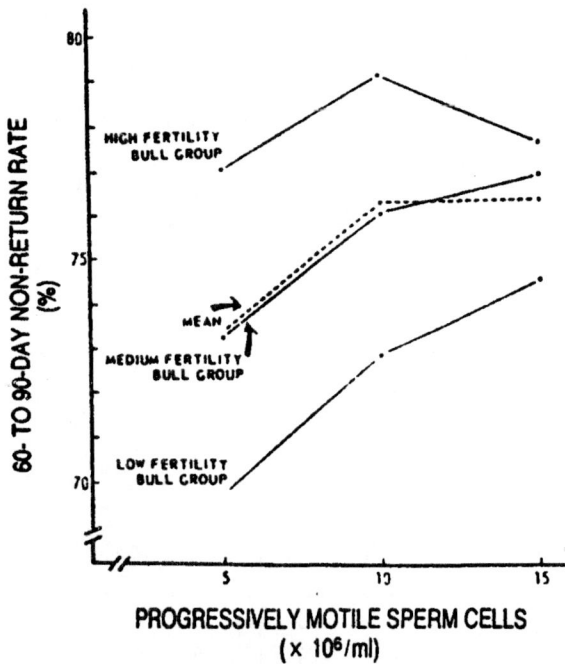

**Figure 13.5.** Non-return rate as affected by motile sperm concentration and fertility level of Holstein bulls. (J. J. Sullivan. 1970. Sperm numbers required for optimum breeding efficiency. Proc. 3rd Tech. Conf. on Artificial Insemination and Reproduction. NAAB. p. 36)

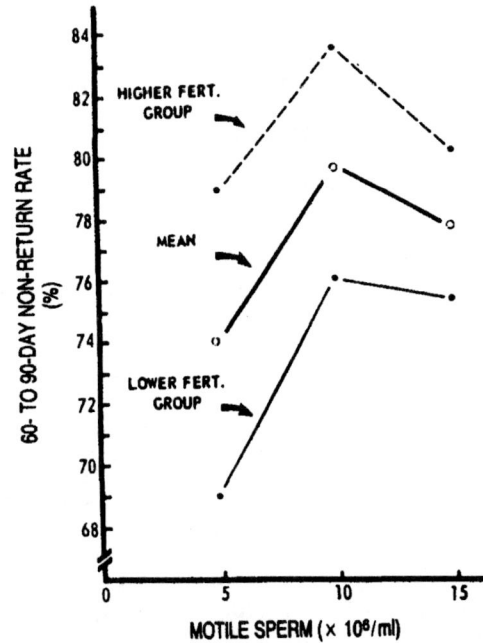

**Figure 13.6.** Non-return rate of dairy cows as affected by motile sperm concentration and fertility level of semen from Angus and Hereford bulls. (J. J. Sullivan. 1970. Sperm numbers required for optimum breeding efficiency. Proc. 3rd Tech. Conf. on Artificial Insemination and Reproduction. NAAB. p. 36)

This concept was supported in a study by Sullivan[9] in which frozen semen was used to inseminate 57,130 cows to Holstein bulls. The 60- to 90-day non-return rate (NR) was significantly lower for insemination doses of 5 million (see Figure 13.5 and 13.6).

Although no industry standards exist for numbers of sperm per insemination dose, each AI organization should determine optimum numbers required for bulls under its own conditions of semen processing and storage. In general, satisfactory results have been achieved when liquid semen contains between 5 and 10 million viable sperm per breeding unit (straw). In the case of frozen semen, it is estimated that from 10 to 40 percent of the sperm may be damaged by the freeze–thaw process; therefore,

considerably more sperm per inseminating unit of semen should be allowed. Many organizations consider about 8 to 12 million viable sperm per breeding unit (straw) to be a minimum level. However, it is well known in the AI industry that some individual bulls can achieve "normal" fertility at lower viable sperm numbers per unit. A knowledge of the fertility level of each bull and of the number of sperm that survive during freezing for each bull is essential. Based on these characteristics it may require 20 to 30 million sperm per unit pre-freeze to result in about 8 to 12 million viable sperm post-thaw. For those bulls below average in fertility, it is advisable to have a higher concentration of viable sperm post-thaw per breeding unit.

A sample semen extension calculation (for frozen semen) follows:

**Background—** Based on fertility history, freezing characteristics, and post-thaw

---

[9] J. J. Sullivan. 1970. Sperm numbers required for optimum breeding efficiency. Proc. 3rd Tech. Conf. on Artificial Insemination and Reproduction. NAAB. p. 36.

recovery, the semen laboratory has determined that this particular bull's semen should be extended to 20 million total sperm per breeding unit (0.5 ml straw).

### Ejaculate Characteristics

Volume: 7 ml
Concentration: 1.6 billion sperm per ml
Total sperm per ejaculate: 11.2 billion
Total sperm per breeding unit desired: 20 million

Theoretically, 560 breeding units (11.2 billion sperm divided by 20 million sperm per unit) could be produced from this ejaculate. However, not all of the sperm cells are recoverable, as there are losses on the surfaces of the semen-processing equipment and in the cotton/powder plug of the semen straws. About 10 percent of the sperm are lost, and consequently semen laboratories must account for such losses in their calculations. Therefore, in this particular example, 504 straws (560 straws minus 10 percent loss) are calculated.

In this case the semen is partially extended (4:1) with the non-glycerol extender (A fraction) as follows:

| | |
|---|---|
| 7 ml | semen |
| 28 ml | non-glycerol extender (A fraction) |
| 35 ml | semen and initial A fraction extender |

After cooling to 41°F (5°C) over a two- to three-hour period, the remaining A fraction extender is added:

| | |
|---|---|
| 35 ml | semen and initial A fraction extender |
| 105 ml | remaining A fraction extender |
| 140 ml | semen and total A fraction extender |

An equal volume of glycerol-containing extender (B fraction) is added incrementally in the coldroom over a 30-minute period. This results in a total extended semen volume of 280 ml:

| | |
|---|---|
| 140 ml | semen and total A fraction extender |
| 140 ml | total B fraction extender |
| 280 ml | semen and total A fraction extender, plus total B fraction extender |

The fully extended semen is then loaded into 0.5-ml straws by vacuum, and after an appropriate equilibration period, straws of semen are frozen in liquid nitrogen vapor and stored in liquid nitrogen. In this particular example, the original 7 ml of semen is extended 40 times (40×) on a total volume basis, resulting in 504 breeding units.

*Note:* Because extended semen is drawn into the straw plug during the filling process, it actually requires more than 0.5 ml of extended semen to fill the straw (e.g., an average of 0.555 ml per straw, depending upon filling machine vacuum setting).

Generally, semen laboratories will allow a certain deviation in numbers of straws produced from an ejaculate (i.e., number of straws calculated, plus or minus 5 to 10 straws). If the deviation is greater than this number, an investigation will be made to determine the reason for any discrepancy. If a discrepancy cannot be resolved, the semen in question is discarded.

Semen extension calculations can be easily programmed into a laboratory programmable calculator or personal computer.

## Antibiotics

In commercial AI centers, strict health programs and hygienic housing and semen collection conditions have vastly reduced the potential for disease transmission through bull semen. As discussed in Exercise 24, Certified Semen Services, Inc., provides a comprehensive program that outlines *minimum* health requirements for bulls producing semen for artificial insemination. In this program, AI center bulls and mount animals are continuously monitored for tuberculosis, brucellosis, leptospirosis, persistent BVD infection, trichomoniasis, and campylobacteriosis (vibriosis). Maintaining healthy, disease-free bulls in a risk-reduced environment can be considered as a "first line" of defense against disease transmission through semen. Also, however, the CSS-required incorporation of antibiotics into neat semen and semen extender provides additional security through the effective microbiological control of specific pathogenic organisms of concern that potentially could be present.

In the early development of commercial artificial insemination, semen primarily was stored and distributed at 41°F (5°C) or warmer as liquid semen. It was necessary to identify compounds that would control bacteria in the nutrient-rich semen extender but not harm the fertility of the sperm cells. Many antibacterial compounds, such as sulfanilamide, penicillin, and streptomycin have been used with varied success (see Foote, 1976; Foote, 1978 for reviews). Early results with antibiotics generally demonstrated an improvement in non-return rate or fertility. This was believed to be due to control of organisms such as *Campylobacter fetus* (vibrio).

In 1961, Elliott, et al.,[10] demonstrated that *Campylobacter fetus* in bull semen was not being adequately controlled by the levels of penicillin and streptomycin routinely used in semen processed for freezing. Sullivan, et al.,[11] later

showed that polymyxin B sulfate with dihydrostreptomycin and penicillin controlled *Campylobacter fetus*, particularly when neat semen was treated with antibiotics followed by extension with semen extender containing antibiotics. Hamdy and Miller[12] and Hamdy[13] provided evidence that lincomycin and spectinomycin also provided control against *Campylobacter fetus* as well as mycoplasmas. In 1979, CSS adopted the use of penicillin, dihydro-streptomycin, and polymyxin B sulfate as the minimum requirement for use during semen cryopreservation. The addition of antibiotics to neat semen and extender was included in these requirements. Some organizations also included the use of lincomycin and spectinomycin.

Because of evidence that ureaplasmas and mycoplasmas could be isolated from bovine semen and because some associations between these types of organisms and infertility were being claimed, NAAB and its member organizations conducted research from 1983 to 1986 to evaluate newer antibiotics for the control of mycoplasmas, ureaplasmas, *Haemophilus sommnus,* and *Campylobacter fetus* subsp. *venerealis* in cryopreserved bovine semen. Effective control of these organisms was demonstrated using a combination of gentamicin, tylosin, lincomycin, and spectinomycin (GTLS) when added during processing for cryopreservation to the neat semen and in the nonglycerol fraction of extenders. In addition, concurrent studies demonstrated that this combination of antibiotics was not detrimental to semen quality and had no significant effects on fertility (non-return rate). Consequently, in 1988, CSS revised its minimum health requirements to include the new GTLS antibiotic

[10] F. I. Elliott, D. M. Murphy, and D. E. Bartlett. 1961. The use of polymyxin B sulfate with dihydrostreptomycin and penicillin for the control of *vibrio fetus* in a frozen semen process. Proc. 4th International Congr. Animal Reproduction. (The Hague). p. 539.
[11] J. J. Sullivan, et al. 1966. Further studies on the use of polymyxin B sulfate with dihydrostreptomycin and penicillin for control of vibrio fetus in a frozen semen process. J. Dairy Sci. 49:1569.

[12] A. H. Hamdy and C. C. Miller. 1971. Antibiotics for bovine mycoplasmas. J. Dairy Sci. 54:1541.
[13] A. H. Hamdy. 1972. Linco-spectin as a bovine semen additive. Proc. 4th Tech. Conf. on Artificial Insemination and Reproduction. NAAB. p. 54.

combination (see Appendix 1 of CSS Minimum Requirements—Exercise 24). In the above research, CSS antibiotic efficacy was demonstrated in five specific extenders. These are listed as tested and approved extenders in the CSS Minimum Requirements. Other semen extender formulations could possibly alter the efficacy of CSS antibiotics. Therefore, any deviation from tested and approved extenders needs to be evaluated by CSS to determine whether efficacy testing is required.

Additional research conducted by Kim and Shin[14] has also demonstrated that the GTLS antibiotic combination, in conjunction with the effects of glycerol concentration and freezing/thawing, results in complete control of the five species of Leptospiras that are important in North America.

## Color Coding

Although the information that is printed on the straw is what is most important for identification purposes, several organizations also utilize color coding of extended semen or straws mainly to differentiate particular breeds. This is useful information for field recognition of breeds by AI technicians within an organization. Colors for the major dairy breeds were originally recommended by the Purebred Dairy Cattle Association (PDCA) and later adopted by NAAB and the National DHI program. These colors are fairly uniform among the organizations that use color coding; however, the shade of a particular color may vary. Commonly used dairy semen color codes are: Ayrshire—purple; Brown Swiss—brown; Guernsey—yellow; Holstein—green; Jersey—red. Some of the certified food and vegetable dyes have been sat-

isfactory for coloring extended semen with no apparent detrimental effects. In pure dye percentages, the following give adequate coloring to extended dairy semen: purple grape shade, 4.1 percent; brown, 3.7 percent; emerald green, 2.7 percent; and strawberry red shade, 5.2 percent. One drop of dye to 10 ml of extended semen is usually employed.

*Note:* Uncolored egg yolk extender has been used for Guernsey semen. Alternatively, colored semen straws (about 20 different colors) are commercially available from AI equipment suppliers and may be used for appropriate color coding.

Color codes for the beef breeds are much less uniform across organizations.

Identification tabs on the top of the canes (racks) that hold the semen straws in storage are also frequently color coded as to the breed or progeny-proving status. This facilitates quick identification of semen in storage and in the field. Numerous combinations of background and print colors are possible. Again, these systems are useful within a particular organization and are not uniform across organizations.

Color coding is primarily a convenience for use within an AI organization. It should also be emphasized here that the identification information printed on the package (straw) is the only way to accurately and positively identify the sire.

## Storage of Semen at Ambient Temperature

Before the introduction of frozen semen, and particularly liquid nitrogen as a refrigerant (see Exercise 14), many efforts were made to develop methods that maintained the fertility of bull semen at ambient (room) temperature. Even though the transportation and equipment making frozen semen a practical reality are now readily available throughout most of the world, there are some countries and circumstances where ambient temperature stor-

---

[14] S. G. Kim and S. J. Shin. 2001. Glycerol and GTLS effect leptospira species in bovine semen. Proc. 18th Tech. Conf. on Artificial Insemination and Reproduction. NAAB. p. 63.

age is useful and desirable. For example, in New Zealand liquid semen is used extensively to inseminate a high percentage of the cow population during a short breeding season.

The storage of semen at ambient temperature requires a satisfactory nutrient media and the control of bacterial growth. Various combinations of the antibiotics sulfanilamide, penicillin, streptomycin, and polymyxin were shown to be effective in controlling bacterial growth in bull semen extended with yolk-citrate and other extenders[15] and stored at 77°F (25°C).

In 1957 the Illinois Agricultural Experiment workers developed an ambient temperature extender known as IVT by gassing the extended semen with $CO_2$ and sealing the storage vial to preserve the proper $CO_2$ levels. Using the IVT method, semen stored for seven days at ambient temperature resulted in a fertility rate comparable to that of semen stored at a lower temperature. However, the IVT method has not been extensively used for bull semen.

The CUE, a somewhat related extender containing glycine, that does not require gassing with $CO_2$, has given good sperm survival at 77° F (25° C). The presence of glycine, it is reported, promotes the formation of $CO_2$ as a result of sperm metabolism.

Coconut milk extender has also been used as a medium for preserving sperm fertility at ambient temperatures. The coconut milk is boiled for 10 minutes and filtered before use. The formula for the complete extender follows:

### Coconut Milk Extender

| | |
|---|---|
| Coconut milk | 15 ml |
| Sodium citrate dihydrate | 2.2 g |
| Sulfanilamide | 0.3 g |
| Egg yolk | 5 ml |
| Distilled water to make | 100-ml |

---

[15] R. H. Foote and R. W. Bratton. 1950. Motility of bovine spermatozoa and control of bacteria at 5E and 25EC in extenders containing sulfanilamide, penicillin, streptomycin, and polymyxin. J. Dairy Sci. 33:842.

Included in the coconut milk extender (CME) are 135 mg dihydrostreptomycin, 10 mg polymyxin B sulfate, 1,000 units nystatin, and 15,000 units of sterile catalase per 100 ml.

CME-processed semen has given conception rates of 55 to 72 percent after one to five days of storage at ambient temperature. Fertility generally drops greatly after the fourth day of storage.

**Caprogen Extender**— The greatest use of semen stored at ambient temperature is made in New Zealand. Liquid semen is used to inseminate a high proportion of the cattle in the AI program because the main breeding season is short. Of approximately 3 million inseminations annually, the vast majority occur from mid-September until December. Every effort is made to take advantage of the lush grazing season during the spring months.

The New Zealand workers have developed an ambient temperature storage extender by gassing the citrate-buffered egg yolk extender with nitrogen and adding caproic acid. The extender is known as caprogen (see Foote, 1978). The general formula is:

| | |
|---|---|
| Sodium citrate dihydrate | 2.0% |
| Glucose | 0.3% |
| Glycine | 1.0% |
| Glycerol | 1.25% |
| Caproic acid | 0.03125% |
| Sulfacetamide | 0.01% |
| Sufficient double distilled water to make | 100 ml |

Egg yolk, penicillin, and streptomycin are added to the extender before use. Twenty percent egg yolk is used for the premix of semen and extender, but in the final dilution only 5 percent egg yolk is used. The New Zealand workers generally extend semen to 2 million sperm per dose, and 0.5 ml is generally used per insemination. However, the use of semen packaged in 0.25-ml straws (known as "long last liquid") is gaining in popularity. Extended semen can be used over a three-day period. Catalase, at the rate of 20 μg per milliliter of extender, has been found to increase conception rate about 1 to 2 percent and is routinely used in New Zealand. The catalase decomposes the $H_2O_2$ that is formed as a result of sperm cell metabolism.

Caprogen can also be used as a liquid extender for frozen semen. The frozen semen is thawed, mixed with caprogen extender, and used at ambient temperatures. The New Zealand AI centers freeze extended semen in "blood bags" from top bulls when the demand is low, then thaw and redilute it in the ambient temperature extender for use during the peak breeding season. It is used for one to two days with good results.

The optimum temperature range for caprogen-extended semen is 65° to 75°F (18° to 24°C).

By using liquid semen in the caprogen extender, the New Zealand AI centers inseminate many thousands of cows per sire in full use. In 1991, a well-known Holstein sire, Crocketts Trevor, was credited with over 380,000 services during the three-month breeding season.[16]

---

[16] B. Gobin. 1992. Antipodean genetics. Typex (No. 34, October). p. 59.

## QUESTIONS

1. What is the purpose of extending semen?

2. What are the basic requirements for a satisfactory semen extender?

3. How do sperm viability examinations compare for extended and neat semen?

4. What is osmotic pressure, and why is it of importance in extenders?

5. What is an isotonic solution, and how is this characteristic of importance in extenders?

6. What precautions are followed in cooling semen from the time of collection to final extension?

7. What is the purpose of egg yolk, glycerol, sugar, and various salts in a semen extender?

8. Name two basic semen extenders or diluents.

9. If a sample of semen, 8 ml in volume, had an estimated 1.5 billion sperm per milliliter and good viability, how much could it be extended so as to provide 20 million sperm per breeding unit for insemination?

10. Where might semen preserved at ambient temperature be useful? What are two extenders used for semen at ambient temperature?

11. What is a typical number of sperm per unit of semen (straw) used for one insemination? What factors determine the semen extension rate?

12. What is the purpose of antibiotics in semen extenders? What antibiotics are used and in what levels per milliliter of extended semen?

13. Why is extended semen colored or packaged in colored straws? What colors are commonly used for the major dairy breeds?

# REFERENCES

Foote, R. H. 1976. Antibacterial agents for bull semen: Do they help? Proc. 6th Tech. Conf. on Artificial Insemination and Reproduction. NAAB. p. 23.

Foote, R. H. 1978. Extenders and extension of unfrozen semen. In: G. W. Salisbury, N. L. Van Demark, and J. R. Lodge (Eds.). Physiology of Reproduction and Artificial Insemination of Cattle (2nd Ed.). p. 442. W. H. Freeman, San Francisco.

Hafez, E. S. E. (Ed.). 1987. Reproduction in Farm Animals (5th Ed.). Lea & Febiger, Philadelphia. (Ch. 28.)

Lorton, S. P. 1992. Antibiotic combinations for frozen bovine semen: Efficacy and extender interactions. International Workshop on Veterinary Constraints for the Exchange of Bovine Semen (The Hague). August. p. 29.

Marshall, C. E. 1986. Bulls and processing procedures. Proc. Ann. Conf. on Artificial Insemination and Embryo Transfer in Beef Cattle. NAAB. p. 5.

Maule, J. P. 1962. The Semen of Animals and Artificial Insemination. Commonwealth Agr. Bureau, Farnham Royal, Bucks, England. (Chs. 6, 7, 8.)

Mitchell, J. R., and P. L. Senger. 1982. Temperature measurement for the AI laboratory: Theory, devices and applications. Proc. 9th Tech. Conf. on Artificial Insemination and Reproduction. NAAB. p. 22.

Sorenson, A. M., Jr. 1979. Animal Reproduction: Principles and Practices. McGraw-Hill, New York. (Chs. 5, 6.)

# SOURCES OF COMMERCIAL SEMEN EXTENDERS

Continental Plastic Corp.
*http://www.continentalplastic.com/*

IMV International Corp.
*http://www.imvusa.com/*

Minitube of America
*http://www.minitube.com/main.html*

Viam Pac Inc.
1026 280th St.
Glenwood City, WI 54013
email: hgraham@baldwin-telecom.net

# EXERCISE 14

# Frozen Semen; Cryogenic Storage;
# Transportation; Handling

## OBJECT

To become familiar with the processing and use of frozen semen, cryogenic storage methods, transportation, and semen handling.

## DISCUSSION

Frozen semen refers to semen that has been processed with a cryoprotective agent in the extender and is cooled to and stored at very low temperatures. Liquid nitrogen (LN) is the most commonly used refrigerant for the storage of frozen semen at $-320°F$ ($-196°C$). In the early days of AI (1951 to 1956), dry ice and alcohol and mechanical refrigeration were used for frozen semen. These systems were capable of producing and maintaining a temperature of about $-110°F$ ($-79°C$). Liquid nitrogen however, has simplified the entire frozen semen process, because it is stable, it is nonexplosive, and storage containers, depending upon type, need to be replenished with the refrigerant only every 6 to 30 weeks. Worldwide shipping of frozen semen stored in LN containers is routine. Liquid air has also been employed as a refrigerant for frozen semen in some parts of the world. However, since it may permit oxygen build-up and become explosive, the use of liquid air has been quite limited.

Some of the main advantages of frozen semen are:

1. With frozen semen, selective mating is possible. A cattle breeder can use the sire of choice at any time.

2. Frozen semen is valuable in extending the influence of sires over a long period of time. Semen stored in the frozen state for 10 to 25 years has produced living calves. However, since genetic progress in AI occurs at a rapid rate, it is more desirable to utilize newer proven sires that represent continuous genetic advancement. Nevertheless, the storage of frozen semen as a repository of genetic lineages for DNA (genomic) research may be quite valuable.

3. Frozen semen permits almost total utilization of the semen. No frozen semen need be discarded because of age, as was true with liquid semen.

4. Costs of transporting semen from the AI center to area technicians are greatly reduced. Instead of daily or every-other-day shipments, as was the case with liquid semen, a technician may have a supply of semen from selected bulls replenished every few weeks.

5. Dairy and beef cattle breeders can maintain a supply of frozen semen on their own premises and inseminate cows to selected bulls as a part of routine herd management.

6. Selected matings to sires in widely located areas (anywhere in the world) are possible.

7. A herd owner may have semen from a valuable bull "custom collected," frozen, and stored for use in his or her own herd. Frozen semen also permits joint

use of a partnership bull, even though the owners' herds are hundreds—even thousands—of miles apart.

8. Appropriate quantities of antibiotics incorporated into the neat semen and semen extender, as outlined in the CSS Minimum Requirements (Exercise 24), provide for control of potential pathogenic microorganisms in frozen semen.

## Equipment for Processing Frozen Semen

In addition to the laboratory containers and equipment for the extension and cooling of semen (described in Exercise 13), a semen package labeling machine, a semen package filling and sealing machine, an LN freezing tank, temperature-monitoring/recording instrumentation, and LN storage refrigerators are items needed in a frozen semen operation. There are LN refrigerators with a capacity for holding a few hundred semen units for field use by inseminators or storage in breeders' herds, as well as larger refrigerators that hold 100,000 or more breeding units for central storage and distribution purposes. The processing of frozen semen is well mechanized in modern AI centers. Figures 14.4 and 14.7 depict examples of equipment frequently utilized by AI organizations. The names of various North American manufacturers/suppliers of AI equipment can be found in Appendix C.

## Semen Packaging

Plastic straws have become the predominant package for processing frozen bull semen throughout the world. Since their commercial introduction in the late 1960's, straws of various size configuration have been employed, with a continuing trend toward the use of lower semen volumes (Rajamannan, 1970; Pickett and Berndtson, 1978; Pickett, et al., 1978; Cassou, 1983; Kroetsch, 1992). Currently, the 0.5-ml straw is the most commonly-used semen package in the United States, while the 0.25-ml straw is used more frequently in several other countries. It is likely that the 0.25 ml straw will become more prominent in the United States in the future. Before the conversion to the use of plastic straws, semen was frozen exclusively in glass ampules of various size (0.5 to 1.2 ml). However, the AI industry gradually changed to straws because of several important advantages: (1) Less storage space is required for straws. (2) There is minimal loss of sperm cells during the insemination process with the straw system compared to ampules. (3) Automated systems for the labeling as well as the filling and sealing of straws are very efficient. (4) The geometry of the straw (i.e., greater surface area to volume ratio) provides for a faster rate of heat transfer, thus allowing for more uniform freezing and rapid thawing, which is advantageous from the standpoint of semen quality. After the freezing process, straws of semen can be held at $-320°F$ $(-196°C)$ in bulk fashion for central storage or in small goblets configured with metal canes or racks containing identification tabs for field distribution (Figure 14.1).

Other well-known methods have included the freezing of semen in pellets and the packaging and freezing of semen in artificial insemination pipets. Frozen semen in pellets has a definite storage efficiency, but identification of individual pellets has not been very successful, and there is also a possibility of pellet contamination (or cross-contamination). Use of pelleted bull semen has not been widely accepted in North America or in Western Europe. Semen frozen in the insemination pipet has been used with varied success in the United States. This method was convenient for the user since it eliminated the loading of

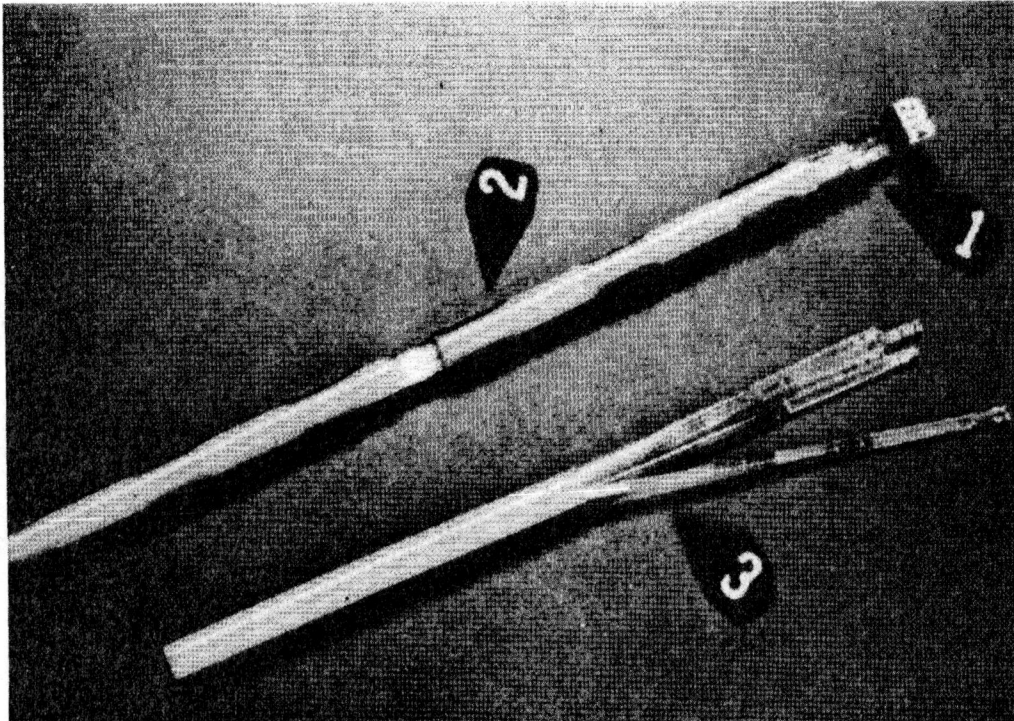

**Figure 14.1.** Straws of frozen semen (3) are typically placed in small plastic goblets (2) that are clipped to metal canes or racks (1) for cryogenic storage.

the insemination equipment. Identification was printed directly on the insemination pipet. However, a major disadvantage of this method was storage inefficiency.

## Extenders for Frozen Semen

The preparation of semen extenders and the extension of semen are outlined in Exercise 13. As indicated, egg yolk–citrate, milk, and egg yolk–tris are the most popular semen extenders in North America. AI organizations often conduct in-house research to identify optimum levels of various extender components for use with their particular processing and semen-freezing methods. This is because research has demonstrated that extender composition can interact with other variables, such as the freezing method and the individual bull, affecting the overall semen quality.

## Procedures for Freezing Semen

With the accidental discovery[1] that glycerol provided protection for sperm cells cooled to very low temperatures (Polge and co-workers in Cambridge, England, 1950), the commercial freezing of bull semen became a distinct possibility. Subsequently, several AI organizations undertook investigations into various methods of freezing semen and the development of equipment for the storage and handling of frozen semen. Eventually there was virtually a total conversion to the use of frozen semen with glycerol as a cryoprotectant.

A method of freezing semen as adapted by British workers was described by Polge.[2] Over

---

[1] C. Polge. 1968. Frozen semen and the AI programme in Great Britain. Proc. 2nd Tech. Conf. on Artificial Insemination and Reproduction. NAAB. p. 46.
[2] Ibid.

125

the years there have been many modifications as technologies have improved. In North America it is fairly common to process bull semen for freezing by using the following general steps:

1. Immediately after collection, transport the properly identified semen to the laboratory, make quantitative/qualitative measurements, add appropriate antibiotics, and allow necessary time for the antibiotics to be in contact with the neat semen before extension. (*Note:* From the time of collection, semen must be protected thermally to avoid cold shock.)

2. Add the initial increment of 90° to 95°F (32° to 35°C) non-glycerol extender. (The ratio of extender to semen may vary with the sperm concentration, or a standard volume of extender may be used.) Slowly cool

to 41°F (5°C). The partially extended semen is cooled in a refrigerator, cold cabinet, or coldroom (a minimum of two hours suggested). The non-glycerol fraction of extender also contains antibiotics.

3. Add the remaining non-glycerol fraction of extender at 41°F (5°C).

4. Add the glycerol fraction of extender by slow dripping or in increments (Figure 14.2). The glycerol fraction of extender is added to the non-glycerol fraction of extender plus semen at a 1:1 ratio. The glycerol fraction is added slowly to avoid osmotic shock.

5. Package the fully extended semen into straws that have been properly labeled (see Appendix I) and cooled to 41°F (5°C). See Figures 14.3 and 14.4.

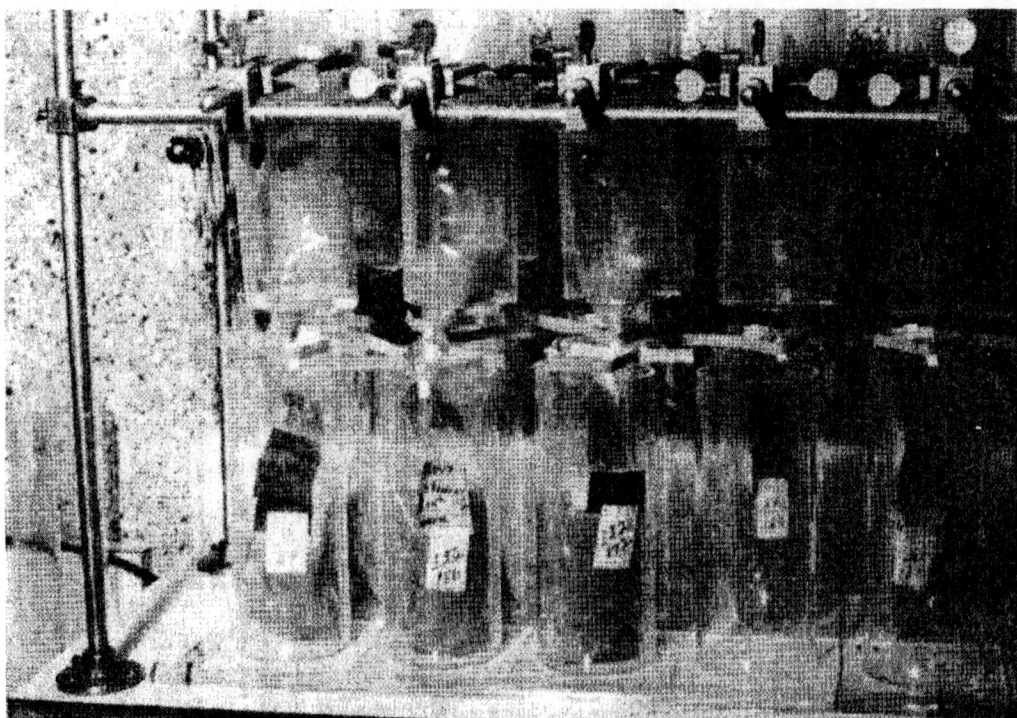

**Figure 14.2.** After the partially extended semen is cooled for at least two hours to about 41° F (5° C), the glycerol fraction of extender is added slowly. (Courtesy, Select Sires, Inc., Plain City, OH)

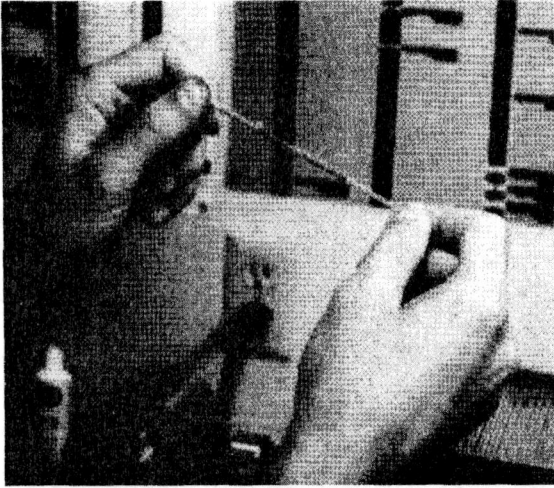

**Figure 14.3.** Identification is printed on straws before they are filled and sealed. Information includes AI center code, breed code, bull's AI center number, registration name and number, and collection code. (Courtesy, Select Sires, Inc., Plain City, OH)

6. Freeze straws of semen after an appropriate "equilibration" period (typically 3 to 6 hours). The equilibration period refers to the time from adding the glycerol fraction of extender until freezing. Changes occurring in the sperm cell membranes during this period increase sperm survival in the freeze-thaw process.

## Freezing

Several methods and freeze rates have been used for satisfactorily freezing the packaged semen. A primary objective of any of these methods is to prevent crystallization of

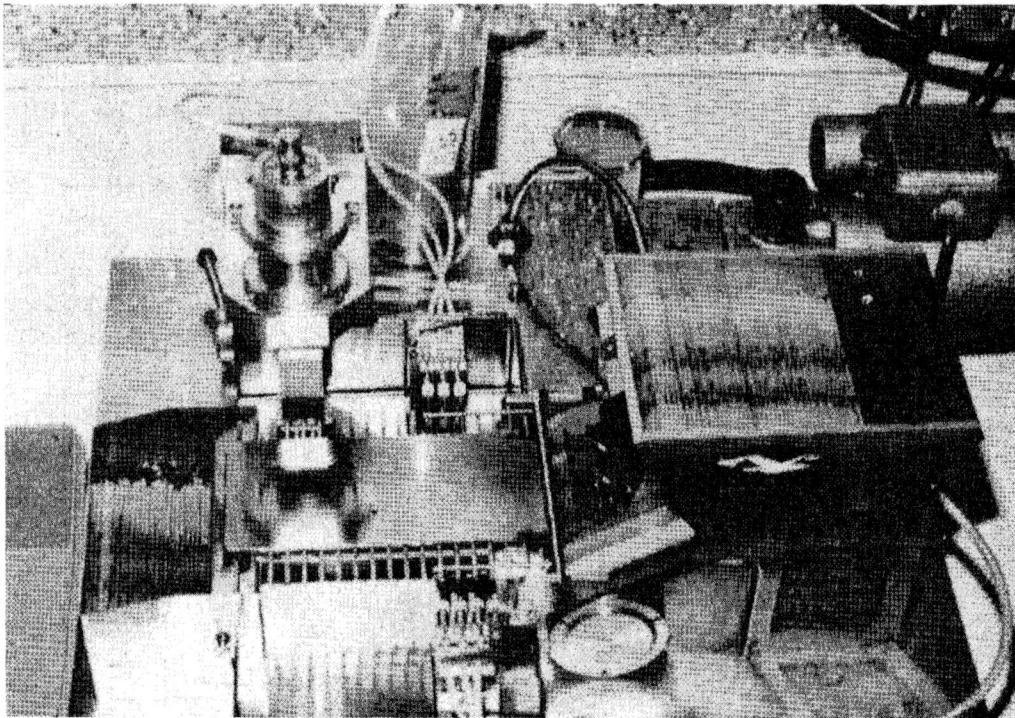

**Figure 14.4.** In the coldroom (41° F [5° C]), labeled straws are automatically filled with extended semen and sonically sealed. (Courtesy, Select Sires, Inc., Plain City, OH)

water within the sperm cells and to freeze rapidly, with glycerol acting as a protective agent.[3]

1. ***Dry ice and alcohol*—** This method was used in the early days of freezing semen. Ampules of semen placed in a bath of alcohol (or acetone) and dry ice were cooled at a rate of about 1.8°F (1°C) per minute from 41°F (5°C) to 5°F (−15 C) and at a rate of about 5°F (−3°C) to 7°F (−4°C) per minute from 5°F (−15°C) to −110°F (−79°C). Cooling rate was controlled by the manual addition of dry ice to the alcohol bath. The ampules of frozen semen were stored in containers of dry ice and alcohol (−110°F [−79°C]) or in electric refrigeration units (−119°F [−84°C]).[4] Although these methods were used successfully for some period of time, they were largely supplanted by other methods after the adoption by the AI industry of liquid nitrogen as a refrigerant. Also, later studies demonstrated that semen stored at dry ice/alcohol temperatures (about − 110° F [− 79° C]) sustained greater deterioration in viability than that stored at cooler LN temperature (− 320° F [− 196° C]).[5]

2. ***Mechanical*—** Automatic temperature controlled LN freezing chambers have been used to freeze both ampules and straws of semen. Liquid nitrogen is introduced by solenoid valve, and cold nitrogen vapor is forced throughout the freezing chamber by use of fans. Freezing rates are programmable. Depending upon chamber configuration, straws may be frozen horizontally on racks or vertically in goblets on metal canes/racks (Figure 14.5). This method allows for many straws of semen to be frozen per batch and can be very labor efficient.[6,7]

3. ***Nitrogen vapor*—** Freezing semen in static or moving vapor above the liquid nitrogen is common for semen packaged in straws. However, it was also shown to be acceptable for freezing semen in ampules.[8] Nitrogen vapor freezing is typically carried out in the upper portion of a large LN refrigerator. Following the required equilibration period in the coldroom, straws of semen are placed on horizontal metal racks (usually 58- or 100-straw capacity) for freezing. Up to five racks of straws (a freeze load) are quickly transferred from the coldroom/cabinet into the vapor portion of a wide-mouthed LN refrigerator. The racks are positioned separately on a screen support so that straws are uniformly about 3 cm above the surface of the liquid nitrogen (Figure 14.6). Freezing is monitored by a thermocouple placed either in the vapor at the level of the straws or in a dummy straw. Depending upon starting vapor

[3] G. L. Rapatz. 1966. What happens when semen is frozen? Proc. 1st Tech. Conf. on Artificial Insemination and Bovine Reproduction. NAAB. p. 45.

[4] H. A. Herman. 1981. Technical developments: Past and future. In: Improving Cattle by the Millions. Ch. 5. Univ. of Missouri Press, Columbia.

[5] B. W. Pickett, A. K. Fowler, and W. A. Cowan. 1960. Effects of continuous and alternating storage temperatures of − 79° and − 196° C on motility of frozen bull semen. J. Dairy Sci. 43:281.

[6] C. H. Allen and J. O. Almquist. 1981. Effect of bulk freezing straws of bovine spermatozoa in a programmed freezer on post thaw survival. J. Anim. Sci. 53:1432.

[7] C. E. Marshall and C. M. Cowan. 1984. Experiences with programmable freezers. Proc. 10th Tech. Conf. on Artificial Insemination and Reproduction. NAAB. p. 47.

[8] E. D. Clegg, B. W. Pickett, and E. W. Gibson. 1965. Non-mechanical Nitrogen Vapor Freezing of Bull Semen. Conn. Ag. Exp. Sta. Rep. No. 5.

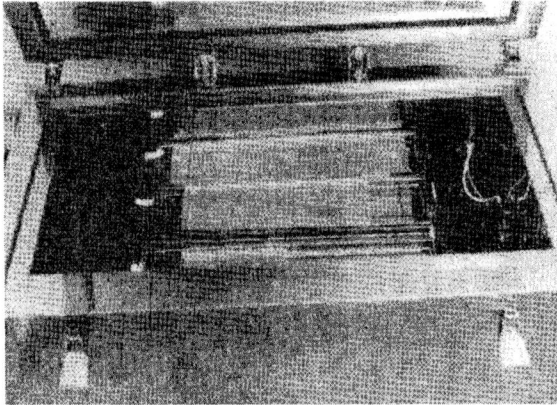

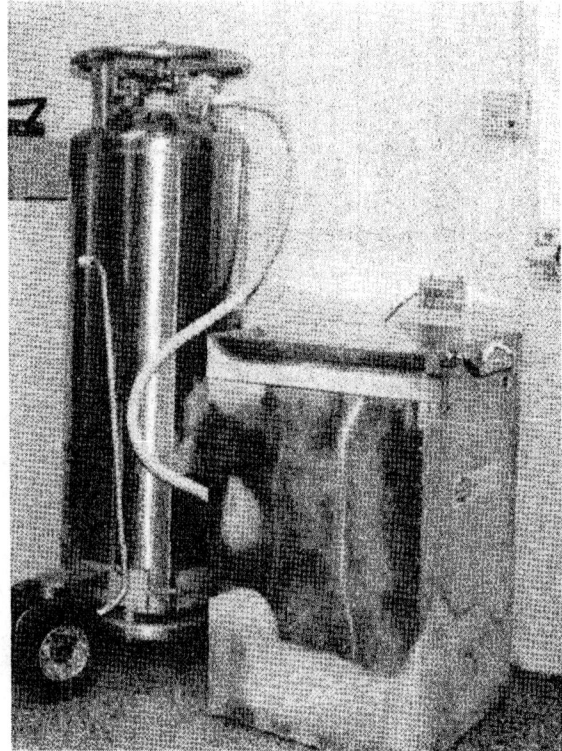

**Figure 14.5.** Automatic mechanical LN freezing chambers for *(top)* horizontal freezing of straws on racks (Courtesy, Accelerated Genetics, Westby, WI) or *(right)* vertical freezing of straws in goblets on canes (Courtesy, the former Atlantic Breeders Coop., Lancaster, PA)

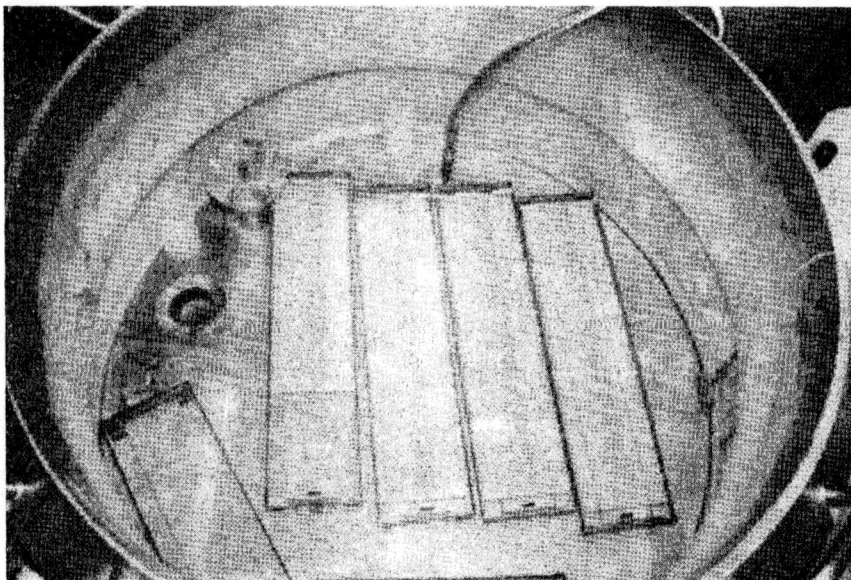

**Figure 14.6.** Freezing semen in static or moving vapor above the liquid nitrogen. Straws are "racked" in the coldroom and quickly transferred into the upper portion of a wide-mouthed LN refrigerator for freezing. After semen reaches −148°F (−100°C), straws are plunged into liquid nitrogen.

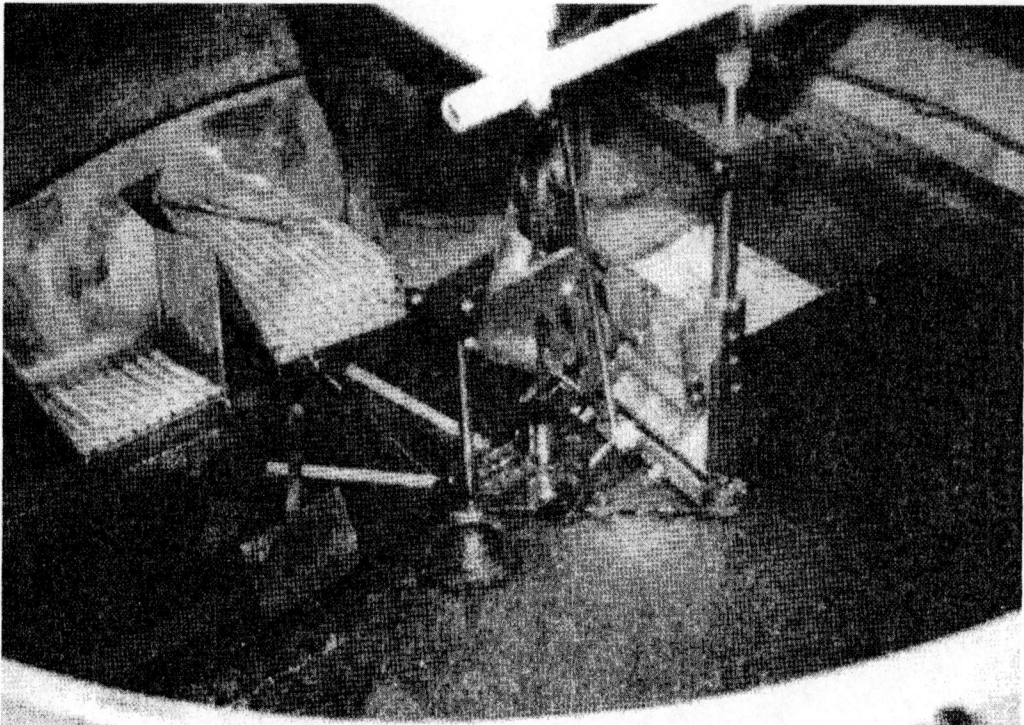

**Figure 14.7.** After freezing and quality control, straws are automatically inserted into small plastic goblets in nitrogen vapor at − 292° F (− 180° C). Filled goblets are then clipped to metal canes/racks.

temperature, refrigerator size, and introduced heat load, the freezing is accomplished in about 7 to 10 minutes. Higher initial vapor temperatures and slower cooling rates have been recommended for 0.25-ml straws compared to those for 0.5-ml straws.[9] Generally, after the frozen semen reaches −148°F (−100°C), the straws are plunged into liquid nitrogen, where they are temporarily held until further evaluation and packing. Various modifications of nitrogen vapor freezing procedures are applied throughout the AI industry.

Individual AI organizations have developed specific freezing techniques and proce-dures to insure a uniform quality product based on the particular characteristics of their extender composition, semen package, and freezing configuration.

## Storage

Frozen semen is stored in liquid nitrogen at −320°F (−196°C) or in LN vapor at about −292°F (−180°C). After the semen has been quality checked, straws may be stored in bulk fashion or may be placed in plastic goblets attached to labeled metal canes/racks for central storage and/or field distribution (Figure 14.7).

A variety of LN refrigerators are available for various storage and shipping purposes (Figures 14.8 and 14.9). If stored and transferred properly, frozen semen can be kept indefinitely without losing its fertilizing capacity. It is important to routinely monitor the LN level and to insure that the refrigerator is filled on a regular basis.

[9] P. L. Senger, J. R. Mitchell, and J. O. Almquist. 1982. Freezing semen in the .25 ml French straw. Proc. 9th Tech. Conf. on Artificial Insemination and Reproduction. NAAB. p. 32.

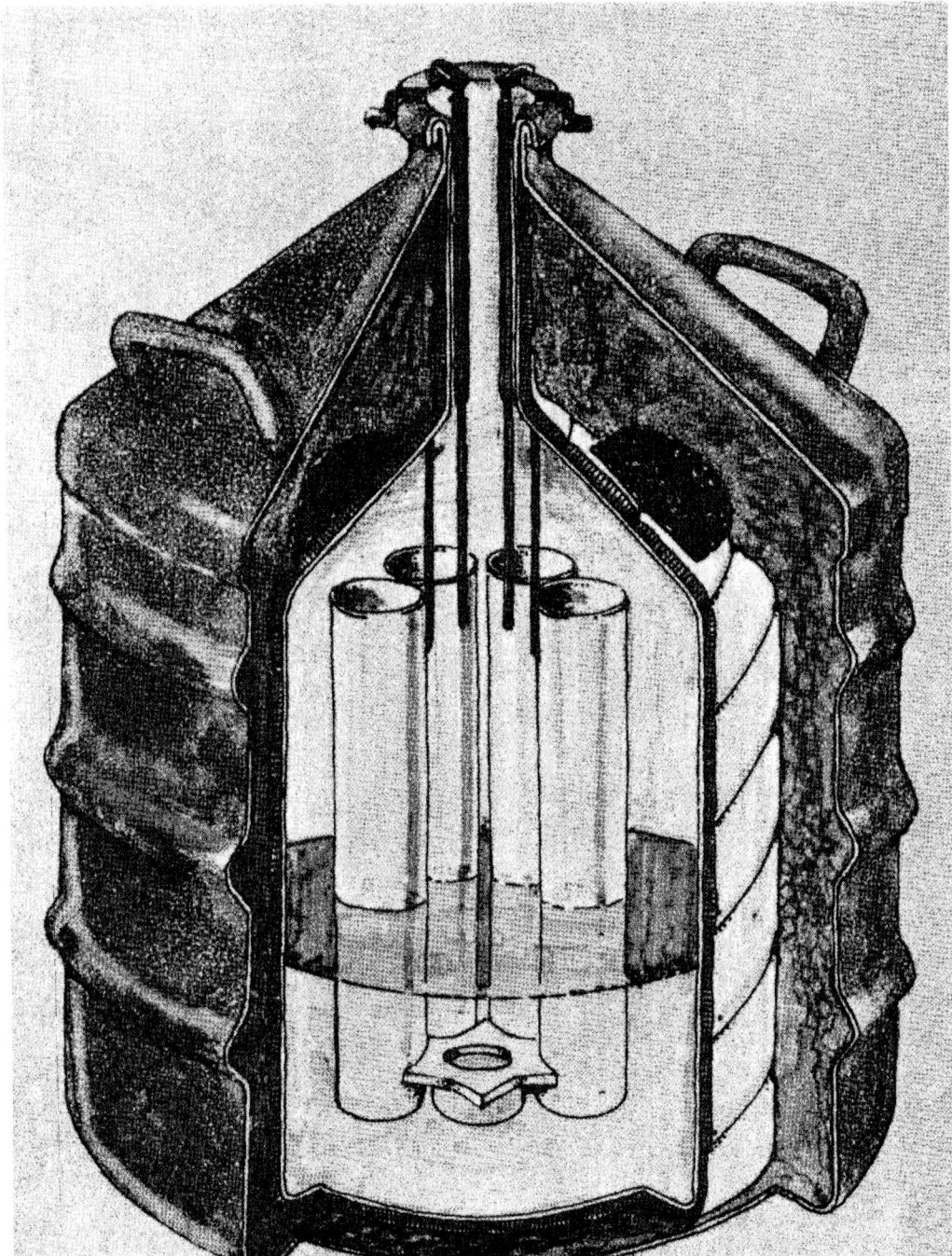

**Figure 14.8.** Liquid nitrogen refrigerator (cutaway section) showing construction and canisters for storing canes/racks of frozen semen. Liquid nitrogen level is shown at bottom of interior of container, and cryogenic vapor surrounding canisters in upper portion. The outer shell and the inner liner of the LN refrigerator are joined only at the neck tube. A vacuum between the inner liner and the outer shell provides proper insulation for maintaining cryogenic conditions. (Courtesy, R. D. Brunt, Union Carbide, Indianapolis)

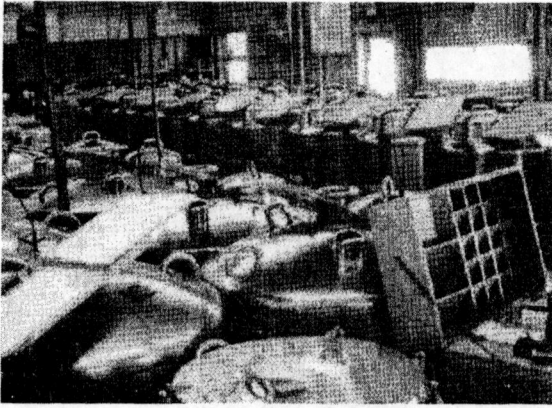

**Figure 14.9.** Frozen semen storage and distribution center, where millions of semen units are stored in large LN refrigerators. Domestic and export orders are packed and shipped from such centers on a routine basis. (Courtesy, ABS Global, DeForest, WI)

## Liquid Nitrogen Safety

Nitrogen is one the earth's most available resources, making up approximately 80 percent of the atmosphere. As a gas, nitrogen has no color, odor, or taste. It is non-toxic and, for all practical purposes, chemically inert.

The liquid nitrogen used in AI refrigerators is made by compressing air into the liquid state and distilling it until it is 98 percent pure. Since liquid nitrogen in nonflammable, it is not a fire hazard. In fact, it can be used to put out a fire. Because it is extremely cold ($-320°F$ [$-196°C$]), liquid nitrogen provides a safe, economical refrigerant for maintaining frozen semen.

Even though liquid nitrogen is relatively safe, there are potential hazards because of two properties: (1) It can cause burns due to the extreme cold temperature, and (2) large amounts spilled or released in a closed area will vaporize rapidly, displacing oxygen, and can cause suffocation.

Because of its extremely low temperature, liquid nitrogen can cause a freezing injury or frostbite. Eyes can be seriously damaged by coming into contact with liquid nitrogen. Therefore, safety precautions must be taken seriously and followed closely:

1. Always handle liquid nitrogen carefully so that it will not splash or spill.

2. Protect eyes with glasses, safety goggles, or a face shield whenever filling a refrigerator or removing semen from it.

3. Wear protective gloves that can be removed quickly and easily in case nitrogen should splash into them.

4. Protect arms by always wearing long sleeves.

5. Wear trousers outside boots to shed any accidently spilled liquid.

6. Don't let children play around an LN refrigerator.

As long as LN refrigerators are kept in ventilated areas, there should be no problems. However, a leak or even the normal venting process could displace oxygen if a room or area is sealed off. If this happens, a person can quickly lose consciousness without sensing the lack of oxygen. (Therefore it is prudent to monitor oxygen levels in LN storage areas. Portable as well as stationary oxygen monitoring instruments are commercially available.)

When liquid nitrogen is transferred from bulk tanks into smaller storage units and then later into field units, chances of an accident can be reduced by performing the operations outdoors.

Liquid nitrogen is classified as a hazardous material under the Code of Federal Regulations, Title 49. The identification number and shipping name for liquid nitrogen is "UN 1977—Nitrogen Refrigerated Liquid." The transportation of hazardous materials is regulated by the U.S. Department of Transportation, which requires proper identification number and shipping name on various types of shipping containers.

## First Aid

Asphyxiation

1. If a person seems dizzy or loses consciousness while working with liquid nitrogen, get him or her to a well-ventilated area immediately.

2. If breathing stops, give artificial respiration and supplemental oxygen.

3. Summon medical assistance.

If you suspect an area is nitrogen enriched or if someone has lost consciousness, use a self-contained breathing apparatus before entering the area.

Cryogenic Burns

1. Rewarm the affected area by immersion in warm water (100° to 110°F [38° to 43°C]), use of body heat, or exposure to warm air. Do not use hot water or an open fire.

2. Avoid trauma. Treat for shock if necessary. Do not rub or massage the affected part. If the injury involves the feet, do not attempt to walk.

3. Prevent infection by cleansing the area with a bland soap. Dressing is not necessary if the skin is intact.

4. Burns that result in blistering or deep tissue damage should be examined by a doctor immediately.

5. Elevate the affected part slightly to control swelling.

## Care and Maintenance of an LN Refrigerator

1. On the farm, keep the LN refrigerator in a clean, dry, and well-ventilated area where it can be observed frequently. To avoid corrosion, set the refrigerator on wooden boards or on a pallet. To maximize its holding time, the refrigerator should be kept in a cool location out of direct sunlight and away from sources of warm air. The area should also be well lighted.

2. Keep the insulated stopper in the refrigerator at all times when not in use, with the dust cover closed. The stopper fits loosely and is vented to permit the escape of nitrogen gas. This practice avoids a pressure build-up and possible bursting. The LN refrigerator must not be more tightly stoppered than when it comes from the supplier.

3. Handle the LN refrigerator carefully! Rough treatment and jarring impacts may cause a break in the junction between inner liner and outer shell, resulting in the loss of vacuum, nitrogen, and valuable frozen semen. Avoid dents and scratches in the outer shell that may degrade the refrigerator's holding time.

4. If the LN refrigerator is transported in a vehicle, secure it tightly so that it cannot tip over (a ventilated box is recommended). If the refrigerator is moved by car, place it in the trunk. In a pickup truck, secure the refrigerator in a front corner of the truck bed. Park in the shade so the refrigerator is not exposed to the sun.

5. Check the level of liquid nitrogen weekly by removing the insulated stopper and lowering a measuring stick to the bottom of the container. Remove the dipstick after 8 to 10 seconds, and then wave it in the air. Frost condensation will appear on the part that was submerged, indicating how

much liquid nitrogen remains in the refrigerator. It is the user and not the AI organization that is responsible for checking the nitrogen level and making sure the LN refrigerator is filled on a regular basis. It is a good practice to keep a record of the dates the LN refrigerator was filled and the weekly level of liquid nitrogen measured to monitor its usage. Vigilance is important since even new refrigerators can have defects and can fail.

6. Frost or sweat on the LN refrigerator or rapid loss of liquid nitrogen indicates the refrigerator may have developed a leak or has lost its vacuum. If this occurs, contact your semen supplier or service organization immediately. The semen may need to be transferred out of the suspect refrigerator. Develop a plan to have an alternative refrigerator available for this purpose.

## Handling and Use of Frozen Semen

Temperature control is the most important aspect of semen handling. To preserve the fertilizing integrity of sperm, straws of semen should not be exposed to temperatures above −148°F (−100°C) except during thawing of the semen. Each exposure above this temperature level may kill numerous sperm within the straw due to ice crystal movement (recrystalization). If frozen semen has been mishandled (i.e., allowed to reach temperatures above −148°F [−100°C]) once or several times, its fertilizing potential may be greatly diminished or lost. Once a straw of semen has been removed from the refrigerator, it must be used or discarded. Frozen semen cannot be warmed and then refrozen! If the supply of LN refrigerant runs low due to neglect or refrigerator failure, if the transfer of semen from one container to another slows down, or if there is a delay in tran-

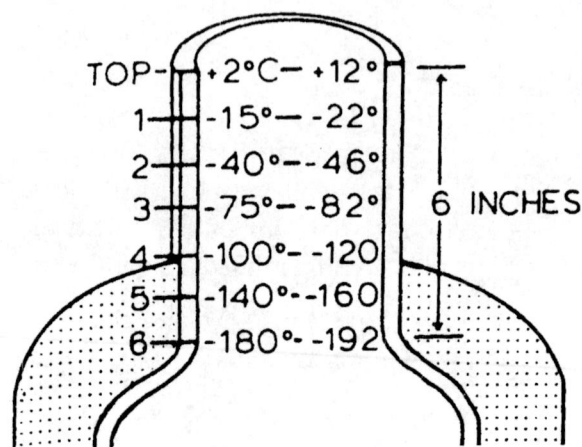

**Figure 14.10.** Typical temperature range in the neck tube of an LN refrigerator. The relatively high temperatures in the neck of the refrigerator make it apparent that units of semen should be removed from canes and lifted into the neck in a matter of seconds. (R. G. Saacke. 1974. Concepts in semen packaging and use. Proc. 8th Conf. on Artificial Insemination of Beef Cattle. NAAB. p. 11)

sit, a consequent rise in temperature can occur, resulting in damaged sperm cells.

Improper handling of semen under field conditions undoubtedly accounts for low conception in many instances. However, problems can be easily avoided by understanding and exercising proper frozen semen temperature control. The inseminator and the direct herd customer should learn the correct methods for handling frozen semen and follow them carefully at all times. Inside the LN refrigerator, semen that is submerged in liquid nitrogen has a temperature of −320°F (−196°C), while semen that is in the vapor above the liquid has a temperature of about −292°F (−180°C). The "neck tube" of the refrigerator ranges in temperature from about −292°F (−180°C) at its bottom to about +50°F (+10°C) at its top (Figure 14.10).

When frozen semen is raised into the neck tube, it warms up very rapidly. The key to successfully handling frozen semen and preserving sperm integrity is generally to avoid raising semen any higher than the lower portion of the neck tube. However, when it is absolutely necessary to raise the semen higher (e.g., when transferring semen to another refrigerator or when removing a single straw for thawing), the operation must be carried out as rapidly as possible (in 10 seconds or less) so that the cane/rack of semen being transferred or the remainder or semen on a cane/rack from which a straw was thawed never reaches the critical temperature of −148°F (−100°C).

There are at least two situations in the usual field practice of artificial insemination in which opportunities exist for damaging frozen semen by improper handling: transferring semen and thawing semen.

**Transferring Semen**—When you transfer frozen semen into your LN refrigerator, you must take the responsibility for proper handling. Usually, when you buy semen, you also refill your refrigerator with liquid nitrogen. Therefore, it's also a good idea to fill your refrigerator with liquid nitrogen before you start transferring semen. It's recommended that you purchase whole canes of semen instead of trying to split canes. This avoids handling of individual straws or ampules, which can lead to thermal damage. Transfers should be made out of wind and sunlight. Have LN refrigerators side by side, with two people making the transfers when possible. One person selects the cane to be transferred, while the second person brings the canister to receive the cane into the neck of the second refrigerator. As soon as a cane is transferred, lower each canister into the bottom of the refrigerator. Follow this transfer routine, one cane at a time, until the job is completed.

Transferring entire canisters containing the canes or goblets of semen is fairly simple. Place the two LN refrigerators side by side, and quickly transfer each canister. Some liquid nitrogen may drip off the canister or boil out the neck of the refrigerator, so you should wear gloves and shatterproof goggles and should wear your pant legs over your boots. *Again, the frozen semen should not be exposed to warm temperatures (i.e., above −148°F [−100°C]) for more than a few seconds.*

**Thawing Semen**—When thawing semen it is important to obtain the maximum recovery of sperm from the frozen state (in the unit of semen selected for insemination) and at the same time to protect the integrity of the frozen semen that remains in the LN refrigerator. It is also important to protect the thawed sperm from thermal shock or contamination prior to deposition in the female reproductive tract. These objectives can be achieved with the following procedures.

For optimum sperm recovery results, the thawing procedures recommended by the semen-processing organization should be followed. This is because there are interrelationships between freezing and thawing rates, composition of semen extenders, and semen package size that may vary between the individual AI organizations. Recommendations of the semen-processing organizations are based on research, using their particular processing characteristics.

If the supplier's recommendations are not available, however, we recommend thawing semen as follows:

For straws:

> Thaw in warm water 90° to 95° F (33° to 35° C) for a minimum of 40 seconds.

For ampules:

> Thaw in iced water about 41° F (5° C) for 10 minutes (1.0-ml size) or 5 minutes (0.5-ml size). After the appropriate thaw period, the ice coat around the ampule should slide off easily.

The thawed semen should remain in the thawing bath until just before inseminating. This period should not exceed 15 minutes.

## PROCEDURE

1.  Be sure the breeding kit is clean and supplies are well organized and stored in a manner that prevents contamination from dust and debris.

2.  Place the breeding kit next to the LN refrigerator. Have sleeve, sheaths, AI gun, scissors (straw cutter), and paper towels available for thawed semen.

3.  Place the thaw container next to the LN refrigerator, and open. Check for proper temperature.

4.  Determine the location of the semen in the LN refrigerator. (Always use a semen inventory record to keep track of semen location. This can be a diagram displayed above the refrigerator listing the contents of each canister[10] or a simple canister tally sheet indicating current number of semen units stored on each bull. An up-to-date semen inventory record eliminates excessive handling and searching in the LN refrigerator to find the semen of choice, avoiding exposure of the semen to damaging temperatures.)

5.  Raise the canister into the lower portion of the neck tube, and locate the desired cane/rack. Grasp the desired cane/rack, and hold it in the neck tube while lowering the canister to the bottom of the neck tube. Bend the top of the cane/rack up slightly to facilitate straw removal. Using forceps (tweezers), remove a straw and quickly transfer it to the thaw container. Lower the cane/rack into the canister, and return it to its storage

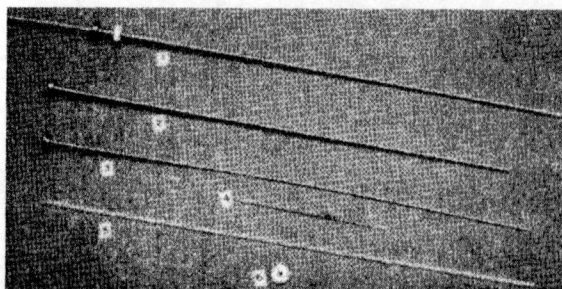

**Figure 14.11.** Insemination gun for French straw system (1) assembled, loaded AI gun. Component parts include (2) barrel, (3) plunger, (4) 0.5-ml straw, (5) disposable plastic sheath, and (6) "O" ring.

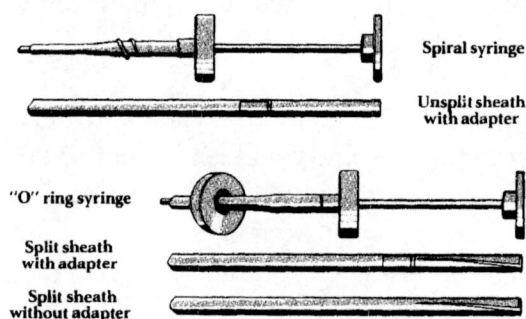

**Figure 14.12.** Illustration of types of AI guns (spiral and standard "O" ring) and sheaths (unsplit; split with and without adapter). (Courtesy, ABS Global, DeForest, WI)

position. At no time should the canister or cane stay in the neck tube over 10 seconds. If the cane/rack cannot be located and the straw removed within 10 seconds, the canister should be lowered to the bottom of the refrigerator and allowed to cool down for a minimum of 30 seconds before another attempt to remove a straw is made.

6.  After thawing: Dry the straw, check identification, properly cut the straw, and load it into the insemination gun. *If you have not inseminated cows recently, rehearse your routine for handling straws and loading the insemination gun. See Figures 14.11 and 14.12 for descriptions of insemination equipment for straws.*

---

[10] P. L. Senger, J. K. Hillers, and W. N. Fleming. 1980. On-the-farm management of semen tanks. Proc. 8th Tech. Conf. on Artificial Insemination and Reproduction. NAAB. p. 25.

7. Protect the insemination gun from a harsh environment.

8. Prepare to inseminate the cow.

Additional pointers you should consider when handling and thawing semen are the following:

1. Occasionally check the accuracy of the thaw bath thermometer.

2. Thaw each unit of semen individually.

3. Shake the straw as it is taken from the LN refrigerator to remove any liquid nitrogen that may be retained in the cotton plug end of the straw. This can prevent straw plug "blow-outs."

4. Thoroughly dry each straw or ampule of thawed semen. Even a small drop of water can be lethal to sperm.

5. Check the bull identification code on every unit of semen.

6. Shake the air bubble from the middle of the straw to the sealed end.

7. Cut the tip of the straw squarely and through the air space below the seal. An angle cut may prevent the straw from fitting securely into the sheath. Check to see that the straw is firmly seated into the plastic adapter or tip of the sheath, depending on the type of inseminating device you use.

8. Clean the scissors or straw cutter after each use.

9. When assembly of the insemination gun is complete, gently depress the plunger to remove the air space at the upper end of the straw. This avoids picking up contamination that could be introduced into the uterus.

10. Wrap the assembled insemination gun in a clean, dry paper towel, and tuck it within your clothing for transport to the cow.

11. Never experiment on your own. The recommendations made are supported by valid research.

Figure 14.13 (A–H) depicts the procedures for thawing semen processed in straws and for loading insemination equipment. Figure 14.14 (A–J) is included to describe these procedures for ampules. Although semen has not been processed in ampules for several years, there are still ampules in storage (particularly custom-collected semen) that are used occasionally.

## Transporting and Shipping Semen

**Liquid Semen—** Obviously most semen is shipped frozen; however, there may be occasional shipments of liquid semen. Procedures followed in the past for the shipment of liquid semen in vials are included here for reference:

1. After the semen has been tested for quality, extended, and cooled to about 41°F (5°C), place the amount to be shipped in a sterile vial, properly labeled and sealed. Shipping vials must be full to obtain the best sperm survival. If there is insufficient semen to fill a vial, add enough mineral oil to fill to the top of the vial.

2. To insulate, wrap the vial in several thicknesses of paper and place it alongside a partially inflated balloon or a small can filled with ice.

3. Wrap the vial and the balloon or ice container together tightly in heavy insulating paper, such as Jiffy Wrapper.

4. Insert the wrapped package into the shipping container with sufficient corrugated paper or packing to hold it firmly in place. Seal and address the container, and either mail it or have it delivered by truck or parcel service.

For short-distance transportation by car, bus, etc., the insulated vials of semen may be '

**Figure 14.13.** Steps for thawing straws of semen and loading insemination equipment.

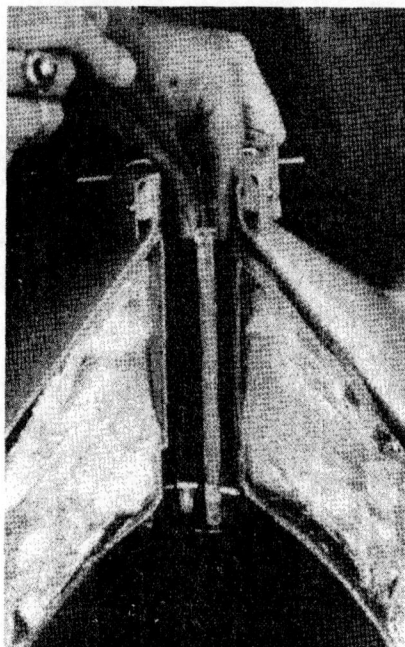

**Figure 14.13A.** *Step A.* Locate the desired semen in the LN refrigerator, keep the cane/rack low in the neck tube, remove the straw carefully, and quickly lower the cane/rack back into the refrigerator.

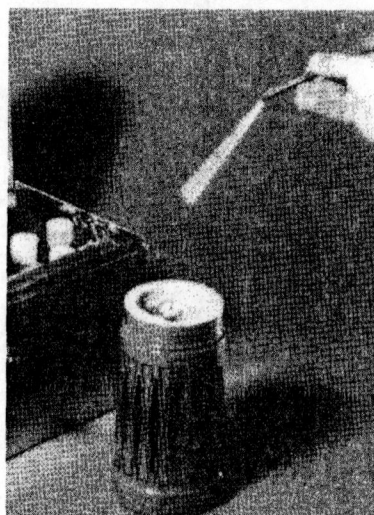

**Figure 14.13B.** *Step B.* Shake the straw two or three times (to remove any liquid nitrogen in the end of the straw plug and avoid plug blow-out) while transferring it directly into the AI kit thaw bath (thermos bottle or commercial thawing unit) that has been checked for proper temperature. Keep the straw in the thaw bath for the required minimum thawing time and until the inseminator is ready to load the AI gun.

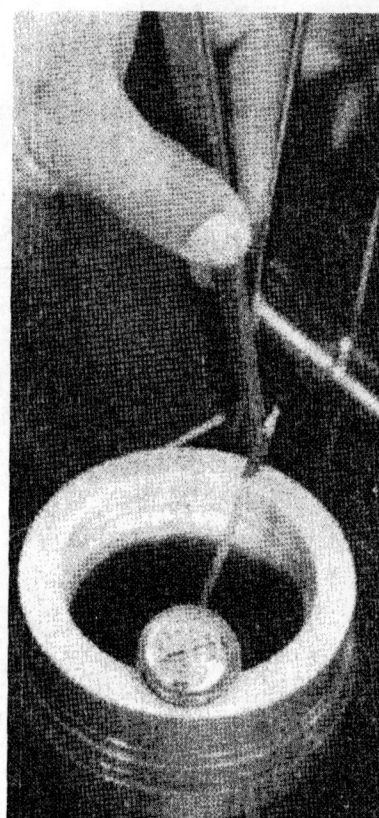

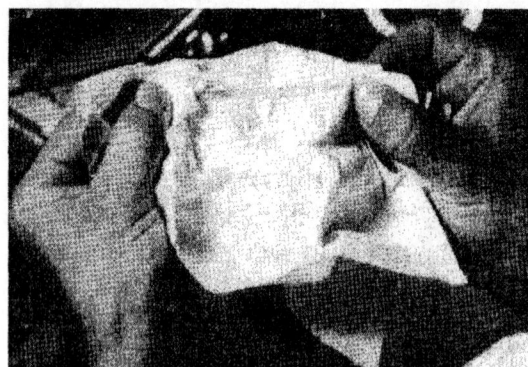

**Figure 14.13C.** *Step C.* After thawing the straw, remove it from the bath, thoroughly dry it with a paper towel, and read the label to insure proper sire identification. A protected area should be used if the ambient temperature is below 70°F (21°C).

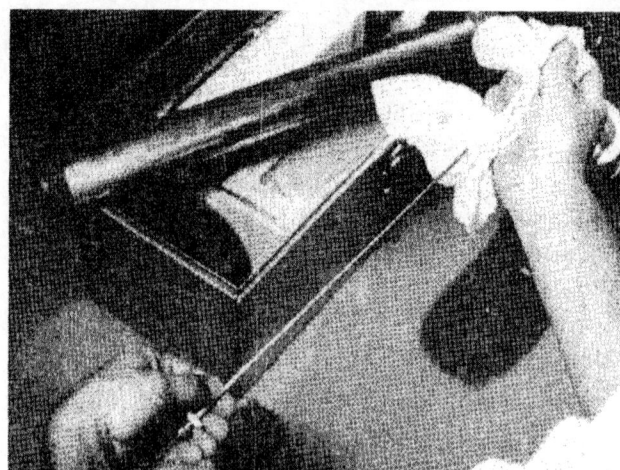

**Figure 14.13D.** *Step D.* Keep the thawed semen straw protected from temperature shock (wrap in a paper towel), and friction-warm the AI gun by rubbing it with a paper towel.

**Figure 14.13.** Continued

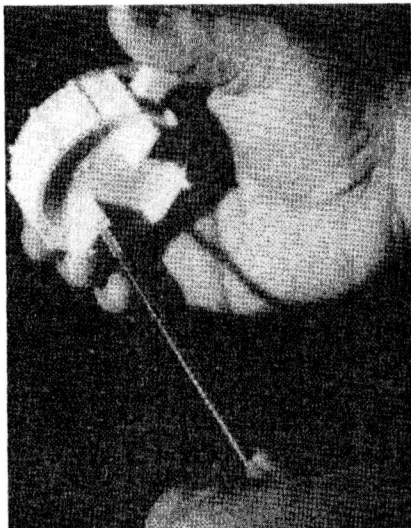

**Figure 14.13E.** *Step E.* After inserting the straw into the AI gun with the seal and air space exposed, cut off the sonic seal using scissors or a commercially available straw cutter (shown). Be sure the cut is made squarely through the air space below the seal.

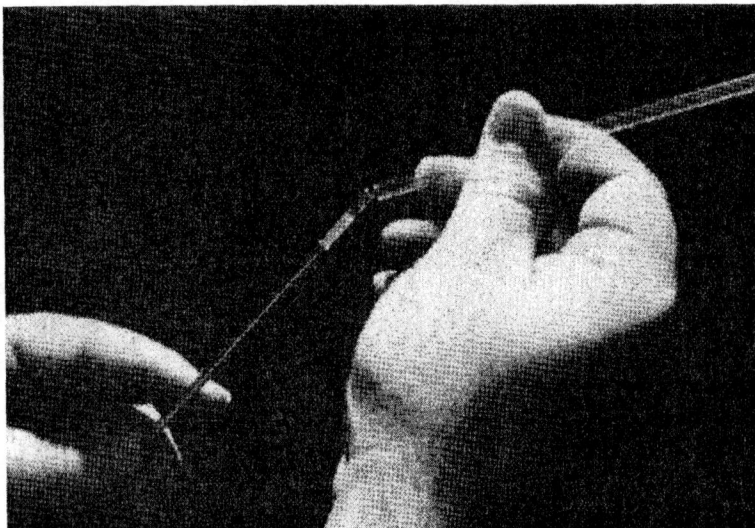

**Figure 14.13F.** *Step F.* Slip a disposable plastic sheath over the entire AI gun. *Note:* Other types of sheaths (not shown) contain a plastic adapter into which the cut end of the straw is inserted prior to slipping the sheath over the AI gun. The adapter allows use of all types of straws and insures a good seal between straw and sheath to avoid back-leakage, which can result with poorly cut straws (Figure 14.12).

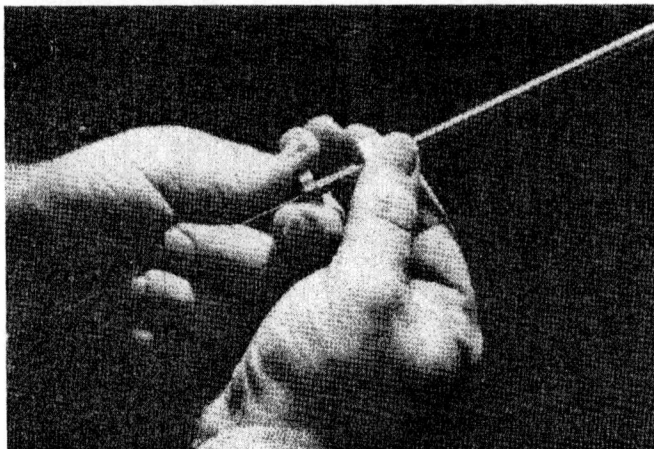

**Figure 14.13G.** *Step G.* Tighten the sheath securely by sliding the "O" ring down and giving it a slight twist. *Note:* A spiral type AI gun is also available that eliminates use of the "O" ring to secure the sheath. This type of AI gun uses unsplit sheaths that also contain a plastic adapter (Figure 14.12).

**Figure 14.13H.** *Step H.* After moving the plunger slowly forward until the semen is just about to emerge from the AI gun tip, wrap the loaded AI gun with a couple of clean, dry paper towels and proceed to the breeding chute or stanchion. (Courtesy, Select Sires, Inc., Plain City, OH)

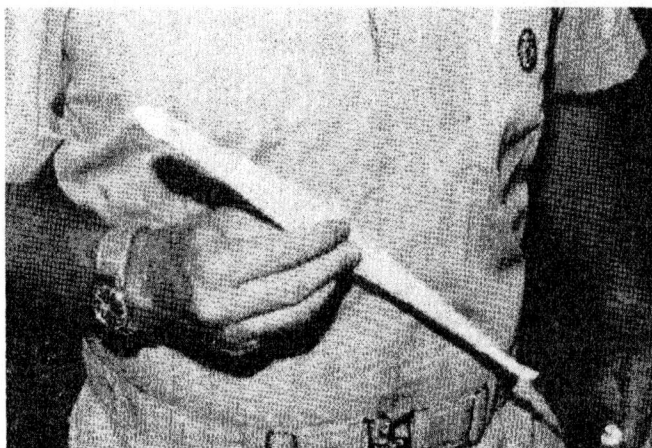

**Figure 14.14.** Steps for thawing and utilizing frozen semen ampules. (Courtesy, B. W. Pickett, Colorado State University)

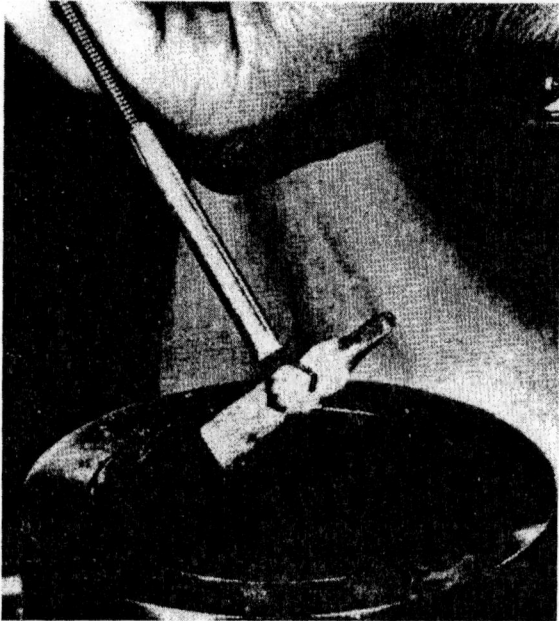

**Figure 14.14A.** *Step A.* Remove the ampule of frozen semen from bulk storage.

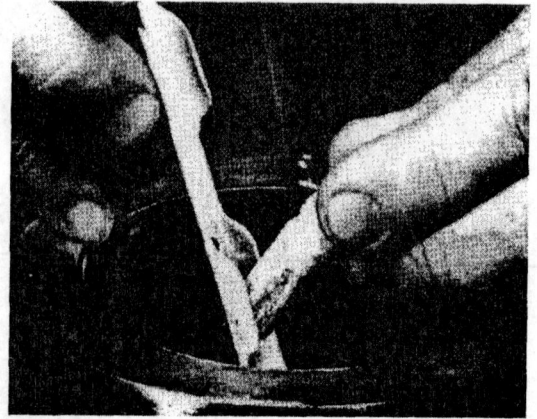

**Figure 14.14B.** *Step B.* Remove the ampule of frozen semen from a cane. Be careful to expose only the ampule being removed.

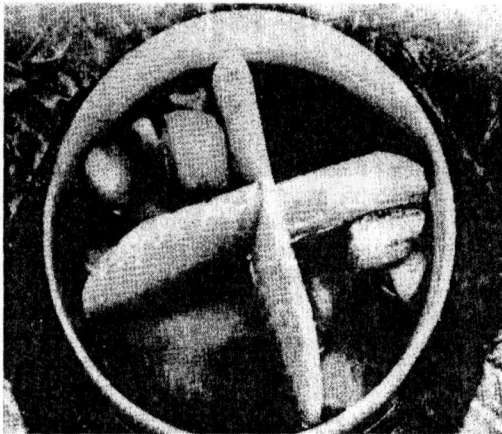

**Figure 14.14C.** *Step C.* Place the ampule in a thaw bath, and keep the ice cubes separated from thawing ampules.

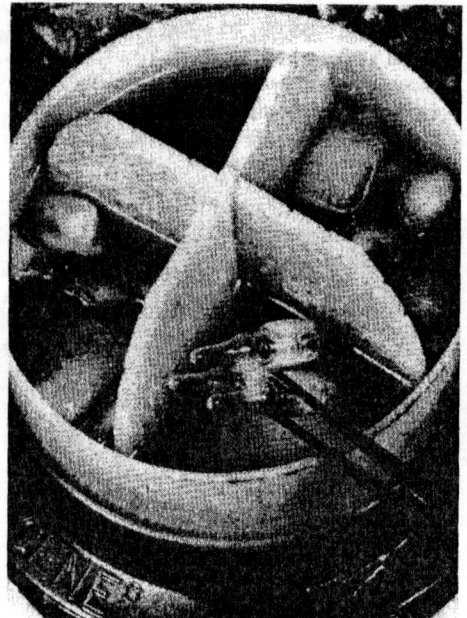

**Figure 14.14D.** *Step D.* Do not permit ampules to freeze together during thawing.

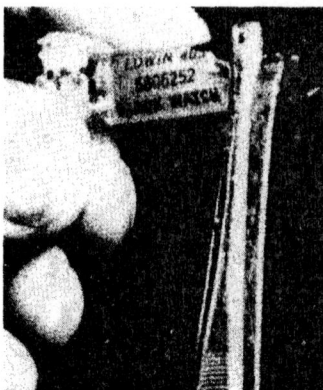

**Figure 14.14E.** *Step E.* Do not remove the ice coat to hasten thawing of the ampule.

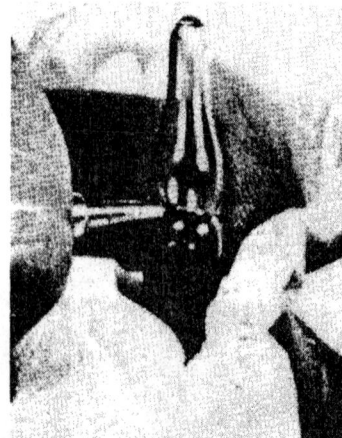

**Figure 14.14F.** *Step F.* Score the neck of the ampule with a scribe.

**Figure 14.14.** Continued

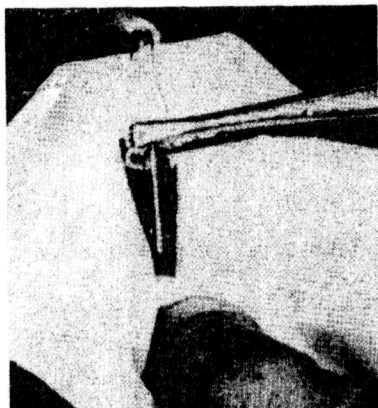

**Figure 14.14G.** *Step G.* Water is spermicidal. Dry the ampule carefully before opening.

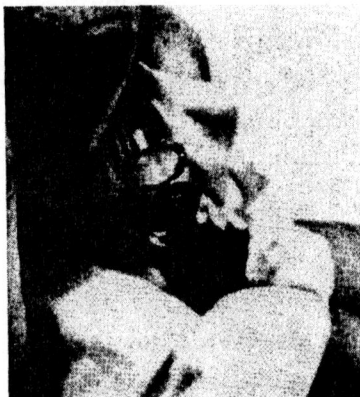

**Figure 14.14H.** *Step H.* Snap open the ampule in an upright position.

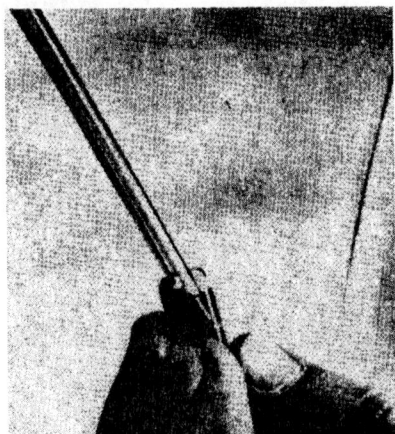

**Figure 14.14I.** *Step I.* Insert the catheter slowly, withdrawing semen as you lower the catheter into the ampule.

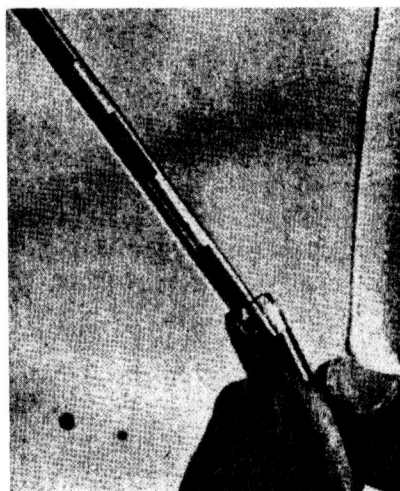

**Figure 14.14J.** *Step J.* Do not break the fluid column when withdrawing semen. A procedure such as shown here will result in a much greater loss of semen.

placed in a thermos bottle filled with cracked ice. The thermos bottle should be well packed in a large container to prevent breakage.

For long-distance shipments en route for 60 to 80 hours, it is essential that the package be adequately refrigerated; that the semen be protected from the intense cold of the refrigerant; and that the refrigerant be insulated against the external temperature.

Semen has been kept alive at a temperature of 40° to 45°F (4° to 7°C) for over 20 days. In general, liquid semen should be used within about 48 hours after collection.

Liquid semen processed in straws can be shipped in containers that are insulated with polystyrene foam. The straws of semen placed in goblets or other containers can be maintained at about 41°F (5°C) using commercially available refrigerant gel packs (refer to Appendix C for information on manufacturers/suppliers).

**Frozen Semen**— Shipping frozen semen is accomplished by the use of LN containers with semen refrigerated at −320°F (−196°C). Domestic and international air shipment of semen in such cryogenic containers is routine for AI organizations. Such shipping containers may carry from several hundred to several thousand insemination doses. By using liquid nitrogen as a refrigerant, the dangers of delay in transit are largely overcome, as the containers usually carry sufficient refrigerant to last for several weeks.

Domestic shipment of frozen semen is also frequently made by bus or truck. In recent years, there has also been increased use of dry shippers (LN refrigerators that contain a material that absorbs the liquid nitrogen when they are filled, producing dry cryogenic containers), which can be delivered directly to the farm or ranch by various commercial package services. Dry shippers have mainly been used for small shipments of frozen semen and they typically have a much shorter working time (about one to three weeks depending on size) compared to most "wet" cryogenic refrigerators.

*Note:* Because of concerns over hazardous materials transport, particularly for air shipments, larger-capacity dry shippers have been developed and are seeing greater usage for semen shipments.

AI organizations also utilize large-storage refrigerators and bulk tanks for banking frozen semen and replenishing the technician and direct herd supply of semen and liquid nitrogen every few weeks. Distribution trucks are used to make the deliveries. Some large AI organizations have nationwide coverage of their technicians and direct herd customers in the field by this plan.

## QUESTIONS

1. What are the chief advantages of frozen semen?

2. Indicate the equipment needs for processing frozen semen.

3. Explain the evolution of semen-packaging systems. What package is commonly used today in the United States?

4. Explain what semen extender components have to do with freezing and thawing methods.

5. What is a cryoprotective agent and how does it function? What is the cryoprotective agent commonly used in freezing semen?

6. What is the purpose of equilibration of semen during the processing period?

7. What are the basic steps in processing and freezing semen?

8. How is frozen semen stored? At what temperature? Is a straw of semen stored at −76°F (− 60°C) safe to use for insemination? Explain.

9. How may frozen semen best be stored on the farm?

10. What is the most important aspect of semen handling? How should frozen semen in straws and in ampules be thawed?

11. List the steps required in thawing semen and loading the insemination equipment.

12. What precautions should be exercised in the use and handling of the LN refrigerator?

13. How would you ship 500 units of semen to a cattle breeder in South America?

14. How would you ship straws or a vial of semen to a breeder in an adjoining state?

# REFERENCES

Cassou, B. 1983. The French Paillette Technique. IMV Corp. publication. p. 5. The Integrity of Frozen Spermatozoa. Proc. of a Round Table Conf. 1978. National Academy of Sciences, Washington, DC.

Kroetsch, T. 1992. Experiences with mini-straws. Proc. 14th Tech. Conf. on Artificial Insemination and Reproduction. NAAB. p. 64.

Pickett, B. W., and W. E. Berndtson. 1978. Principles and techniques of freezing spermatozoa. In: G. W. Salisbury, N. L. Van Demark, and J. R. Lodge (Eds.). Physiology of Reproduction and Artificial Insemination of Cattle (2nd Ed.). p. 494. W. H. Freeman, San Francisco.

Pickett, B. W., W. E. Berndtson, and J. J. Sullivan. 1978. Influence of seminal additives and packaging systems on fertility of frozen bovine spermatozoa. J. Anim. Sci. 47 (Suppl. 2):12.

Rajamannan, A. H. 1970. A method of packaging semen—The straw. Proc. 3rd Tech. Conf. on Artificial Insemination and Reproduction. NAAB. p. 49.

Saacke, R. G. 1974. Concepts in semen packaging and use. Proc. 8th Conf. on Artificial Insemination of Beef Cattle. NAAB. p. 11.

Senger, P. L. 1986. Field handling of frozen semen and insemination technique. Proc. Ann. Conf. on Artificial Insemination and Embryo Transfer in Beef Cattle. NAAB. p. 14.

# EXERCISE 15

# Custom Freezing of Semen

## OBJECT

To become familiar with the custom freezing of semen as carried out in the United States.

## DISCUSSION

The custom freezing sector has become an integral part of the AI industry in the United States. Custom freezing involves the collection, freezing, and storage of semen from sires owned by private individuals or concerns. During 2001, reports from NAAB-member AI organizations indicate that over 2.8 million insemination doses of bull semen were custom collected, about 10 percent of the total semen activity they reported. In addition, another 1.3 million units of semen were custom collected by CSS-only (non-NAAB) participating AI businesses. The fact that custom collection services are available for individual herd owners' bulls is a further tribute to the free enterprise system under which the AI industry in the United States operates.

There are reasons why private breeders may wish to utilize custom freezing services. Following is a brief outline of advantages, disadvantages, and recommendations pertaining to the custom freezing of semen.

### Advantages of Custom Freezing

1. Custom freezing makes it possible for the owners of valuable sires to have semen frozen, stored, and made available for use in their herds over a period of years. It is a form of "insurance" on valuable sires.

2. Through custom freezing, several owners of a sire, even though located hundreds of miles apart, can utilize his services in a routine and systematic manner.

3. Custom freezing permits breeders to own bulls in partnership and to have offspring in many herds. This also helps in sampling and proving young sires for developing a dependable, reliable proof.

4. The owners of valuable sires may add to their incomes through the sales of semen to other breeders. The owners will handle the marketing of the semen, and the custom freezing business will handle storage and shipping.

### Disadvantages of Custom Freezing

Nearly every disadvantage of custom freezing involves the matter of sire health. In some cases, it also involves the collection and storage of semen by unreliable parties, and this scenario can result in the consequent disappointment to the sire owners and their patrons.

1. Any sire in contact with the cow herd and used for natural breeding as well as for furnishing semen for AI use has the potential to transmit certain diseases through his semen, unless he is

145

subjected to a health testing program for those diseases important for AI.

2. From the standpoint of improving cattle by utilizing the best sires available, which AI organizations strive to do, herd owners may, based on their esteem for a less-highly productive sire, supplant the inheritance available from progeny-proven sires of above-average merit. It is the prerogative of all herd owners to use the sire of their choice. Custom collection and sale of semen by individual breeders in many cases just "puts the bull back on the farm."

3. While most custom freezing businesses are established AI organizations and most private owners are legitimate operators, there have been cases of individual operators going into the custom collection business with limited equipment and capital and with very little sense of responsibility. The sire owner has no recourse for unsatisfactory results, such as low quality, poorly labeled semen. Needless to say, unreliable operators of this kind do not last long. On the other hand, there are several privately owned organizations that participate in the CSS program and do a highly commendable job in custom freezing. Any herd owner who contemplates having semen custom frozen should try to find such reliable organizations and individual operators.

4. Some custom freezing services travel to the ranch or farm, collect semen from one or more bulls, evaluate the semen after collection, freeze it if the quality is satisfactory, store it, and provide a supply as is necessary to the owner. However, adequate facilities for handling bulls during collection are lacking on many farms, and ob-

taining a good quality specimen for freezing is more difficult.

5. One of the chief disadvantages of custom collection, as practiced in many instances, is the fact that collections of semen are made at very infrequent intervals and that there is little opportunity to establish a profile of semen quality for a given bull. All too often the bull may be in declining health, or if he is not used to being handled, he may become frightened. Either situation could result in the collected semen being of lower quality than what the bull is capable of producing.

## General Considerations and Recommendations

Breeders who desire to have semen collected from their sires should observe the following suggestions:

1. The nearest established, reputable, custom freezing service should be contacted. At the present time, there are a few AI organizations that offer custom freezing services, as well as market semen from their own bulls. In addition, there are 12 to 20 individual operators, with established records of dependability, engaged in the collection, processing, and storage of frozen semen on a custom basis. Generally speaking, a breeder should not deal with unknown parties.

2. If semen from the bull is to be offered for sale, it is strongly recommended that the sire be taken to the housing facilities of the custom freezing service. This will allow the bull to undergo recommended health testing and provide for more conducive surroundings for collection of high quality

146

semen. While this option involves more time and expense, the possibility of disease being transmitted through the semen is reduced.

3. If the bull is kept on the owner's premises and semen is collected for freezing, these practices should be followed:

    a. The bull should be kept in a separate housing facility and not used for natural breeding.

    b. The health tests as outlined by Certified Semen Services, Inc., should be conducted and satisfactorily passed before semen is collected for freezing. As long as semen is being collected and frozen, particularly for use outside the owner's herd, the bull should be isolated and natural service prohibited.

4. Semen should be collected at a time when the bull is active and healthy. In too many cases, herd owners postpone custom processing until a bull is crippled or too old to produce highly fertile semen.

5. In the case of registered cattle, the bull must be recorded in the association herd books, he must be blood typed, and his semen must be labeled properly and stored in an approved manner. The regulations governing the use of frozen semen for dairy cattle are outlined in Exercise 26. Breeders and herd owners are urged to study this section carefully.

## QUESTIONS

1. What are the advantages of the custom freezing of semen?

2. Should custom collected semen be permitted to be used outside the owner's herd? If so, under what conditions?

3. How would you select an organization or individual to do custom collecting from bulls you own?

4. What advantages are there in housing at the custom freezing service a bull to be custom collected?

5. How does the custom collecting and semen freezing program aid in the progeny testing program?

6. What are the general requirements of breed registry associations for custom collection and storage of semen used for purebred cattle?

## REFERENCES

CSS Minimum Requirements for Disease Control of Semen Produced for AI. 2002. Certified Semen Services, Columbia, MO.

Kellgren, H. C., et al. 1966. Panel discussion on custom collection and electroejaculation. Proc. 1st Tech. Conf. on Artificial Insemination and Bovine Reproduction. NAAB. p. 35.

# PART THREE

# Insemination of Dairy and Beef Cattle;

# Insemination Training;

# Pregnancy Determination and

# Reproduction Problems

# EXERCISE 16

# How to Inseminate Cattle—Techniques

## OBJECT

To learn the proper techniques and develop knowledge and skill in the artificial insemination of cattle.

## DISCUSSION

Timely insemination of cows and heifers, using the correct techniques, is one of the most important aspects of successful AI. Insemination of the female at the proper stage of the estrous cycle and the skillful deposition of fertile semen in the body of the uterus are the two most essential requirements for a high conception rate. The correct insemination techniques can be learned by any person who so desires and who has reasonable manual and mental dexterity. Skill in insemination techniques comes with practice and study.

### When to Inseminate

Generally, cows and heifers should be inseminated from about the middle to not over six hours after the end of the heat period.

The heat period (estrus) is that portion of the estrous cycle when the female is sexually receptive. During this time, increased levels of estrogens from ovarian follicular cells cause profound physiological and behavioral changes in the female. These include swelling of the vulva; discharge of clear cervical mucus; bawling and restlessness; smelling, licking, and rubbing other cattle; and standing to be ridden by herdmates. In addition to prompting the cow to seek out sexual partners for an opportunity to mate, the hormonally induced changes also affect the function and activity of cells lining the genital tract. These changes help insure successful transport and survival of sperm after mating or AI.

Cows normally cycle every 18 to 24 days (21-day average) and usually remain in heat from a few to over 30 hours. Individual cows show considerable variation. Note Figure 16.1, "Timing Guide for the Average Cow." For many years it was believed that the average duration of estrus was about 18 hours. However research conducted in the 1990's, using a radiotelemetric system to monitor estrus behavior continuously, has demonstrated that estrus lasts on average only about eight hours in dairy cows but somewhat longer in beef cattle. The ideal time to inseminate is determined by when the cow will stand solidly for other cows to mount. This is commonly called "standing heat." Identifying standing heat is important because it is the best indicator of "true" estrus and it relates to ovulation (ovulation occurs approximately 24 to 30 hours after the animal first stands to be mounted). Even though the cow will stand solidly during this period, the duration of each stand lasts for only a few seconds (about four to six). Thus, the individual assigned to watch for signs of heat needs to be attentive and a keen observer. The intensity and duration of standing heat is also affected to a great extent by environment. Allowing cows to interact in an uncrowded area with secure footing (nonconcrete surface) is important for maximizing chances of observing mounting behavior. It is

151

| | Viable Sperm | | |
|---|---|---|---|
| Early | Optimal time to inseminate | Fair | Too late to inseminate |

| Hours | 0 | 4 | 14 | 24 | 28 |
|---|---|---|---|---|---|

Onset of Estrus                                    Ovulation

| BEFORE HEAT (6-10 Hours) | STANDING HEAT (8-18 Hours) | AFTER HEAT (10-20 Hours) | LIFE OF EGG 6-10 Hours (after ovulation) |
|---|---|---|---|
| 1  Smells other cows | 1  Stands to be ridden | 1  Will not stand | |
| | 2  Bawls frequently | 2  Clear mucous discharge from vulva | |
| 2  Attempts to ride other cows | 3  Nervous and excitable | | |
| | 4  Rides other cows | | |
| 3  Vulva moist, red, slightly swollen | 5  Off feed and milk | | |
| | 6  First cow up | | |
| | 7  Vulva moist and red | | |
| | 8  Clear mucous discharge | | |
| | 9  Eye pupils dilated | | |

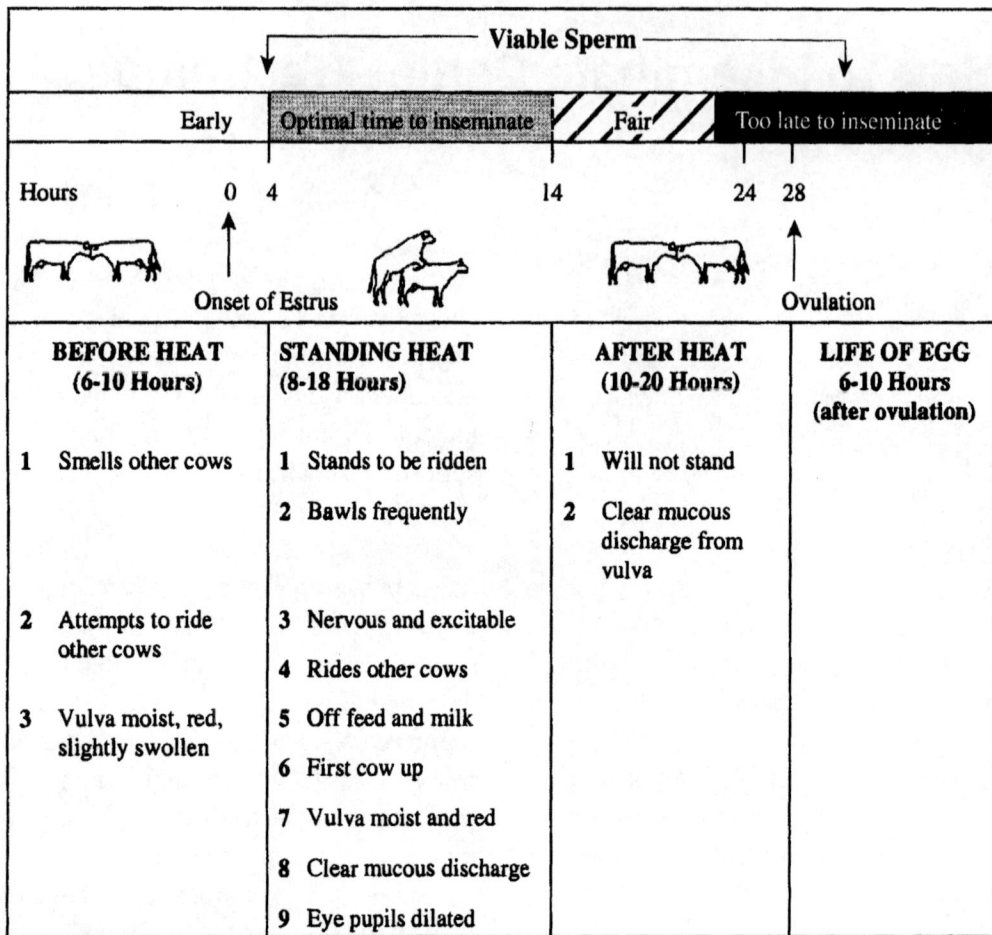

**Figure 16.1.** Insemination timing guide.

recommended that specific times be set aside for heat observation. The herd should be checked three or more times daily for cows in heat (the 20-minute observation periods should be from six to eight hours apart). Historically, cows observed in heat in the morning have been inseminated the afternoon of the same day. Cows observed in heat in the afternoon or evening have been inseminated the next morning. This method is known as "AM–PM breeding" and has been used successfully for many years. However, inseminating cows using the AM–PM schedule is not always practical, and several recent studies have demonstrated little difference between a once-a-day breeding schedule and the AM-PM method.

In fact, various reports have indicated that conception rates similar to twice-a-day (AM–PM) breeding can be obtained when cows are inseminated using a once-a-day schedule.[1,2,3] Table 16.1 shows the results of a field trial comparing the once-a-day and AM-PM breeding for 166 Pennsylvania dairy herds.

Overall, cows should be bred within 24 hours of the onset of standing heat, since sev-

[1] R. H. Foote. 1978. Time of artificial insemination and fertility in dairy cattle. J. Dairy Sci. 62:355.
[2] F. C. Gwazdauskas, J. A. Lineweaver, and W. E. Vinson. 1981. Rates of conception by artificial insemination of dairy cattle. J. Dairy Sci. 64:358.
[3] R. Fogwell. 1990. Scheduling AI in dairy cattle. The MABC/Bullhorn 40 (October):7.

**Table 16.1.** 75 day non-return rates for once-daily and AM–PM artificial insemination[a]

| AI Program | Cows (no.) | Non-Return Rate |
|---|---|---|
| Once daily | 3659 | 60.1 |
| AM–PM | 3581 | 60.6 |

[a]R. L. Nebel, et al. 1994. Timing of artificial insemination of dairy cows: Fixed time once daily vs morning and afternoon. J. Dairy Sci. 77: 3185.

eral studies show a sharp decline in conception after this point. The individual herd management practices will likely determine whether AM–PM or once-a-day breeding is employed.

The objective in timing insemination is to insure that a population of viable sperm is present in the female genital tract before the ovum is released. The fertile life of the ovum is much shorter (a few to about 10 hours after ovulation) than the life of the sperm cell (about 18 to 30 hours); and since sperm must undergo capacitation before being capable of fertilization, they should be present in the genital tract several hours prior to ovulation. During the capacitation process, changes in the acrosomal and plasma membranes of the spermatozoa result in release of enzymes that enable the sperm to immediately penetrate the ovum.

While there may be a fairly broad range in the time to inseminate after the beginning of estrus, a preponderance of data indicates that the best conception rate occurs when the cows are inseminated from about 4 to 14 hours after the beginning of the heat period. Another factor that should be considered in determining the best time to AI is embryo quality. Virginia research has revealed that early breeding after onset of estrus results in higher quality embryos but also lower fertilization rates (i.e., due to lower accessibility of sperm to the ovum), while later breeding following the onset of estrus (~24 hours) results in higher fertilization rates but lower embryo quality (i.e., due to aging of the ovum or insufficient viable sperm).

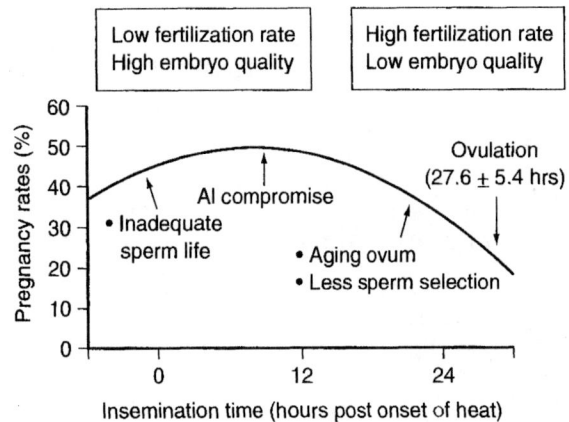

**Figure 16.2.** AI as a compromise based on early inseminations being inadequate due to high levels of unfertilized ova and late inseminations characterized by poor embryo quality. However, high embryo quality appears to be associated with early insemination and high fertilization rates are associated with late insemination. (R. G. Saacke. 1998. AI fertility: Are we getting the job done? Proc. 17th Tech. Conf. on Artificial Insemination and Reproduction. NAAB. p. 6)

Thus, acceptable pregnancy rates appear to represent a compromise between embryo quality and fertilization rates (see Figure 16.2).

Nevertheless, the optimal time to inseminate depends upon the frequency of accurate heat detection. Nebel and Mowrey[4] have recommended that: 1) when visual observations for estrus are frequent (every 2 to 4 hours) cows should be inseminated approximately 12 hours following detection (the AM–PM method), 2) when cows are visually observed

---

[4] Nebel, R. L. and C. M. Mowrey. 2000. When to breed—Have we been wrong all these years? Hoard's Dairyman. December 2000. p. 801.

for estrus less than six times daily, insemination should be performed about 6 hours following visual detection, since onset of estrus is not known, 3) with systems that record specific mounts, the first mount of standing estrus can be accurately identified, making the best time to inseminate 4 to 14 hours after onset of standing activity.

Study Figure 16.1 carefully, noting the behavior and conditions of a cow "Before Heat" (Items 1–3), during "Standing Heat" (Items 1–9), and "After Heat" (Items 1 and 2). The experienced herd operator becomes adept at observing the "signs" of a cow coming into heat and, throughout the period, then times the insemination accordingly.

## Practices and Aids in Heat Detection

Estrus detection efficiency is certainly a major factor influencing herd reproduction goals. Management practices should be such that cows and heifers are systematically checked for heat. Research data have indicated that upwards of 50 percent of all eligible ("breedable") heats go undetected and that between 10 and 30 percent of cows bred are not actually in heat. Obviously such errors need to be minimized. Management for good reproduction involves at least three factors: (1) accurate and easy identification of each animal while in the exercise lot or pasture; (2) an accurate, up-to-date record of breeding, calving, and observed heat dates; and (3) eternal vigilance on the part of herd operators and their employees to regularly observe cows and heifers for heat. See to it that the information is recorded, and if in order, arrange to have the animal inseminated.

Cows come into heat equally during all hours of the day. Although the precise time a cow comes into heat is difficult to determine based on visual observations, it is critical to schedule as many observations periods as possible to detect the highest proportion of cows and heifers in heat. Proper timing of insemi-

nation is impossible if heat periods are not observed. The trend toward larger herds and mass handling of cattle has increased problems associated with heat detection. Some practices and aids used to assist in heat detection are:

1. **Heat expectancy charts**—These charts are calendars that indicate when the female is expected to return to estrus, based on previous cyclicity. Information may be recorded, such as various signs of estrus and results from estrus detection aids. The use of heat expectancy charts helps farm employees assigned to estrus detection focus on when individual females should be coming into heat. This certainly improves detection of short or weak heat periods that might be missed if attention were not focused on these females.

2. **Twice-daily turnout during the winter months**—Cows continually confined to stalls may not exhibit heat but often do so if turned out in contact with other cows. New York studies indicate a 6 percent higher non-return rate for cows turned out twice daily as compared to cows not turned out at all. Also, as has been demonstrated in the collection of semen from bulls used in AI, mounting activity can be enhanced with a change in collection room location or a change in the animals that are interacted with. Presenting novel stimuli to cows is apt to be equally as effective in creating an atmosphere conducive to improving mounting activity during heat observation.

3. **Heat-mount detector pad**—A pressure-sensitive device called a "heat-mount detector pad" has been found to be helpful to both dairy and beef

operators in detecting heat. The heat-mount detector pad is glued to the cow's rump about midway between the pin bones. The unactivated pad is white in color and contains non-toxic chemicals in two small separate chambers. When a herdmate mounts a cow that is equipped with the heat-mount detector pad, sustained pressure on the device causes the two chemicals to run together and produce a red color (Figure 16.3). The red color indicates that the cow has been mounted and is probably in heat. Partially activated detectors may indicate that the female is coming into heat.

Various reports indicate that the use of heat-mount detector pads, along with visual observation, may enable detection of nearly 100 percent of the heat periods in a herd. Such devices are particularly helpful for detecting heat in heifers in beef herds or in heifers in dairy herds that are often on pasture some distance from the milking herd. Difficulties with the heat-mount detector pad are that low-hanging brush, back scratchers, and cattle oilers can activate the detector, as will mounting by other cows when an animal is in a free stall or is tied and cannot escape. Usually, good management of the breeding herd can reduce the occurrence of such problems.

4. **Chalk, crayon, or paint on tail head**—In large herds, the practice of smearing the tail head and sacral area of open cows with soft chalk (orange, yellow, or blue in color), crayon, or tail paint provides an inexpensive and fairly efficient method to detect those cows that have been mounted. When an animal is mounted by other cows, the chalk, crayon, or paint becomes

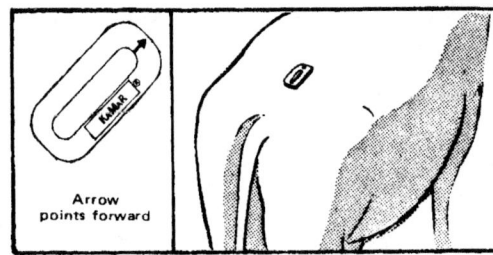

A

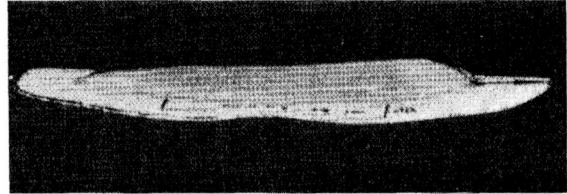

B

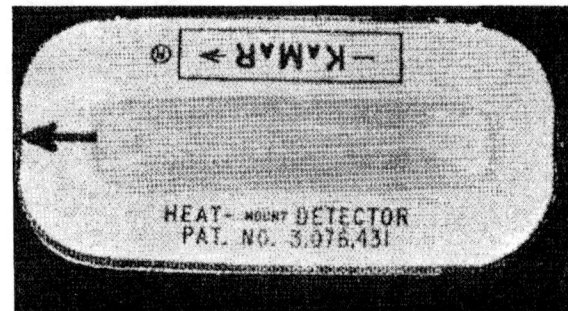

C

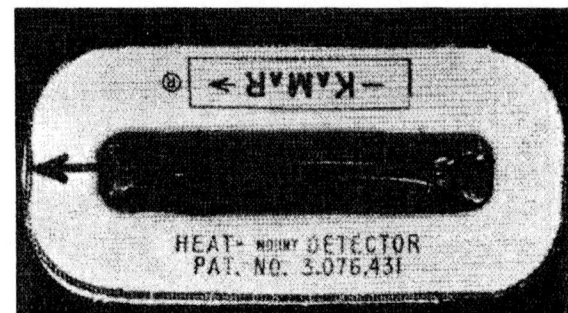

D

**Figure 16.3.** Use of heat-mount detector pads. (A) A heat-mount detector in place on a cow's back. (B) Profile view of a heat-mount detector showing how it sits on an animal's back. (C) Top view of unactivated detector. (D) Heat-mount detector after activation—indicates cow in heat. (Courtesy, KAMAR, Inc., Portland, ME)

smeared and partially rubbed off. The chalk must be applied at frequent intervals (every two to four days); however, this can be done easily while the cows are feeding.

155

5. **Spotter animals**—Since the bull is adept at detecting cows in heat, various methods have been devised to so utilize the bull's detection ability but to prevent natural insemination.

    a. One such method is use of the vasectomized bull, in which a segment of the ductus deferens from each spermatic cord is removed. The blood and nerve supplies are left intact, and the testes function normally; however, sperm are blocked from reaching the urethra. The vasectomized bull has normal sexual behavior. Since sexual contact is made when mounting, it is important that the vasectomized bull be health tested and free of venereally transmitted diseases.

    b. Another method is use of the "gomer" bull, resulting from a surgical procedure called a "penectomy," in which a portion of the penis is removed and provisions are made for urination. No sexual contact is possible with the gomer bull, which overcomes the problem of transmitting venereal disease.

    c. Another method is to block extrusion of the penis by an easy-to-install device for the purpose, the Pen-O-Block, sold by the Pen-O-Block Co., Tallahassee, Florida.

    A chin ball marker is used on spotter bulls. The ink from the chin ball marker leaves a colored streak on the rump of the mounted cow.

6. **Androgenized cows, heifers, or steers**—A low-quality dry cow, heifer, or steer treated with testosterone (or a combination of testosterone and estrogen) will make an effective teaser, or heat detector, animal. The animal chosen for the hormone treatment should have good feet and legs and be large enough to mount cows. Studies at Michigan State University[5] indicate that the use of animals treated with the male hormone is more effective in detecting cows in heat than other methods attempted. However, not every animal responds to hormone treatment, or some may become refractory.

    "Masculinized" cows, heifers, or steers that mount open cows and heifers do not spread venereal disease and need not be surgically altered. They are also quieter and easier to handle than gomer bulls. Hormone treatment should start with gradual doses as recommended by a veterinarian. A testosterone implant, effective for four to six months, may also be used. Booster injections are given when a treated animal becomes less aggressive. If a hormone-treated animal is disposed of, the necessary withholding time should be observed before shipment for slaughter. Dairy operators in increasing numbers are utilizing this type of teaser for heat detection. Androgenized detector animals are also fitted with a chin ball marker.

7. **Electronic devices**—Various electronic devices have been used for heat detection.

    a. A commercially available probe that can be inserted into the cow's vagina measures changes in electrical resistance of the mucus. Low probe readings are characteristic of estrus. The device is expensive, and readings must be made frequently. Also, the portion of the

---

[5] J. S. Stevenson and J. H. Britt. 1977. Detection of estrus by three methods. J. Dairy Sci. 60:1994.

156

probe placed in the female genital tract must be meticulously sanitized between uses to avoid spreading disease.

b. Electronic pedometers are available that monitor the amount of a cow's walking activity, which is known to increase (about four times) during the estrus period. A pedometer is usually installed on a leg band, and it can be read manually or automatically in the milking parlor. Fertility based on pedometer readings has been shown to be comparable to that based on visual observation for standing heat. Durability and cost are important considerations.

c. A radiotelemetric system called Heat Watch® (DDx Incorporated, Denver, CO) came onto the market in the mid-1990's. This system uses a miniaturized pressure-sensitive radio frequency transmitter that is affixed to the sacral region of the cow. When the heat mount transducer is activated, it sends a signal to a remote receiver which then transmits data to a personal computer. Data includes transmitter (cow) ID, date (month, day, year), time (hour and minute), and duration of sensor activation. Program software converts data into cow activity reports that herd operators use to make breeding decisions. This system appears to be very accurate and can monitor estrus continuously. Users have reported increased estrus detection efficiency and improved AI conception rates. A major advantage is that the onset of estrus can be determined precisely. Limitations are that the range of transmitters is one-quarter mile (but can be boosted) and the system is costly.

The previously listed aids are helpful under conditions of herd management best suited for their use. Visual observation and management by the herd operator, adequate records, and animal identification should always accompany their use. No one should make the mistake of depending entirely on any one aid as the full answer to effective heat detection.

It should also be noted that conditions such as hot and cold environmental temperatures and lots or paddocks that do not provide good footing for cattle tend to result in decreased mounting activity and increased difficulty in detecting estrus.

## When to Inseminate Following Calving

The reproductive tract of the cow should have time to recover from producing a previous calf before being inseminated again. Normally, although there are often exceptions due to disease or injury in calving, it requires 30 to 40 days for involution (return to normal) of the cow's uterus. Various studies indicate that, on the average, the highest non-return rate is obtained when cows are inseminated about 60 to 80 days following calving; however, in order to maintain a calving interval of about 12 to 13 months for the herd, some cows need to be inseminated between 40 and 60 days following calving. When a cow has fully recovered from a previous freshening and is discharging clear mucus from the vulva when in heat, insemination 40 to 60 days post-partum seems practical.

Many herd operators have a veterinarian routinely check each cow following parturition to determine the condition of the reproductive tract before breeding back. Such a veterinary herd-health program is a good policy and can identify problems and reduce days open for many cows. High-producing cows may come

157

into heat a few weeks later following calving than lower-producing cows, and their first-service conception rates may be as much as 15 to 20 percent lower. Herd operators need to consider these factors in a reproductive management program.

## Heat Cycles Following Calving

Most normal cows come into heat 25 to 40 days after calving. Some may show signs of heat as early as 15 to 20 days after calving, but they should not be bred at that time. Heat periods may vary from 18 to 25 days in length. While the average interval between heats is about 21 days, a cow that has a normal reproductive tract should be inseminated if cycling regularly. Exceptions are the cow discharging pus and the cow in heat every 14 to 15 days, which is probably "cystic" and requires veterinary attention.

## PROCEDURE

### Equipment

AI equipment and supplies are sanitized when manufactured and packaged to prevent contamination. The inseminator should always keep insemination supplies enclosed in the manufacturer's package until ready for use. Most technicians use disposable insemination supplies. These should not be reused and should be collected and destroyed or disposed of immediately after use. The disposable plastic obstetrical sleeve (shoulder-length glove) is the most common type of protection used for the palpating arm. However, reusable rubber obstetrical sleeves may be used and should be washed thoroughly in a disinfectant solution after every insemination.

The inseminator's kit, which is used to organize and carry insemination supplies, should also be kept sanitary by protecting it and its contents from contamination and by regular cleansing with a disinfectant solution.

The equipment and supplies needed to inseminate cattle include:

1. An inventory of frozen semen stored in a liquid nitrogen refrigerator.

2. An inseminator's kit.

3. A thaw container and thermometer for measuring temperature when thawing semen (usually incorporated into the inseminator's kit).

4. Disposable shoulder-length plastic gloves.

5. Paper towels and soap.

6. Lubricant (K-Y jelly or other non-toxic lubricant).

7. Straw tweezers or forceps.

8. Scissors or straw cutter.

9. Insemination gun.

10. Sheaths.

11. Rubber footwear or disposable plastic boots.

12. Bucket and boot brush.

13. Disinfectant solution.

For ampules:

1. Disposable plastic insemination tubes (Figure 16.4).

2. Disposable plastic polybulbs or syringe fitted with rubber tubing (Figure 16.4).

3. Ampule scribe.

All equipment and supplies listed can be purchased from AI organizations or various agricultural supply houses (see Appendix C). Liquid nitrogen is needed on a continuing basis and is routinely available from semen suppliers.

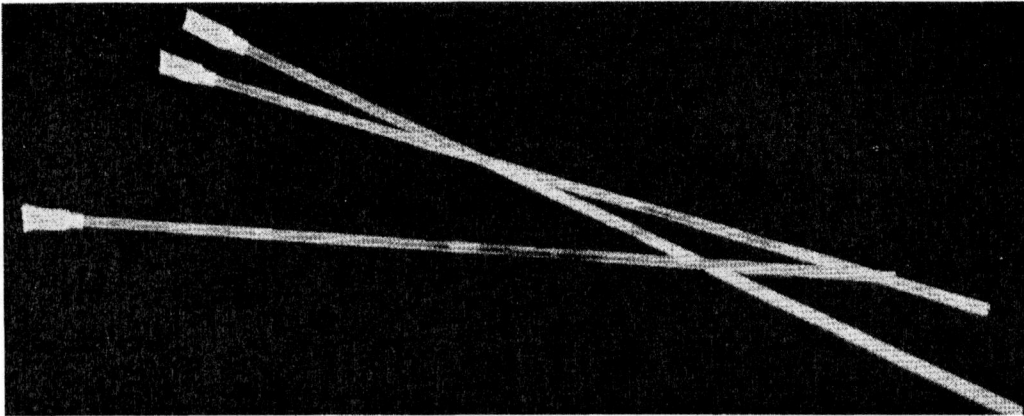

**Figure 16.4.** Plastic insemination tubes, with attached polybulbs, for semen packaged in ampules. (Courtesy, Edwards Agri-Supply, Inc., Baraboo, WI)

One of the chief advantages of artificial insemination is that it allows for the prevention of reproductive diseases that could be spread by bulls in natural breeding. This advantage is made possible by providing semen for artificial insemination from healthy bulls and by using sanitary supplies and techniques in the insemination process. However, this advantage can be negated by failing to maintain sanitary conditions when inseminating cows or heifers.

Inseminators, whether professionals representing AI organizations or persons inseminating cows in their own herds, should keep all equipment in clean, neatly organized kits. Following the insemination, they should properly dispose of used articles (AI shoulder-length gloves, sheaths, soiled paper towels, and so forth) and clean and disinfect their boots and kit before moving to the next herd or location.

It is the mark of a careless inseminator when unsightly used equipment is left lying around. It is also the responsibility of the herd owner to provide receptacles (garbage cans or barrels) for the inseminator's use.

## Insemination

The recto-vaginal technique is the most efficient method for bovine artificial insemination and is in use worldwide. Beginning inseminators should concentrate on developing knowledge and skill in the use of this method. They should study diagrams of the cow's reproductive tract, examine reproductive organs removed from slaughtered cows, and practice inserting and passing an AI tube through the cervix of both the excised reproductive tracts and the reproductive tracts of live cows and/or heifers.

In addition to using proper inseminating techniques, it is important to thaw and utilize frozen semen correctly if high fertility is to be maintained. (Exercise 14 outlines details of handling and thawing frozen semen.)

The recto-vaginal technique is the same whether using liquid or frozen semen packaged in ampules, straws, pipets, or pellets.

Steps in Inseminating the Cow

1. Identify the cow that is to be inseminated. If it is a registered animal, be sure to note the complete name and registration number as well as the ear tag or neck chain number. The inseminator and the herd owner should be knowledgeable of the AI requirements of the particular breed registry association.

2. Restrain the cow in a stanchion or breeding chute as appropriate and, if

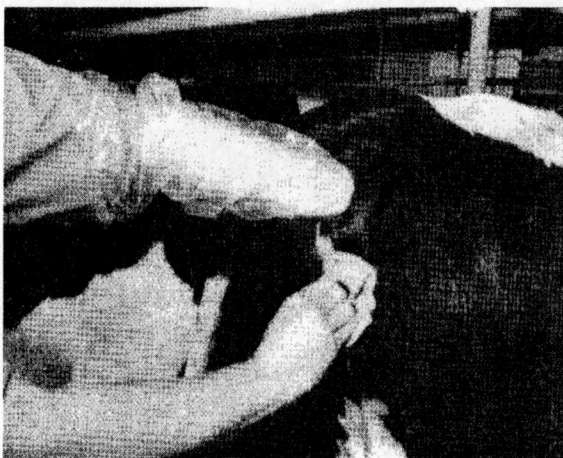

**Figure 16.5.** Cleaning the vulva area of the cow prior to insemination. (Courtesy, ABS Global, DeForest, WI)

needed, clean the vulva and adjacent parts with warm water. Use soap only if the animal is extremely dirty, and wash all soap away before drying with a paper towel (Figure 16.5).

3. After properly thawing the frozen semen and loading the insemination gun (see Exercise 14), wrap the loaded AI gun in a paper towel and tuck it inside the coveralls for protection until breeding.

4. Wearing a sleeved plastic or rubber glove, place the hand (usually the left) into the rectum of the cow, and remove the fecal matter. This is best accomplished by first inserting two or three fingers into the opening of the anus and allowing air to enter the rectum, which usually causes the cow to eliminate feces (Figures 16.6A, 16.6B). Lubricating the gloved hand and arm and the anal region of the cow will make insertion of the hand easier. Mild soap and water are frequently used, as well as K-Y jelly. The cow's tail should be located on the outside of the palpating arm. It may also help to grasp the cow's tail about

8 to 10 inches down from the tail head with the free hand while inserting the palpating hand into the cow's rectum. If the rectum doesn't empty, the feces should be removed manually. Complete removal of feces however, is not to be expected. Once most of the feces are removed, constriction rings of the rectal wall are likely to be encountered. Relax these rings by placing two fingers through the rings and gently massaging back and forth. Next, locate the cervix. Locating and controlling the cervix is essential to the technique of artificial insemination, and this skill must be mastered before further steps are attempted. With the constriction rings relaxed, the cervix, usually lying on the floor of the pelvis, can be located by "sweeping" the fingers across the floor of the pelvic cavity. The cervix has a hard, gristly feel and is easily identified. Once the cervix is found, the body of the uterus and the uterine horns, located forward of (anterior to) the cervix, can be felt. In the open cow in heat, the uterine horns are usually firm and coiled back on each side of the body of the uterus. A schematic view of the cow's reproductive tract is shown in Figure 16.7.

In older cows, the reproductive tract may lie further forward than in young cows. In pregnant cows or in cows with considerable pus in the uterus, the reproductive organs may be far forward in the abdominal cavity. Beginners should practice on as many cows as possible and learn "the feel" of the reproductive organs when grasped with the gloved hand through the wall of the rectum. The fingers become "educated" to the feel of the various parts of the cow's reproductive tract only with experience.

160

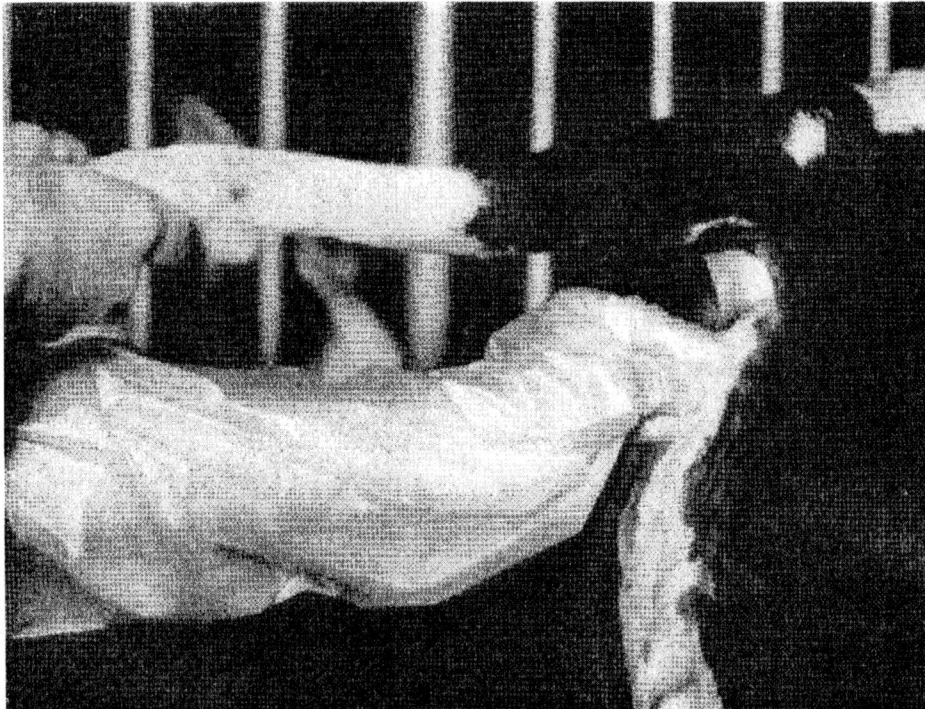

**Figure 16.6A.** Inserting the palpating hand into the cow's rectum prior to recto-vaginal insemination. Lubrication and forming the fingers into the shape of a cone facilitate entry. (Courtesy, Select Sires, Inc., Plain City, OH)

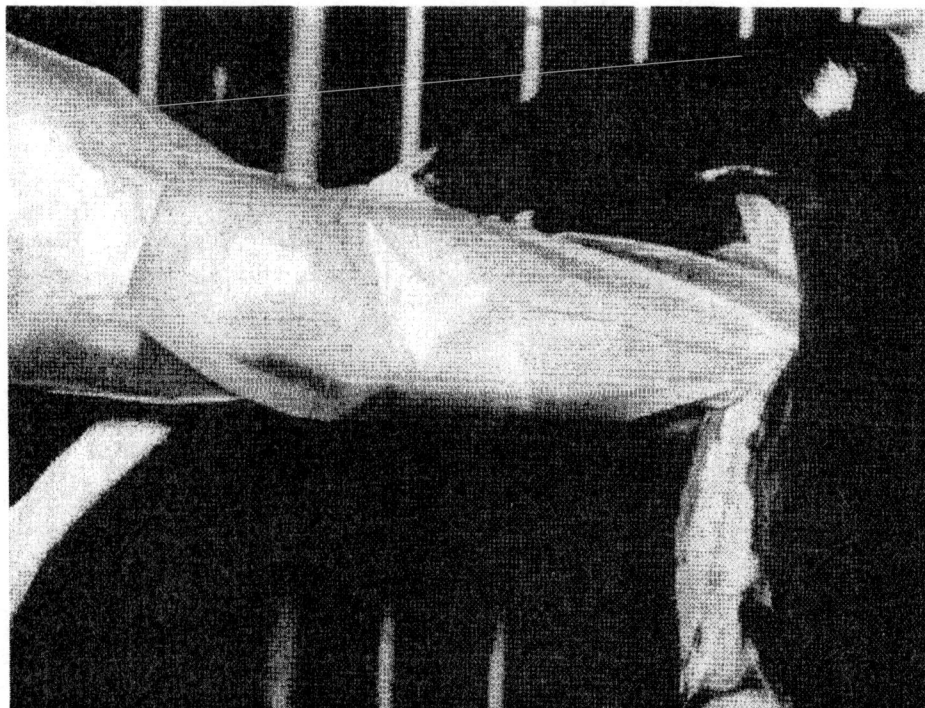

**Figure 16.6B.** After insertion of the palpating hand, remaining fecal matter is removed and the inseminator can locate the cervix. *Note:* The cow's tail is placed on the outside of inseminator's arm to keep it from interfering with the insemination procedure. (Courtesy, Select Sires, Inc., Plain City, OH)

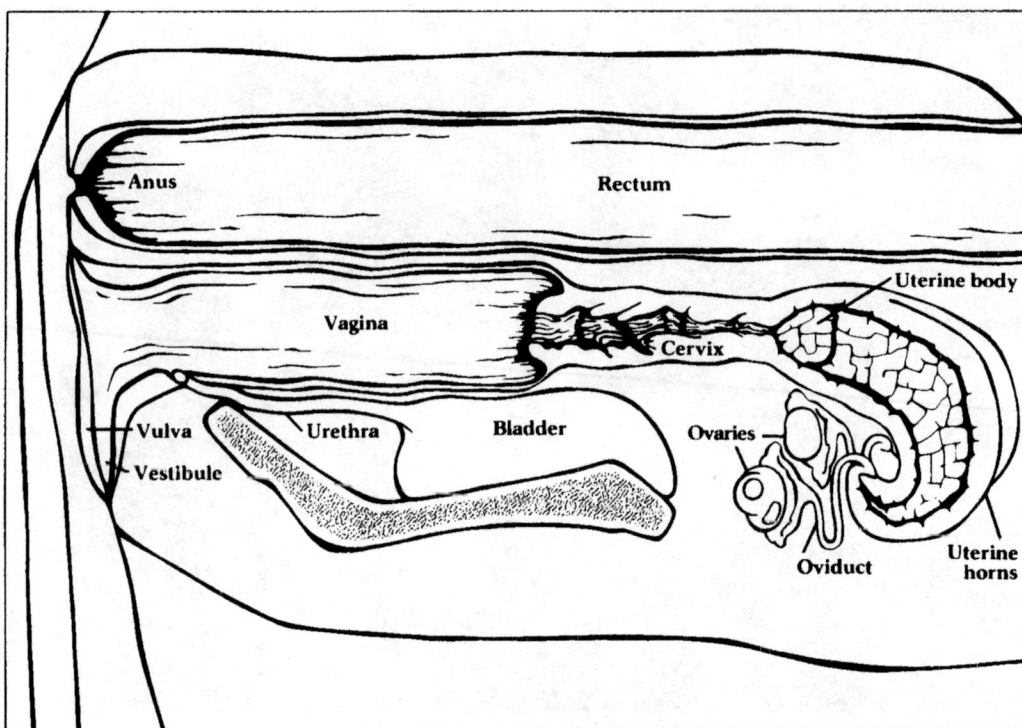

**Figure 16.7.** Schematic view of the female reproductive tract, showing its relationship to other anatomical structures. (Courtesy, ABS Global, DeForest, WI)

5. Having located the cervix, firmly grasp it with the thumb and first two fingers. At this time, with an absorbent paper towel, wipe the vulva clean and dry, particularly the lips, to reduce contamination of the inseminating instrument as it is inserted into the reproductive tract. Spread the lips of the vulva by gently pressing down on the vaginal opening with the palpating hand. Carefully insert the insemination tube or loaded AI gun through the vestibule and into the vagina at an upward angle of about 30 degrees. This avoids entering the opening of the bladder (urethra), which is located on the floor of the vestibule, and facilitates entering the vagina.

The next step is to control the cervix so that the inseminating instrument can be directed into and eventually passed through it. The cervix should be pushed slightly forward at this time to eliminate any folds in the vaginal wall. With the other hand, level the insemination tube or AI gun and gently push it forward until the tip just reaches the external opening of the cervix (Figures 16.8A, 16.8B).

Withdraw the AI tube about an inch, and encircle the back end of the cervix with the thumb and first two fingers. The rest of the palpating hand serves to guide the tube into the cervical canal. The insemination tube or AI gun should be gently pushed forward and worked through the cervix. The thumb and first two fingers are kept just ahead of the tip of the AI tube so as to manipulate the cervix. The cervix should be gently maneuvered over the tube. Don't try to force the tube through the cervix. Severe injury to the

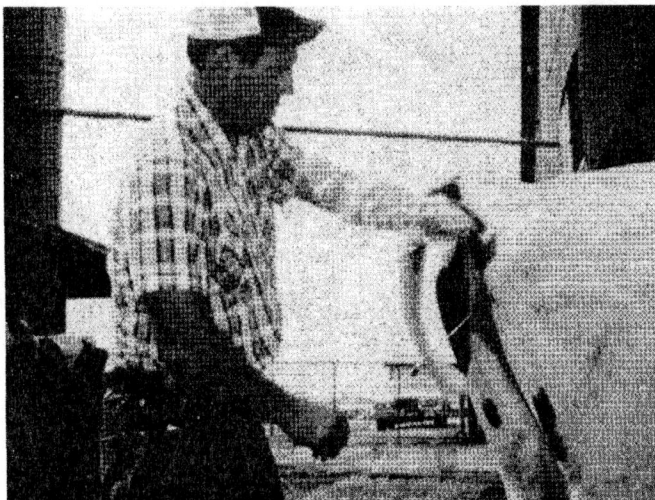

**Figure 16.8A.** Inserting the insemination gun into the reproductive tract at an upward angle. (Courtesy, Select Sires, Inc., Plain City, OH)

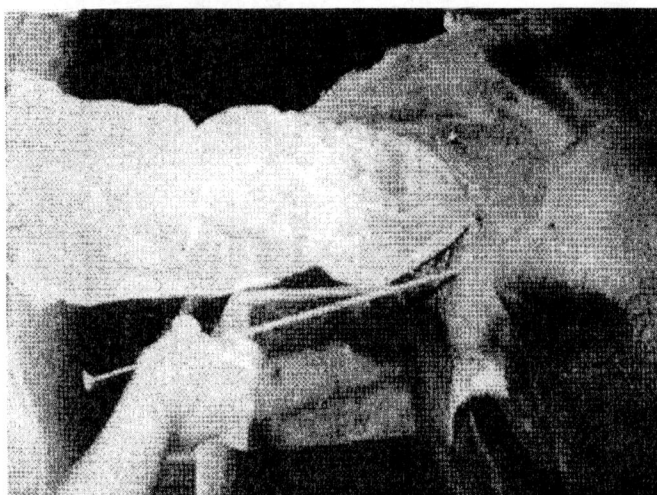

**Figure 16.8B.** The insemination gun is leveled and gently pushed forward into the vagina. (Courtesy, Select Sires, Inc., Plain City, OH)

tissues or perforation may result. Since the cervix has several folds (annular rings), the insemination tube should be manipulated up and down so as to pass through these rings. Sometimes the cervical opening is not in the center of the cervix but is located to either side or on the upper or lower part of the cervix. Use the forefinger of the palpating hand to feel the tip of the tube and to determine when it has penetrated the cervical opening. Guide the tube gently until it has just passed through the cervix into the body of the uterus. The body of the uterus extends only about ¾ of an inch anteriorly beyond the internal cervical opening.

*Note:* To reduce the possible introduction of contaminants into the uterus during the insemination process, some inseminators use disposable sanitary sheath protectors that fit over the AI gun sheath. With the sheath protector in place, as the AI gun is introduced into the cervix, slight forward pressure causes the AI gun tip to break through the sheath protector and into the cervical canal, avoiding any direct contact with the cow's vestibule and vagina.

163

6. Expel the semen slowly, using gentle pressure on the AI gun plunger, bulb, or syringe. Take at least five seconds. This insures expulsion of most of the semen out of the insemination tube or gun. For a first service, it is recommended that semen be deposited in the body of the uterus (or a little may be deposited in each horn). On subsequent services (or in situations in which the cow or heifer may be pregnant), semen should be deposited in the middle portion of the cervix. This prevents any possible damage to the mucus plug in the anterior cervical canal that might interrupt an early pregnancy.

*Note:* There are differences of opinion as to the best site of semen deposition (i.e., body of uterus vs. deep in the uterine horns) for a first service. With horn breeding there appears to be a greater chance for uterine bleeding and possible infection to occur. However, there doesn't seem to be any appreciable difference in conception rate whether semen is deposited in the body of the uterus or in the uterine horns.

Figure 16.9A to 16.9E schematically depicts important steps in the rectovaginal insemination technique.

Beginners usually have trouble at first in "passing" the insemination tube through the cervix. Practice and patience are necessary. In some cows, and particularly heifers, it is impossible to pass the tube all the way through the cervix. In some cases, the semen is simply expelled in the cervix on a first service, and the results are practically equal to those of uterine insemination. At no time should the insemination tube or AI gun be forced.

7. Following semen deposition, slowly withdraw the insemination tube or AI gun and the palpating arm. Holding the used insemination tube or AI gun sheath in the palpating hand, remove the shoulder-length AI glove, turning it inside out over the soiled equipment.

8. Dispose of the used equipment in waste containers, clean and sanitize the scissors/straw cutter and AI gun, and wash hands.

9. Complete the necessary records on the barn chart or the necessary herd breeding and calving records. If needed, supply the appropriate breeding receipt.

10. Clean and disinfect boots and bottom of the AI kit.

Other techniques for artificial insemination that have been used with varied success are the speculum method and vaginal deposition method. These techniques are no longer popular and do not yield results as good as the recto-vaginal method;[6] however, they are briefly described here for general information.

## Speculum Method

1. Identify and restrain the cow to be inseminated.

2. Clean the vulva and adjacent parts, and wipe the vulva dry. Place nontoxic lubricating jelly on the lips of the vulva.

3. Draw the semen into the insemination tube, to which a polybulb is affixed, or use a syringe connected to the insemination tube by means of a rubber tubing connector in place of the polybulb (Figure 16.10). The insemination tube should be about 3 inches longer than the speculum.

---

[6] J. J. Sullivan, et al. 1972. A comparison of recto-vaginal, vaginal and speculum approaches for insemination of cows and heifers. The A.I. Digest 20 (January):6.

**Figure 16.9.** Steps in the recto-vaginal insemination technique. (Courtesy, Select Sires, Inc., Plain City, OH)

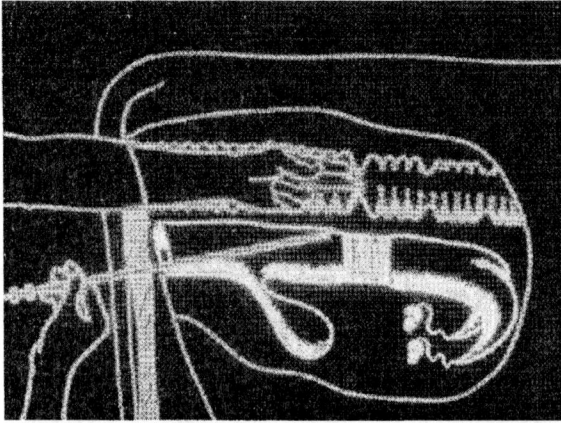

*Step A.* Constriction rings in the rectal wall can be relaxed by placing two fingers through the rings and gently massaging back and forth. The insemination gun is inserted into the vagina.

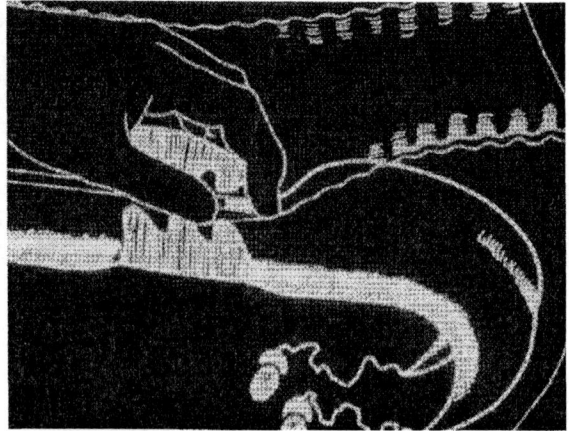

*Step B.* The cervix is manipulated over the insemination gun or AI tube.

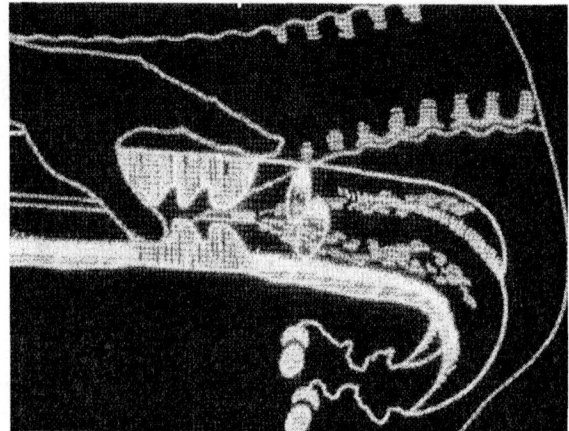

*Step C.* The forefinger is used to help position the tip of the AI gun at the internal cervical opening.

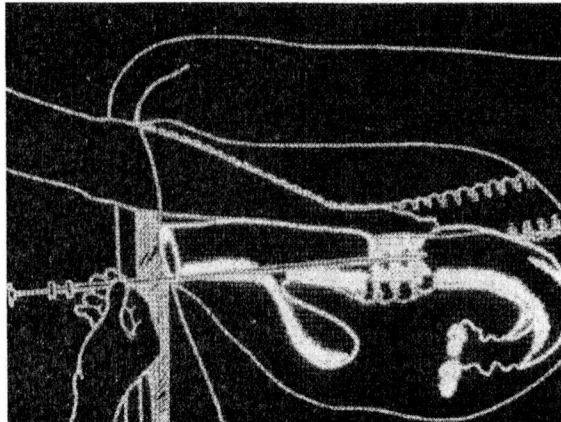

*Step D.* Semen is slowly deposited in the body of the uterus.

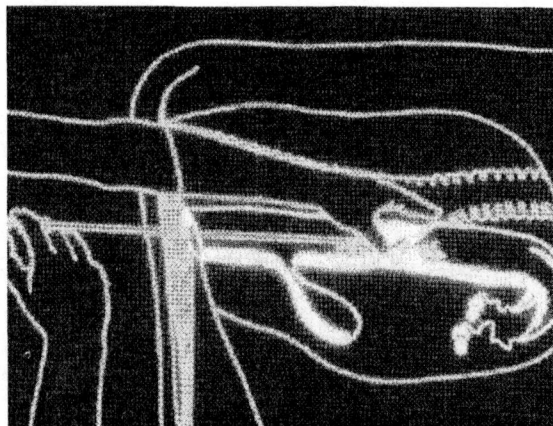

*Step E.* Care must be taken not to pull back on the AI gun while expelling the semen, to avoid withdrawal from the uterus and mis-deposition of any semen in the cervix or vagina.

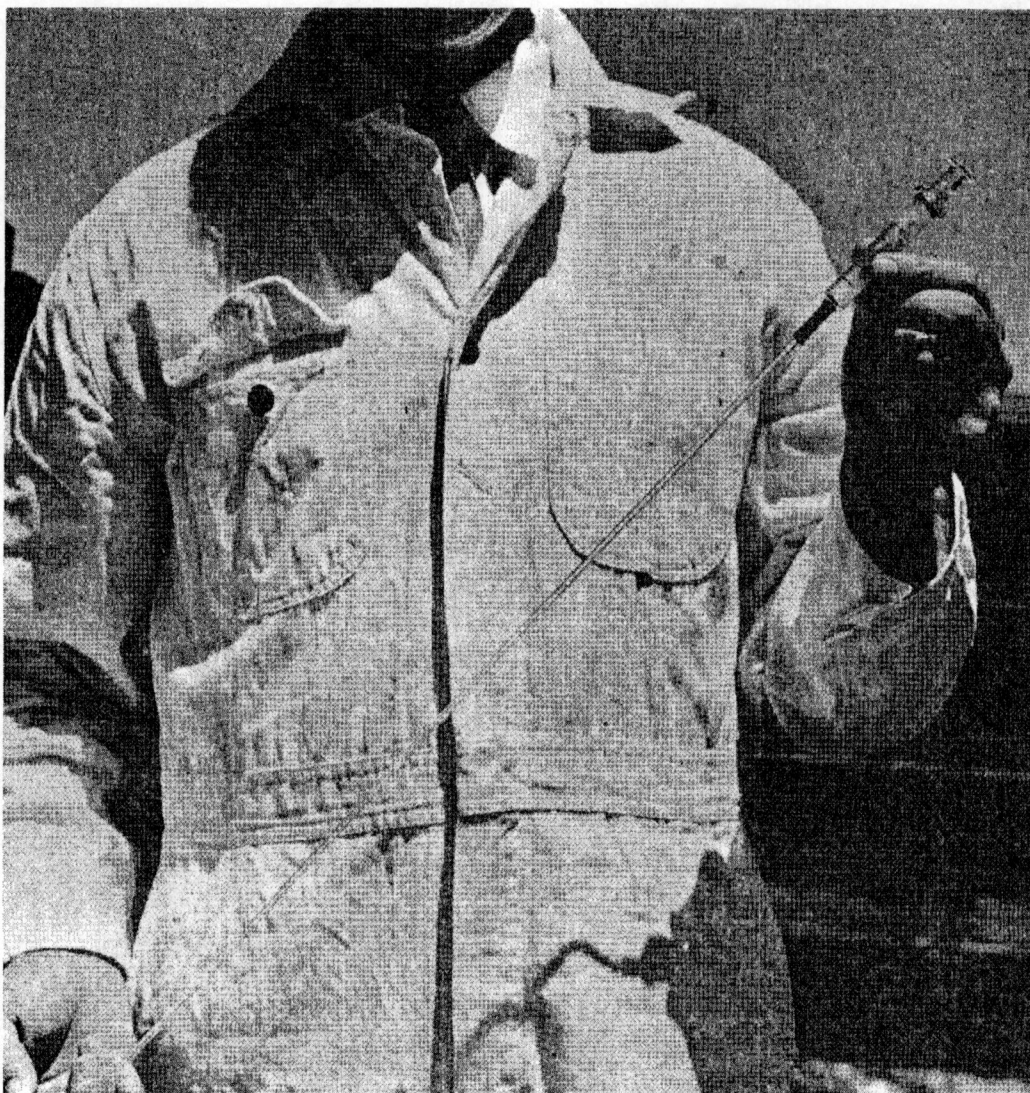

**Figure 16.10.** The insemination tube and attached syringe used for insemination with the aid of a speculum. The insemination tube should be at least 18 inches long, or about 3 inches longer than the speculum.

4. Gently insert a heavy-walled Pyrex glass speculum, about 16 inches long, into the vagina. The cervix is located by means of a pen light inserted into the speculum or by means of a headlight (Figure 16.11).

5. When the speculum is in place (it must be held or the cow will expel it) and the cervix has been located, place the tip of the insemination tube into the external cervical opening. The speculum should be withdrawn about 1 inch so that semen that may run out of the cervix will not be withdrawn when the speculum is removed. The insemination tube can be inserted into the cervix to a depth of about 1 inch. This is not difficult when the cow is in heat. In some cows, the tube may easily penetrate further, but force should not be used. Slowly expel the semen by pressing on the polybulb or syringe (Figures 16.11 and 16.12).

6. Withdraw the speculum and the insemination tube. Record all the necessary information. Keep the used

166

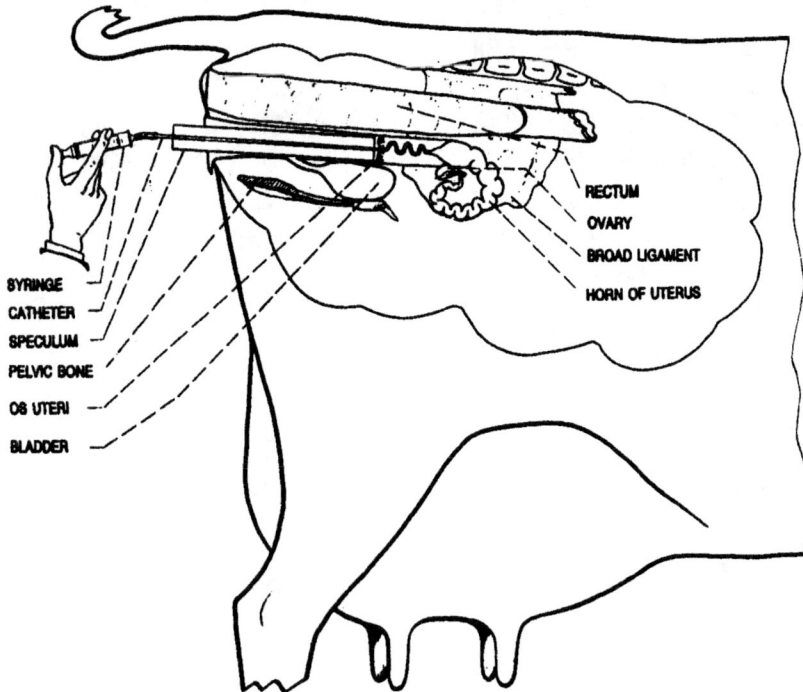

**Figure 16.11.** Schematic drawing of insemination using the speculum method.

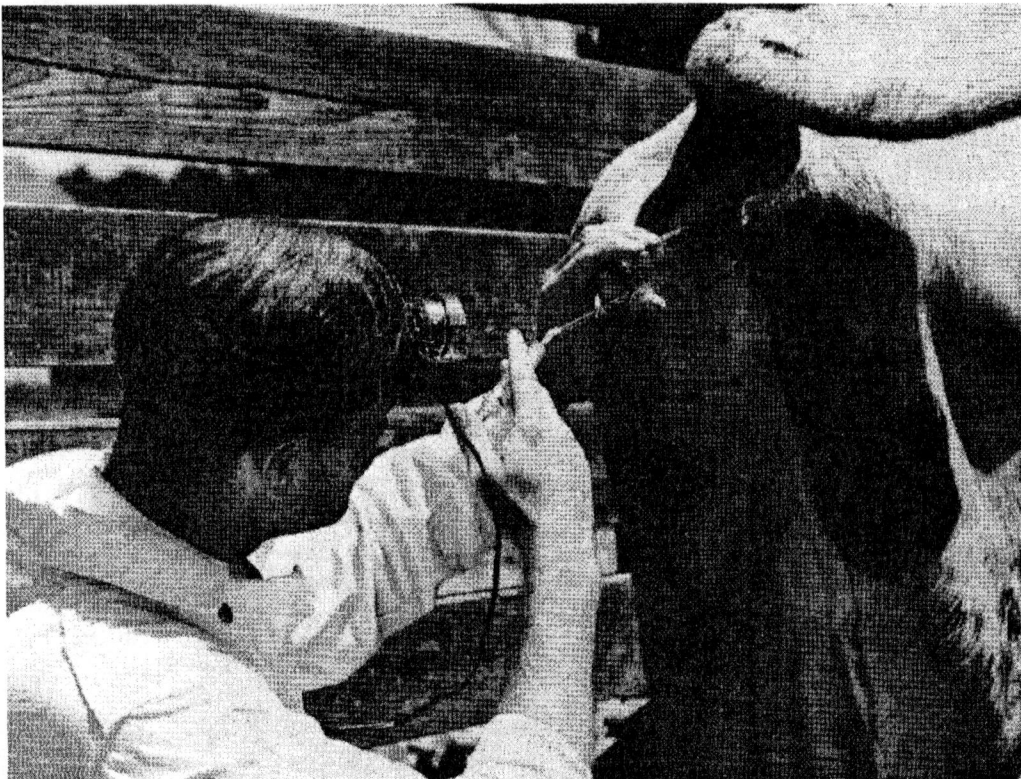

**Figure 16.12.** The speculum in place, the cervix located by headlight, and semen being deposited into the external cervical opening.

speculum and other non-disposable equipment in a separate container, or wrap the items in paper towels, until they can be washed and sterilized.

Objections to the speculum method are the job of washing and sterilizing equipment; the need for a separate speculum for each cow inseminated at a given time; and the fact that, under field conditions, the first-service non-return rate is about 10 percent lower than with the recto-vaginal technique.

**Vaginal Method—** The insemination tube of semen, fitted with a bulb or syringe, is simply inserted into the anterior vagina and the semen expelled near the external opening of the cervix.

Semen contained in gelatin capsules and inserted into the vagina has also been tried in numerous cases. While conception may result, the rate is low. The vaginal method is the least desirable of the three methods of insemination described.

## QUESTIONS

1. At what stage of heat should cows be inseminated? Why? When does ovulation occur in relation to heat?

2. What is the rationale for recommended timing of insemination? What are the usual signs that a cow is in heat? How often should the herd be checked for cows in heat? What aids are available for detecting cows in heat?

3. What is the appearance of the vulva, cervix, and uterus during the estrus period? During the non-estrus period? Explain the physiological reasons for these changes.

4. At what site in the reproductive tract should the semen be deposited? Why?

5. What is the typical volume of semen used per insemination?

6. What are the steps to be followed in preparing the cow and making the insemination?

7. How are cows identified for insemination?

8. What records should the inseminator keep? What records should be left with the herd owner?

9. In regard to AI technique, are there any advantages in using the "straw system" over other semen-packaging methods? Explain.

10. Why should all equipment used for insemination be kept neat, clean, and sanitary? Why should inseminators wash their boots and the bottom of AI kit in disinfectant before leaving the farm?

## REFERENCES

Dransfield, M. B. G., et al. 1998. Timing of insemination for dairy cows identified in estrus by a radiotelemetric estrus detection system. J. Dairy Sci. 81: 1874.

Fricke, P. M., 1998. Assessment of AI and embryo transfer technique using transrectal ultrasonography. Proc. 17th Tech. Conf. on Artificial Insemination and Reproduction. NAAB. p. 63.

Jordan, Ellen R. (Ed.). 1983. Dairy Integrated Reproductive Management. Coop. Ext. Serv., West Virginia Univ. Fact Sheet Nos. IRM-5, 6, 7, 10.

Salisbury, G. W., N. L. Van Demark, and J. R. Lodge. 1978. Physiology of Reproduction and Artificial Insemination of Cattle (2nd Ed.). W. H. Freeman, San Francisco. (Chs. 18, 19, 22.)

Senger, P.L. 1996. Electronic approaches to the solution of the estrous detection problem. Proc. 16th Tech. Conf. On Artificial Insemination and Reproduction. NAAB. p. 12.

Sorenson, A. M., Jr. 1979. Animal Reproduction: Principles and Practices. McGraw-Hill, New York. (Ch. 12.)

Wiltbank, M. C., J. R. Pursley, and J. L. M. Vasconcelos. 2000. What is optimal time for AI? Proc. 18th Tech. Conf. On Artificial Insemination and Reproduction. NAAB. p. 83.

# EXERCISE 17

# Artificial Insemination of Beef Cattle; Controlled Estrus—Beef and Dairy

## OBJECT

To become familiar with the role of artificial insemination in beef improvement and how to make it work.

## DISCUSSION

In January 2002, the USDA reported there were about 33.1 million beef cows and 5.5 million beef replacement heifers in the United States. Most of these (about 95 percent) were kept for the production of commercial beef, and the remainder were registered "seed stock" cattle.

It is generally agreed among beef specialists that the most rapid improvements in economic traits of beef cattle can be achieved through (1) performance testing and the selection of breeding stock on the basis of performance and (2) the high use of outstanding, progeny-proven sires by means of artificial insemination. There must also be a program of sampling and proving young beef bulls. The true economic value of a beef bull, just as is true of a dairy bull, cannot be measured unless a progeny-testing program is followed. It's been stated[1] that "Unless each generation of bulls for artificial insemination is the product of the previous generation on which money has been spent, the profit from all the work on improvement through breeding is limited to expanding the use of good bulls in commercial herds and reducing the use of poor bulls" and that "Rate and direction of change are still influenced by the breeders from whom AI bulls are bought."

Through the use of artificial insemination, above-average, performance-tested bulls can be used on many cows; however, the most desirable route for improving beef cattle is the high use of outstanding *progeny-tested* bulls by means of artificial breeding, permitting such sires to account for as many as 15,000 calves a year rather than 25 to 50 under natural use. An example of a superior progeny-tested AI bull is shown in Figure 17.1.

The economic traits in beef cattle are moderately to highly heritable. Heritability is the proportion of the differences among cattle, measured or observed, that is attributable to genetics (additive gene action). The degree of heritability of a trait is significant because it determines the amount of genetic improvement

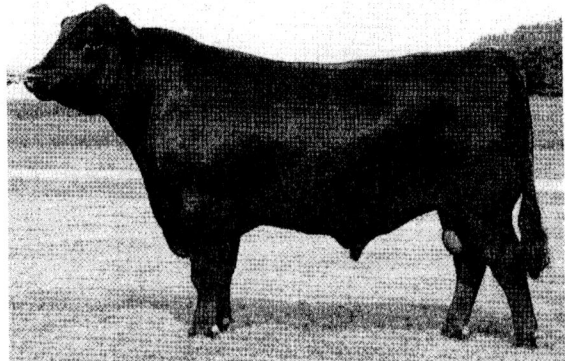

**Figure 17.1.** A popular Angus bull, 29AN1523 BON VIEW NEW DESIGN 878, Registration 13062750, available through artificial insemination. (Courtesy, ABS Global, DeForest, WI)

---

[1] I. M. Lerner and H. P. Donald. 1966. Modern Developments in Animal Breeding. Academic Press, London and New York.

**Table 17.1.** Heritability Estimates of Some Economically Important Traits in Beef Cattle[a]

| Trait | Heritability |
|---|---|
| Conception rate | .10 |
| Calving interval | .08 |
| Birth weight | .33 |
| Weaning weight | .28 |
| Cow maternal ability | .30 |
| Feedlot gain | .45 |
| Pasture gain | .28 |
| Efficiency of gain | .45 |
| Yearling weight | .40 |
| Conformation score | |
| Weaning | .28 |
| Yearling | .38 |
| Carcass traits | |
| Carcass grade | .33 |
| Ribeye area | .55 |
| Tenderness | .45 |
| Fat thickness | .33 |
| Retail product (%) | .30 |
| Retail product (lb.) | .65 |
| Cancer-eye susceptibility | .30 |

[a]A. L. Neumann and K. S. Lusby. 1986. Beef Cattle (8th Ed.). John Wiley & Sons, Inc., New York.

that can be made over time. Heritability estimates are expressed on a scale of 0 to 1.0. Selection of breeding stock for economic traits, particularly weaning weight and yearling weight, puts selection on a sound and scientific basis. Heritability estimates for several of the important economic traits in beef cattle are summarized in Table 17.1.

Beef producers stand to profit by the use of artificial insemination when bulls that transmit high rates of gain and high weaning weights are used. Some of the advantages of beef AI are:

1. Offers superior gains and more profit per feeder and, likewise, per finished steer (Figure 17.2).

2. Builds better inheritance for performance in the cow herd.

3. Controls the spread of disease by the bull.

4. Helps to maintain better breeding and calving records.

5. Makes the identification of cattle easier.

6. Produces calf crops nearly all at once, produces more uniform feeders, and will likely make the calving season shorter.

7. Permits the practice of crossbreeding without a great investment in bulls of a second breed.

8. Aids beef producers in reducing by 75 to 80 percent the number of bulls needed. If the majority of eligible cows and heifers can be inseminated at least once, or twice if necessary, only a few "clean up" bulls are needed.

9. Reduces the likelihood of inherited defects. Due to rigid sire selection, progeny testing, and screening of bulls used in artificial insemination, the risk of harmful recessives, such as dwarfism, osteopetrosis, and syndactylism and lethals is reduced to a minimum.

10. Allows the use of outstanding sires that transmit superior economic traits, thus yielding higher herd profits compared to use of natural service sires. (See "Artificial Insemination versus Natural Service" later in this exercise)

11. Encourages improved herd management.

## How to Make Beef Artificial Insemination Work

Artificial insemination of beef cattle has been used steadily since the 1960's. In 1963, some 235,000 beef cows were reported as serviced by AI organizations. Today, it is esti-

172

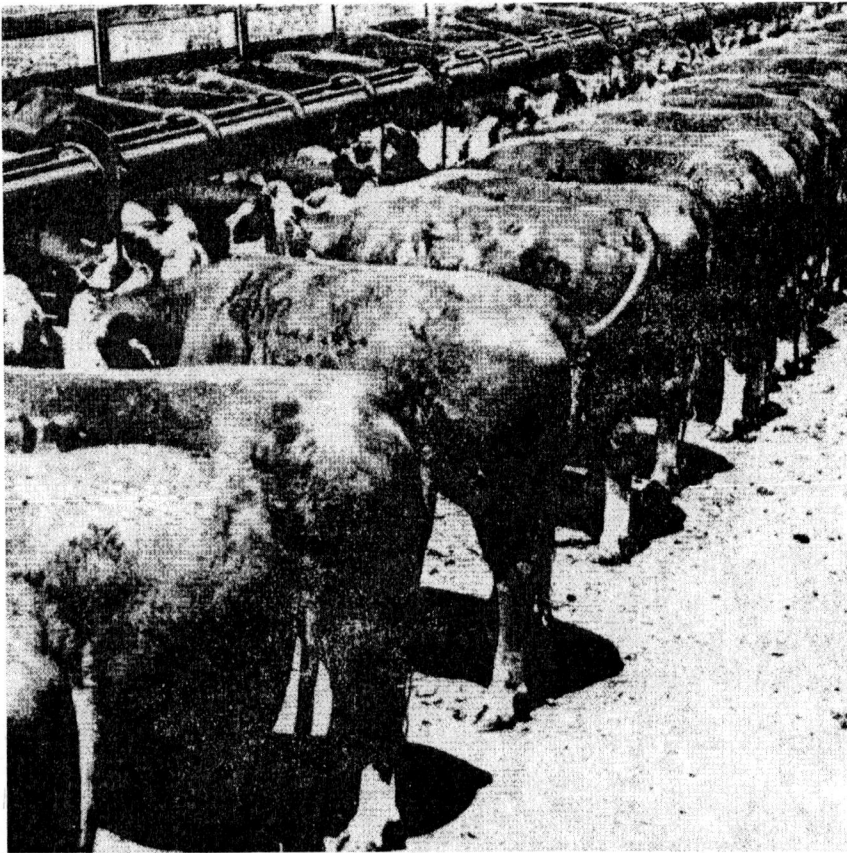

**Figure 17.2.** A uniform group of AI-sired steers in the feedlot. Sired by L9 Domino 7, 12601, a registered Polled Hereford bull, bred and tested at the U.S. Range Livestock Experiment Station, Miles City, MT.

mated that about 5 to 7 percent of the total beef cows and heifers of breeding age are bred using AI. This figure may be considered low, however, because it does not include a large number of privately owned bulls whose frozen semen is for sale.

One of the most important factors in making artificial insemination work is the attitude of herd operators. Once they decide that they must increase the dollar returns from their herds, they will generally find means to utilize artificial insemination and better sires for all or part of the herds. The following items are essential in making artificial insemination work.

## Management of the Herd

1. There should be a well-defined calving period. Most beef producers depend

heavily on grass and roughage for their herds during all but severe winter weather. In the western part of the country, government-owned ranges, where cattle are grazed for a fee, play an important part in ranchers' production programs. Therefore, the breeding season for artificial insemination is usually from 25 to 65 days. In many cases, cows are inseminated once and turned out on the range with "clean-up" bulls of a different breed to service cows that return.

2. It is very difficult, especially under range conditions, to set breeding dates ahead of those established in preceding years. A change in the breeding dates can best be accomplished with the heifers, although if

yearling heifers are bred, they should be adequately grown out at the time of breeding. Desired 14-month weights for breeding are:

English breeds       650 lbs.
Exotic breeds        750 lbs.

3. The cows and heifers to be inseminated should be held in as small an area as possible to facilitate heat detection and rounding up the cows to be bred. Patterning the behavior of cows and heifers by providing feed, water, or shade in an area to be used for heat detection and breeding will substantially reduce the labor and time required for gathering them. Breeding pastures should be large enough to provide ample forage for the breeding season (unless pasture rotation is practiced). On the other hand, pasture size should not be so excessive that the cows cannot be readily observed. It is a common practice in large herds to divide the cows into lots of 200 to 300 each to facilitate heat detection and breeding.

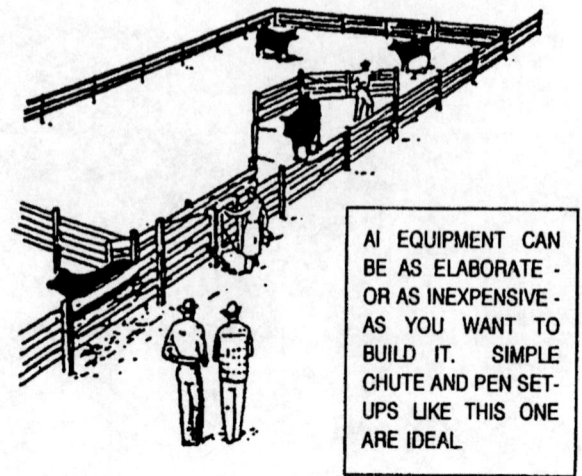

AI EQUIPMENT CAN BE AS ELABORATE - OR AS INEXPENSIVE - AS YOU WANT TO BUILD IT. SIMPLE CHUTE AND PEN SET-UPS LIKE THIS ONE ARE IDEAL

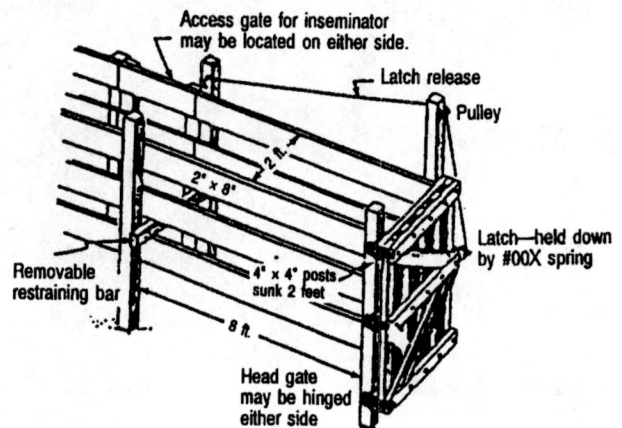

Access gate for inseminator may be located on either side.

Latch release

Pulley

2" x 8"

Removable restraining bar

Latch—held down by #00X spring

4" x 4" posts sunk 2 feet

8 ft.

Head gate may be hinged either side

**Figure 17.3.** Holding pens and breeding chute arrangement. Note design of head gate. (Courtesy, former Curtiss Breeding Service, Elburn, IL)

## Where to Breed

Corrals should be strategically located in that portion of the pasture where it is easiest to corral cows, preferably near a water facility or along well-established cattle travel paths. Wire construction should not be used unless "bumper" poles are provided. Holding pens adequate for as much as 10 percent of the herd are needed.

Holding pens, crowding pens, and the breeding chute may be constructed from poles or lumber (Figure 17.3).

From a holding pen, cows are moved into the crowding pen. If cows will be held for a long time in the holding or crowding area, their calves should be able to get to them to minimize stress. Also to reduce

stress, plan cattle movement so that it is done quietly.

It is recommended that chutes for confining the cows for insemination be about 56 to 60 inches high and 26 to 28 inches wide. About 8 feet of length is needed for large cows. A walk-in gate is needed at the back of the chute for the inseminator. A roof over the breeding chute is needed in some localities and is useful for any unit.

Wood is preferred for chutes and holding pens to reduce noise. Cattle should be worked quietly and gently.

A simplified holding pen and breeding chute for the rancher with many cows and another for the small herd operator are shown in Figure 17.4.

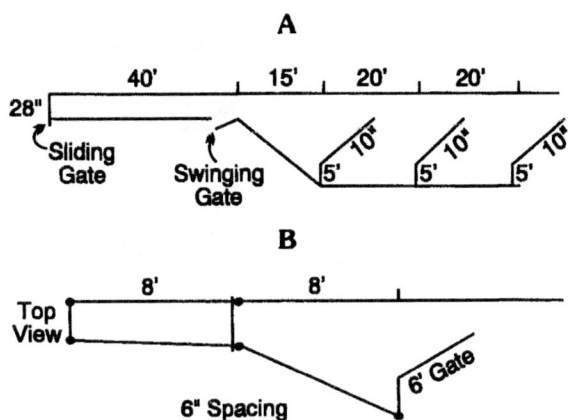

Figure 17.4. (A) Corral unit and breeding chute 28 inches wide and long enough for four to eight cows. A squeeze chute should be avoided. In a breeding chute, sliding gates are optional. It is better to keep a cow from backing up with a bar or pole inserted behind her and just over her hocks. A gate should be placed in the side of the chute behind the last cow so that the technician can conveniently enter the chute. The two holding pens should each be large enough for 20 to 25 cows. (B) Breeding chute and holding pen for a small herd. (Courtesy, ABS Global, Inc., DeForest, WI)

Specifications for the small herd operator include a chute 28 inches wide, 8 feet long, and 5 feet high. (Cows will enter a longer chute more readily, but added length is added cost.) Lumber used should be either 2 × 6 inch or 2 × 8 inch, with 6-inch spacing. Boards should be spaced on each side of the chute so that a bar can be inserted easily between them. There should be enough space for a cow to stand with a bar placed behind the animal and just above the hocks. This arrangement prevents the cow from backing up in the chute.

## How to Breed

Cows should not be bred earlier than about 60 days following calving. Detecting cows in heat is the factor that concerns most people in AI. Experience has shown that detection is generally not a problem if the observers have a good knowledge of cattle and want to get the job done and the cows are coming into heat. It is important that observations be made at least early in the morning and late in the evening, if not more frequently during the day.

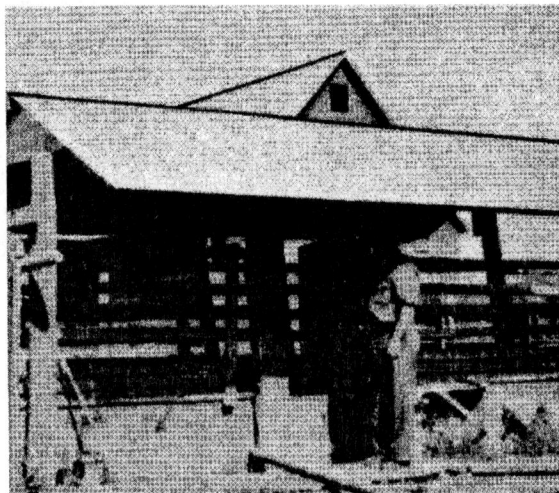

Figure 17.5. A chute for inseminating beef cattle adjoins the corrals.

The length of time a cow herd should be bred is dependent upon individual owners. No shorter period of time than 25 days can be recommended to include cows tending to have a long cycle. Artificial insemination will take an additional few days to start working effectively in herds in which it is being used for the first time.

Many cattle breeders with AI experience are inseminating 100 percent of their herds artificially. Others, however, are using "cleanup" bulls after a minimum 25- to 45-day breeding season.

## Handling

Common-sense management is important in the routine handling of cattle, particularly range cattle, in an AI program. As with any other operation, cattle handled quietly become accustomed to a routine. It is not necessary to bring in the calves with the cows to be bred if they will not be separated very long. Other management activities should be kept to a minimum during the breeding season. The fact that the cows will be placed in a chute to be bred should not be the incentive to initiate other activities such as health programs and branding. The breeding chute (Figure 17.5) should be used only for breeding purposes.

175

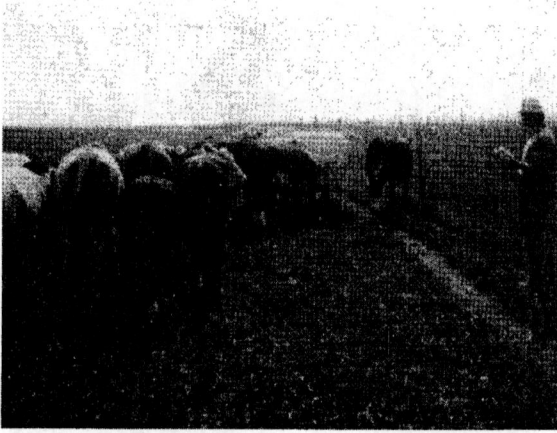

Figure 17.6. Observing for heat. (Courtesy, Select Sires, Inc., Plain City, OH)

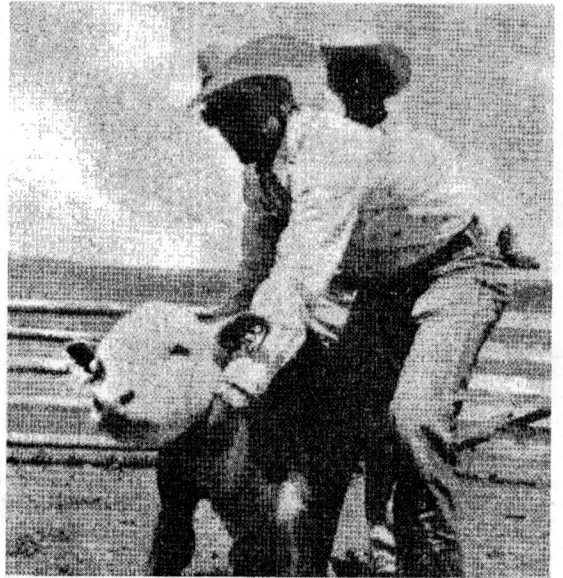

Figure 17.7. Ear tags are used to identify calves.

It must be emphasized that careful planning has been a prerequisite of successful AI programs. Particularly for large operations using artificial breeding for the first time, possible changes in management and nutritional levels should be considered carefully.

## Heat Detection

Various devices have been tried and are being utilized as aids to identifying cows in heat, although experienced operators often depend on visual observation alone (Figure 17.6). Detection aids include hormone-treated steers or cows, sterilized bulls, bulls wearing aprons, bulls with the penis deviated by surgical means, tailhead chalk, crayon, or paint, heat mount detection pads, radiotelemetric systems, and marking harnesses. A chin ball marker arrangement worn by a masculinized cow or a bull surgically treated so that he can mount but not serve the cow has met with favor in many herds. Estrus detection aids are reviewed in Exercise 16.

## Identification

Individual identification of cows in an AI program is strongly recommended because it facilitates heat detection (such as identification of a cow to be brought in later) and it is the basic step in a herd production record system.

Methods of identification include number brands (which need to be clipped in the spring to be read), ear tags, neck chains, and temporary dye brands. Number brands are the most reliable method since they cannot be lost. Most operators depend on ear tags because they are easy to apply. Loss of tags is a common problem that can be reduced by tagging in both ears (Figure 17.7).

## Time to Breed

On ranches and farms in which the inseminator is employed or available full time, a twice-a-day insemination schedule is common. That is, cows detected in the morning are bred in the evening, and cows detected at night are bred the following morning. For small herds in which the cows can be checked easily for heat and on which complete breeding and calving records are kept, insemination once a day has also given good results. Various synchronization programs also utilize timed inseminations where breeding is done at a scheduled time following a synchronization treatment. It is im-

176

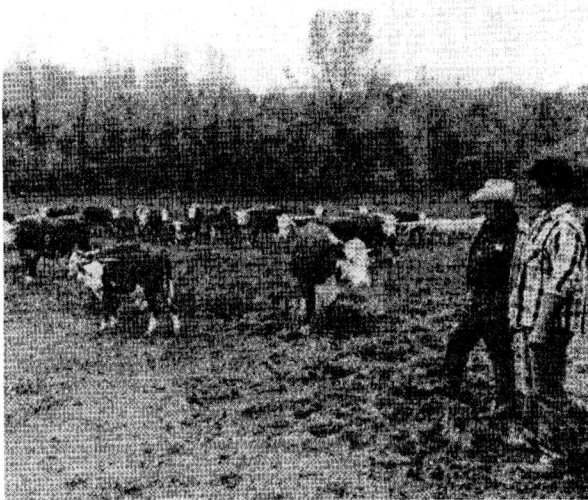

**Figure 17.8.** A Pennsylvania herd owner and the AI representative from COBA/Select Sires look over the beef herd. (Courtesy, COBA/Select Sires, Columbus, OH)

portant to recognize that representatives from AI organizations can be an important resource for herd operators regarding information on semen handling, insemination, management, and genetics (Figure 17.8).

## Nutrition

Good nutrition is fundamental for a cow to come into heat before she can conceive and produce. One of the easiest ways to start a program of good nutrition is to divide the beef cow's year into four periods, each of which is typified by her varying nutritional needs:

|  |  | **Days** |
|---|---|---|
| Period One | Post-calving | 82 |
| Period Two | Pregnant and lactating | 123 |
| Period Three | Mid-gestation | 110 |
| Period Four | Pre-calving | 50 |

Period One is tough for the cow. She is having to meet tremendous demands. She is lactating at her highest level, she is undergoing uterine involution, and she must cycle and rebreed. In a beef AI program, it is es-

pecially important that she do this in a timely fashion.

During Period Two the cow should be in the early stages of pregnancy while still nursing her calf. If she's in a spring calving program, she also should be gaining weight and laying on an energy reserve for the winter. Period Three follows weaning and is referred to as mid-gestation. This is when the cow's nutritional needs are the lowest, because all she must do is maintain the developing fetus and herself.

Period Four is the second most important stage. Seventy to eighty percent of total fetal growth is taking place, and the cow also is preparing for lactation. She should be gaining weight. Inadequate nutrition now can carry over into Period One and negatively affect rebreeding success.

The season of the year during which a cow calves also affects her nutritional requirements.

Bear in mind that in addition to the stage of production and season of calving, nutritional requirements also are affected by cow size, milk production level, weather, and cow age.

Nutritional requirements actually refer to what's needed from four categories: energy, protein, minerals, and vitamins that play a role in beef nutrition.

The National Research Council's guidelines for beef cattle nutrition are listed in Table 17.2.

You can use these figures to help set up a program, but remember that they are only guidelines and that you have to consider your own resources and the factors affecting your cows' requirement levels. You might want to contact your extension agent or a specialist at the closest land-grant university or government research center to help you fine tune your program.

In recent years, beef cattle producers have been using body condition scores (BCS) to monitor effectiveness of their nutrition programs. Post-calving and pre-calving are the most nutritionally critical to cows. Body condition has a significant impact on reproductive performance

177

**Table 17.2.** NRC Requirements[a]—1,000-Pound Beef Cow

| | Management Periods | | | |
|---|---|---|---|---|
| | Post-calving | Pregnant and Lactating | Mid-gestation | Pre-calving |
| TDN/energy (lb./day) | 13-15 | 11-12 | 8.5 | 10 |
| Protein (lb./day) | 2.0 | 1.6 | .9 | 1.1 |
| Digestible protein (lb./day) | 1.2 | .9 | .45 | .55 |
| Calcium (gm/day) | 27 | 24 | 13 | 5 |
| Phosphorus (gm/day) | 27 | 24 | 13 | 15 |
| Vitamin A (IU/day) | 24,000 | 24,000 | 20,000 | 24,000 |

[a]Compiled from NRC Nutrient Requirements of Beef Cattle (6th Revised Ed.). 1984. National Academy Press, Washington, DC.

(cyclicity) and productivity during these times. BCS systems use numbers to describe cattle condition. For example, a score of 1 represents extremely thin condition and a score of 9 extremely fat condition. It is recommended that mature beef cows should be at least BCS 5 at time of calving, whereas two-year-old heifers should be at least BCS 6 at calving (because of their additional growth requirements). Table 17.3 lists descriptions of body condition for a commonly used BCS system.

### When to Condition Score Cows

*Weaning*—Pay particular attention to young cows weaning their first calves; they're most likely to be thin at this time.

*30 to 45 days after weaning*—Gives a good idea how fast cows are bouncing back after weaning. Thin cows should be gaining back condition if cow type is matched with the feed resources.

*90 days before calving*—Last opportunity to get condition back on cows economically. This would be a good time to separate thin cows from cows in good condition.

*Calving*—If cows are thin, you may want to change the feeding program. It is difficult, economically, to put condition on cows after calving. It takes large amounts of high-quality feed.

*Breeding season*—If cows are thin at this time, you may need to implement an early weaning strategy to enhance the pregnancy rate of cows.

## Requirements for Beef Artificial Insemination

1. Cows must be in good condition with a high percentage of them cycling normally.

2. The feeding program should be meeting your cows' nutritional needs.

3. Sufficient catch corrals with well-built breeding chutes should be provided to handle cows with minimum stress.

4. Trained personnel must be available to detect heat, to handle the cows, to care for the semen, and to inseminate.

5. Heat detection and insemination are time consuming and confining. They have to be done correctly, and they have to be done on a schedule.

6. Cows must be visibly identified.

7. Accurate and complete records must be kept.

**Table 17.3.** Description of Body Condition Scores

| Score | BCS Description |
| --- | --- |
| 1 | Animal is severely emaciated. Tailhead and ribs are prominent and the animal appears weakened. No fat can be palpated over the ribs, spinous processes, or hip bones. A BCS 1 animal is near death. |
| 2 | Cow is emaciated, but tailhead and ribs are less prominent, individual spinous processes are still sharp to the touch, but some tissue cover exists along the spine. Cow has little visible muscle tissue, but is not weak. |
| 3 | Beginning of fat cover over the loin, back, and foreribs. The backbone is still highly visible. Processes of the spine can be identified individually by touch and may still be visible. Spaces between the processes are less pronounced. There is muscle tissue loss, especially in the rear quarters. |
| 4 | Foreribs are not noticeable, but the 12$^{th}$ and 13$^{th}$ ribs are still noticeable to the eye, particularly in cattle with a big spring of rib and width between ribs. The transverse spinous processes can be identified and feel rounded rather than sharp. |
| 5 | The 12$^{th}$ and 13$^{th}$ ribs are not visible to eye unless the animal is shrunk. The tranverse spinous processes can only be felt with firm pressure and feel rounded but are not noticeable to the eye. Spaces between the processes are not visible and are only distinguishable with firm pressure. Areas on each side of the tailhead are well filled but not rounded. |
| 6 | Ribs are fully covered and are not noticeable to the eye. Hindquarters are plump and full. Noticeable sponginess over the foreribs and on each side of the tailhead. Firm pressure is now required to feel the transverse processes. |
| 7 | Ends of spinous processes can only be felt with firm pressure. Spaces between processes can be barely distinguished. Abundant fat cover on either side of the tailhead with evident patchiness. |
| 8 | Obese, cow is very fleshy and overconditioned. Back is square, brisket is distended, neck thick, and body appears square. Cow has large fat deposits over ribs, around tailhead, and below vulva. Rounds or pones are obvious. |
| 9 | Very obese, with large deposits of fat in the udder, around the tailhead, over the ribs, and in the brisket. Bone structure is not visible and cannot be palpated over the hooks and ribs. The cow appears blocky and mobility may be impaired due to excess fat. These animals are rarely seen. |

Source: Dale Blasi, Extension Beef Specialist, Kansas State University.

8. AI training is a continuous process. Even if you've been to AI school, you will need periodic updating and retraining.

9. You may need to buy a liquid nitrogen refrigerator for semen and AI supplies. You should plan on 1.5 straws of semen per cow you intend to breed AI, and you will need to select your semen supplier carefully.

10. Semen must be carefully chosen to complement the cows. AI calves are worth no more than natural calves unless superior sires are used. Sire selection is not easy; however, the guesswork is removed by using appropriate sire summary information to attain your herd goals (see Exercises 3 and 22).

11. A successful AI program requires a positive attitude.

The success or failure of any AI program is up to the person managing it. For those who make the commitment, the rewards make the effort profitable. One study comparing AI programs showed that conception rates varied from 25 to 100 percent. The difference was management.

## Estrus and Ovulation Synchronization, Programmed Breeding for Beef and Dairy Cattle

Reducing the time and labor costs involved in heat detection should allow greater use of superior bulls through AI. Many studies have been made on control of the estrous cycle in cattle. Synchronization advances estrous cycles so all cycling cows come into heat at a predetermined time. In addition, some protocols induce anestrous females to start cycling.

## The Advantages of Estrus and Ovulation Control

**For the Beef Operator—** Synchronization, properly utilized and with good herd management prevailing, offers these advantages for the beef operator:

1. It increases the use of genetically superior sires through artificial insemination. In addition, it aids in disease control and reduces bull costs for cross-breeding.

2. It greatly reduces, or eliminates, the labor requirements and cost of heat detection and significantly decreases the days needed for AI.

3. It enables the timing of cattle handling and insemination to best fit into the schedule with other required farm work.

4. It groups the animals into desired calving patterns, resulting in a more uniform lot of calves; permits calving time when more labor is available for care of cows and calves, thus reducing losses; and shortens the breeding and calving season.

5. Cows that breed and calve early tend to wean older, heavier calves consistently and have a higher lifetime calf crop percentage.

6. Replacement females will be older and heavier at first breeding.

**For the Dairy Operator—** Synchronization used for non-lactating heifers and lactating cows will enable:

1. Heifers to be bred to a genetically superior dairy bull by artificial insemination rather than to a young bull that will likely never be genetically evaluated or proven or to a beef bull. This procedure alone will add dollar value and production potential to every calf.

2. Heifers to be grouped for breeding to fit the time that herd replacements are most needed.

3. The dairy operator to provide production-tested progeny in young sire-proving programs, in which every dairy operator has a stake.

4. The dairy operator to continue improvement in the herd average for milk production because heifers entering the milking string will be from a bull with superior genetic potential. About one-third of the calvings in the average dairy herd will be first-calf heifers.

5. Cows to be bred back sooner following calving, shortening the calving interval. Systematic breeding programs are convenient, can reduce estrus detection burdens, and can result in higher pregnancy rates.

## Cycling—A Must

No synchronization program can be successful if there is a low percentage of females cycling in the herd. Females must be coming into heat regularly before any treatment.

The estrous cycle can be controlled by the administration of certain drugs. A knowledge of the cycle will make it easier to understand how synchronizing drugs work.

The hormone progesterone essentially predominates during the 21-day cycle of the cow. In a nutshell, as long as progesterone levels are low, the animal will continue her cycling activity. If levels of progesterone increase, this represses cyclicity, prepares the uterus for pregnancy, and, if pregnancy occurs, maintains the uterus for that condition. Traditional estrus synchronization protocols have been geared toward controlling the *corpus luteum* (CL) and consequently the progesterone levels. Newer approaches however have been developed that are aimed at manipulating (synchronizing) ovulation as well. Research using transrectal ultrasound to characterize follicular development in cows has shown that follicle growth occurs in waves throughout the estrous cycle. Most cows will have two or three follicular waves during a 21-day estrous cycle.[2a] Each wave is characterized by rapid growth of several small follicles. One of the follicles in the wave grows larger in size and becomes dominant, restricting growth of the other smaller follicles.[2b] If progesterone levels are high (during presence of a CL) the dominant follicle does not cause estrus behavior, does not continue to ovulation, and normally regresses. When the dominant follicle degenerates a second follicular wave begins at about mid-cycle. Again a dominant follicle is selected from this wave, however this one normally continues to ovulation since its growth corresponds with regression of the CL. Each follicular wave is preceded by an increase in follicle stimulating hormone (FSH) concentration. This is needed to initiate a follicular wave. The subsequent decrease in FSH is also essential for selection of a single dominant follicle.[2c] Understanding control of follicular waves allows approaches that are improving synchronization and fertility (see various synch protocols below).

**For the Normal Estrous Cycle (Figure 17.9)—** The cycle starts with estrus on day 1, when the cow is in heat (the egg is ovulated about 12 hours after the end of heat). During the period of days 2 through 3, the *corpus luteum* (CL, or yellow body) develops on the ovary at the site of ovulation. Progesterone is produced by the CL. Around the time of ovulation, the first wave of follicles emerges, followed by a second wave on day 10. In some cows, a third wave occurs on day 16 to 18. Each wave is preceded by an increase of FSH. The CL will begin to regress about day 16 to 18 if pregnancy does not occur. CL regression is induced by pulses of prostaglandin F2α, released from the uterus beginning around day 15. Subsequent increases in estradiol and LH concentrations cause the large surge of LH at estrus, which results in the next ovulation.

## Prostaglandin

Synthetic prostaglandin products are effective for inducing estrus in mid-cycle cows (days 6 through 17). Several prostaglandin products have been approved for use by the Food and Drug Administration (FDA). They are administered by injection and are available only by prescription from a veterinarian.

---

[2a] Wiltbank, M. C. 1998. Update on synchronization of ovulation and estrus. Proc. 17th Tech. Conf. on Artificial Insemination and Reproduction. NAAB. p. 65.
[2b] Ibid.

[2c] Ibid.

The Estrous Cycle in Cattle

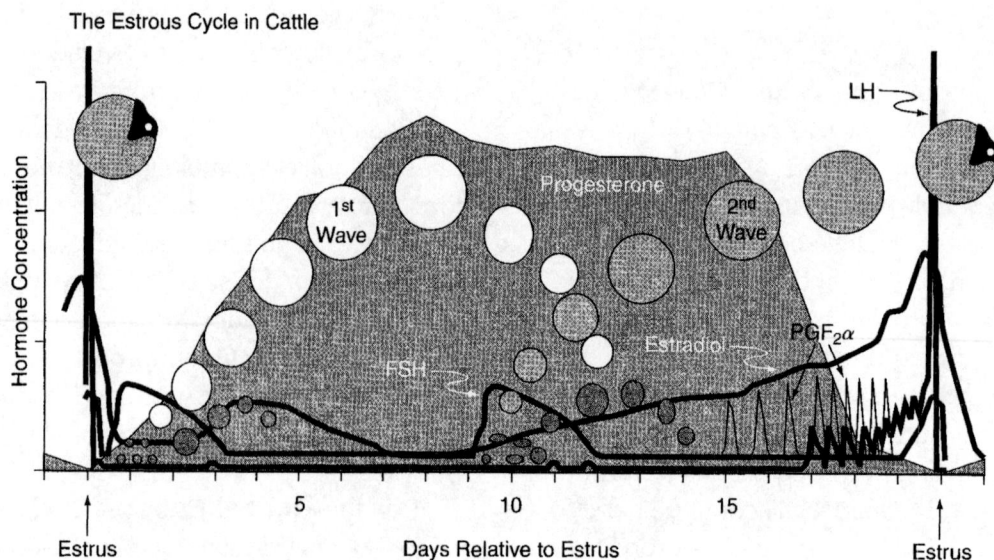

**Figure 17.9.** Illustration of the normal estrous cycle in cattle. Modified from M. Day. 2001. Use of progesterone to induce and synchronize estrus: application of the CIDR. NAAB Symposium on Improving Reproductive Performance at 33rd Res. Symp. and Ann. Mtg. Beef Improvement Federation. San Antonio, TX. pp. 13–25.

The CL will prematurely regress and the cow should come into heat and ovulate within 2 to 5 days. If the cow is in the follicular stage (days 1 through 5 and days 18 through 21), she will not be affected. However, if females are already late in the cycle (days 18 through 21), they should come into heat at about the same time as the treated animals.

Prostaglandin should be used only on non-pregnant females, because it could cause abortion if administered to pregnant cows and heifers, depending on the stage of gestation. There are different systems that may be used when synchronizing with prostaglandin. In the one-injection system, you first detect heat for five days as usual and breed the females detected. If 20 to 25 percent of the animals show heat during that time period, you can assume the herd is cycling normally, and on the fifth day you can give each of the remaining animals a single prostaglandin injection. Animals are then bred as they come into heat, and you should be able to breed almost all cycling animals within 10 days. A main advantages of this system is that it allows you to determine the percentage of the herd show-

ing heat. If the percentage is low, the program can be discontinued, saving additional time, labor, and cost of prostaglandin and semen.

A two-injection system with prostaglandin will allow most animals to come into heat within 5 days after the last injection and be bred accordingly. In this system, all eligible animals are injected on the day you choose to start your program and then 10 to 11 days later (in heifers) or 13 to 14 days later (in lactating cows). Following the second injection, all cycling animals should come into heat within 5 days and they then can be inseminated.

This same two-injection system can be used without heat detection, in which case all animals are bred 76 to 80 hours after the second injection (fixed-time insemination). Results from using fixed-time insemination have been better in heifers than in cows.

## Synchro-Mate B

The Synchro-Mate B (SMB) system has the same goal but differs completely from the prostaglandin system in that Synchro-Mate B is a non-prescription synchronization product that combines the use of a synthetic progesterone and an estrogen. SMB has been approved for use by the FDA. However, currently this product is not available for purchase. Information is included here as background material and also for comparison to other synchronization protocols. The SMB system involves three steps, and all cycling animals will respond at the same time regardless of their cycling status when the program is started.

Step One involves placing a small implant under the skin on the back side of one ear. This is done with all animals on day 1. The implant, which is about ⅛-inch in diameter and ¾-inch long, contains the synthetic form of progesterone (norgestomet). This prevents the ovary from beginning a new cycle until the implant is removed.

Step Two is done at the same time as the implanting and is an intramuscular injection of a combination of hormones, estradiol valerate, and norgestomet. The animal close to ovulation will not ovulate because of the injected norgestomet. The implanted norgestomet prevents ovulation over the next nine days. *Corpus luteum* regression is caused by estradiol in any animals that happen to be in the luteal phase when injected. All cycling stops over a nine-day period.

Step Three is to remove the implant on the ninth day. Following implant removal, animals that respond to SMB will begin a new cycle and be in heat within 24 to 36 hours. Cows can be inseminated at a fixed time (48 to 54 hours) after implant removal or in conjunction with normal observation of estrus.

## MGA

Melengestrol acetate (MGA) is a synthetic progesterone that has been shown through research to successfully suppress heat in feedlot heifers. MGA has been approved for use in re-

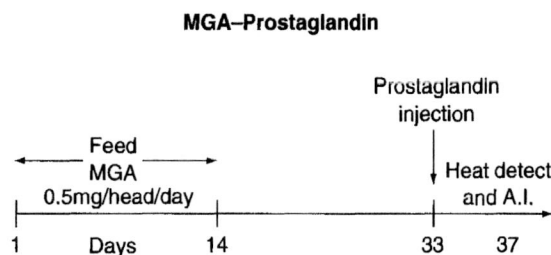

**MGA–Prostaglandin**

**Figure 17.10.** MGA–Prostaglandin synchronization protocol.

productive classes of beef and dairy cattle.[3] Typically after the feeding of MGA (for a 14-day period) is stopped, all cycling heifers will be in heat within one week. However, the heats will not be tightly synchronized. The standard treatment is 0.5 mg of MGA/head/day. A combination of MGA and prostaglandin (Figure 17.10) has the potential to make synchronization more practical for beef producers.

It has been shown that feeding MGA for 14 days then removing it and injecting prostaglandin 16 to 19 days later results in a majority of females coming into heat within 5 days.[4, 5] AI is performed after observation of estrus. The MGA-prostaglandin protocol has become a proven system, particularly for heifers.

In this system, the treatment costs are low and cattle have to be handled only once. In well-managed herds, conception rates can be high. But success depends on all females consuming a consistent quantity of MGA during the 14-day feeding period. A disadvantage of MGA is that the producer must begin feeding

[3] D. J. Patterson, et al. 2001. Emerging protocols to synchronize estrus in replacement beef heifers and post-partum cows. NAAB Symposium on Improving Reproductive Performance at 33rd Res. Symp. and Ann. Mtg. Beef Improvement Federation. San Antonio, TX. pp. 26–51.
[4] M. E. King and K. G. Odde. 1993. MGA-prostaglandin synchronization system: Where we have come from and where we are heading. Proc. Beef Improvement Federation Symp. and Ann. Mtg. (Ashville, NC). p. 1.
[5] W. E. Beal. 2001. Synchronization of estrus in beef heifers. American Red Angus Magazine. April 2001. p. 27.

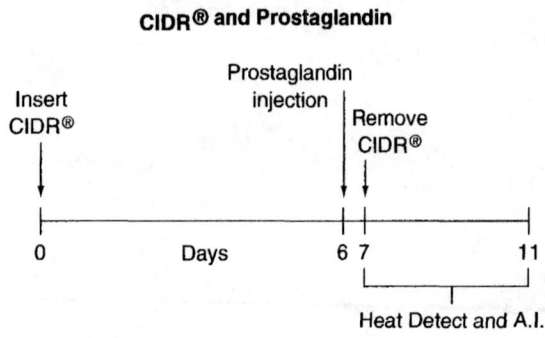

**CIDR® and Prostaglandin**

**Figure 17.11.** CIDR and prostaglandin synchronization protocol.

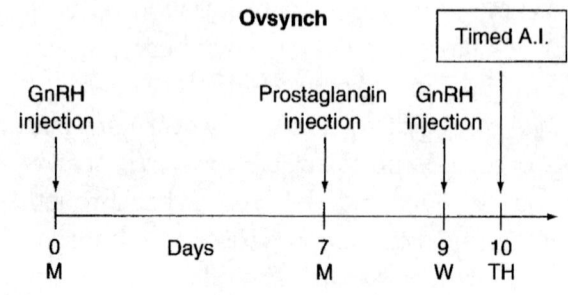

**Ovsynch**

**Figure 17.12.** Ovsynch protocol.

MGA 32 to 34 days prior to the breeding period. This synchronization program should also work well with post-partum beef cows. However, adequate consumption of MGA and percentage of cows cycling are important factors.

## CIDR®

Controlled internal drug releasing (CIDR®) devices are T-shaped intravaginal inserts containing progesterone. CIDR®s have been used successfully in a variety of estrous control programs in other countries resulting in improved heat detection and pregnancy rates. CIDR®s have also been investigated extensively in the U.S. and in 2002 were approved by the FDA for use in dairy and beef heifers and beef cows. Figure 17.11 shows a synchronization protocol for heifers using the CIDR® and prostaglandin. Day[6] has reviewed the use of the CIDR® as a progestin source to jump-start anestrous cows in GnRH-prostaglandin synchronization programs. It is likely that CIDR®s will be used extensively in synchronization programs. For additional information refer to *http://www.cidr.com*.

---

[6] M. Day. 2001. Use of progesterone to induce and synchronize estrus: Application of the CIDR. NAAB Symposium on Improving Reproductive Performance at 33rd Res. Symp. and Ann. Mtg. Beef Improvement Federation. San Antonio, TX. pp. 13–25.

## Ovsynch (for timed insemination in cows)

This protocol (Figure 17.12) actually synchronizes ovulation and was developed for lactating dairy cows.[7] Gonadotropin releasing hormone (GnRH) is injected at any stage of the estrous cycle. This stimulates lutenizing hormone (LH) resulting in the ovulation of old follicles (~85% of cows) and growth of a new wave of follicles within 48 hours (~100% of cows). A second injection, with prostaglandin (PGF2α) is given seven days later. This regresses the original corpus luteum (CL), if one was present, and the CL induced from the first GnRH injection (~95% of cows). A new dominant follicle matures during the next 48 hours. A second GnRH injection 48 hours after prostaglandin initiates ovulation in virtually all cows (~97%) at the same time. Cows then are inseminated 12 to 24 hours later without estrus detection (timed AI). With Ovsynch the number of pregnancies per AI is the same and is similar to when cows are bred after a detected heat. In dairy operations, Ovsynch can reduce the number of days open on average by one estrous cycle (19 to 22 days), which increases profitability. In beef cows, Ovsynch has obtained better results than with Synchro-Mate B. It should be noted that Ovsynch is not as effective in heifers. This may be due to differences in follicular wave patterns between cows and heifers.

---

[7] Ibid.

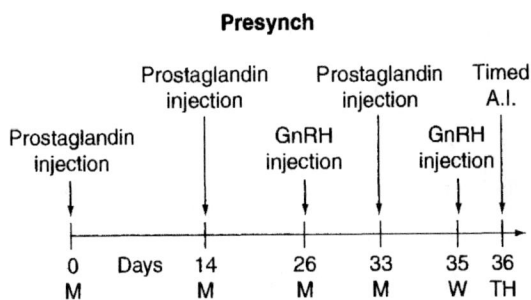

**Figure 17.13.** Presynch protocol.

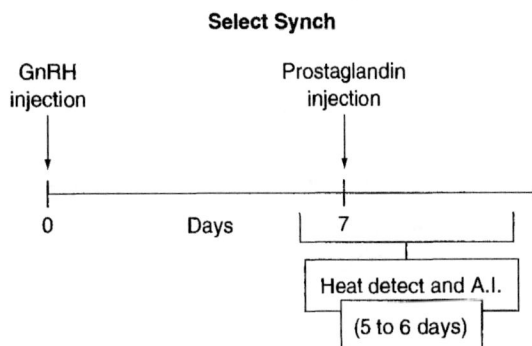

**Figure 17.14.** Cosynch protocol.

## Presynch (for Timed Insemination in Cows)

Another approach that results in higher pregnancy rates than Ovsynch alone is called Presynch. In this protocol (Figure 17.13), cows receive two injections of PGF2α 14 days apart with the second prostaglandlin injection occurring 12 to 14 days before initiation of the Ovsynch program. With this regimen, a higher percentage of cows will be grouped into days 5 to 12 of the estrous cycle by the time of the first GnRH injection of the Ovsynch protocol.

## Co-Synch (for Timed Insemination in Cows)

This protocol (Figure 17.14) is identical to Ovsynch regarding timing of injections of the first GnRH, PGF2α, and second GnRH. The main difference though is that cows are inseminated at the same time that the second GnRH injection is made. Pregnancy rates are usually somewhat better than with the Ovsynch protocol, however an advantage is that the cattle are handled one less time saving on labor.

It should be noted that a 48-hour calf removal between injections of PGF2α and the second GnRH injection has been shown to increase pregnancy rates by 9 percent for

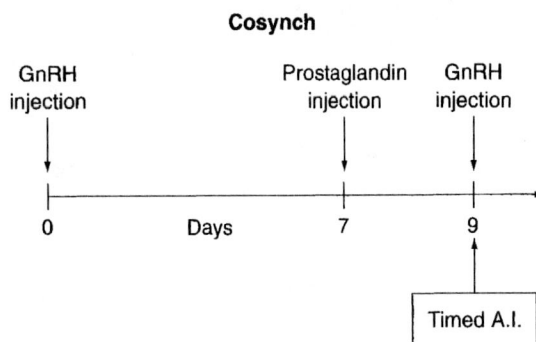

**Figure 17.15.** Selectsynch protocol.

both Ovsynch and Co-Synch protocols in beef cows.[8]

## Select Synch (for Cows)

In this protocol (Figure 17.15), GnRH is injected followed 7 days later by a PGF2α injection. All animals are observed for estrus beginning 1 day before the PGF2α injection (day 6) and continuing for 5 days thereafter. Insemination is performed 8 to 10 hours after first detection of a standing mount. The PGF2α injection is not given to cows that come into heat prior to the scheduled day 7 injection. If timed AI is planned, another GnRH injection

---

[8] T. W. Geary, et al. 2001. Calf removal improves conception rates to the Ovsynch and Co-Synch protocols. J. Anim. Sci. 79:1.

185

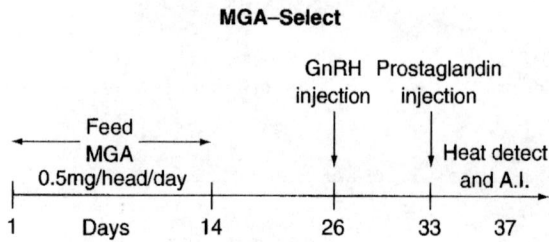

**MGA–Select**

Feed MGA 0.5mg/head/day (Days 1–14)

GnRH injection (Day 26)

Prostaglandin injection (Day 33)

Heat detect and A.I. (Day 37)

**Figure 17.16.** MGA select protocol.

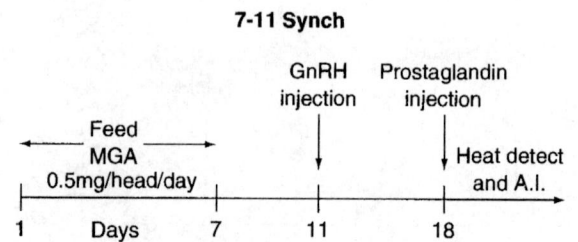

**7-11 Synch**

Feed MGA 0.5mg/head/day (Days 1–7)

GnRH injection (Day 11)

Prostaglandin injection (Day 18)

Heat detect and A.I.

**Figure 17.17.** 7-11 Synch protocol.

is recommended 72 hours after the PGF2α injection (day 10) followed by mass breeding.

## MGA-Select (for Cows)

In this protocol (Figure 17.16), the MGA-prostaglandin system that works well in heifers is combined with a GnRH synchronization for cows. Pretreatment with MGA prior to GnRH and PGF2α injections eliminates any early heats, improves synchronization and improves fertility. Pretreatment with MGA in this protocol also causes some anestrous cows to cycle. MGA (.5 mg/head/day) is fed for 14 days. Twelve days later (day 26) a GnRH injection is given, followed in 7 days (day 33) with injection of PGF2α. Heat detection and insemination follows. If timed AI is planned, another GnRH injection is recommended 72 hours after the PGF2α injection (day 36) followed by mass breeding.

## 7-11 Synch (for Cows)

In this protocol (Figure 17.17), pretreatment with MGA is reduced to 7 days, followed by GnRH on day 11 and PGF2α on day 18. This is followed by heat detection and insemination. 7-11 Synch results in very good synchrony and high pregnancy rates in postpartum beef cows.

Clearly, there are numerous synchronization protocols. To avoid any confusion, it is certainly important to maintain a basic understanding of the estrous cycle and have knowledge of how certain drugs are applied to manipulate or control an outcome (estrus and ovulation). There is much ongoing research to further develop and improve synchronization protocols. You are encouraged to stay abreast of new developments (often reported in the popular press) and to consult with an AI company reproductive specialist and/or veterinarian before embarking on a synchronization program.

## Good Management—An Absolute Necessity

Successful synchronization programs can be achieved only if good management is in place before the program starts. Estrus/ovulation synchronization is not a cure-all for breeding and management problems. It will not replace good management, and it will not be successful under poor management.

In addition to good management, facilities must be adequate to handle the extra activity, and there must be enough trained and experienced personnel to help when breeding starts.

Probably the single most important factor determining success of a synchronization program is the percentage of females that are cycling. Although some protocols can induce cyclicity, if animals are not in good condition and cycling, the program will not be optimal.

## How to Succeed Using Estrus/Ovulation Synchronization and Artificial Insemination

Good herd management; an understanding of the part the synchronizing compound(s) plays in synchronization; preparations for the program before it is attempted; and close cooperation on the part of the herd operator, the veterinarian, and the AI technician are the keys to a successful controlled breeding program. Pertinent factors in planning and carrying out a successful estrus control program are the following:

1. Confer with the veterinarian, and request a check of the health status of the herd. Determine the number of cows to be synchronized and the approximate dates, and make arrangements for the synchronizing compounds.

2. Determine what bulls will be used and the number of units of semen needed. Order the semen well in advance of the breeding season, and have it in the liquid nitrogen tank at the prescribed time.

3. Make sure a well-qualified, experienced person is available to do the inseminating. Large herds, in which many cows will be inseminated in a short time, may need two technicians. This applies particularly to timed AI. Fatigue generally sets in after a technician inseminates 12 to 15 cows in a short time. Conception rates may suffer. Two technicians can alternate between inseminating and semen handling.

4. Provide the necessary facilities to handle the cows to be bred in an efficient manner (described in this exercise).

5. Make sure that each animal is identified by a brand or an ear tag that can be read easily. Keep simple but accurate breeding and calving records.

6. Keep cows to be bred in good physical condition. Heifers and cows with calves should be kept in separate pastures so that their nutritional needs can be taken care of. Extremely thin cows and heifers will not cycle normally. If they are to be bred on schedule, cows need about twice the feed nutrients following calving as they did prior to calving.

## Artificial Insemination versus Natural Service

The cost of artificial insemination per calf will vary with the cost of semen, and with the costs of labor and management and the synchronization protocol prevailing on each farm or ranch. Over the years, various comparisons have been made of the cost per calf born as a result of artificial insemination as compared to natural service.

In 1985, Pace (see references) analyzed costs involved in four synchronization regimes using AI at various calving percentages: (1) SMB using fixed-time breeding, (2) two-injection prostaglandin with fixed-time breeding, (3) SMB with breeding based on heat detection, and (4) one-injection prostaglandin with breeding based on heat detection. Major factors used to determine costs for a synchronization and AI program were labor and AI supplies, drugs for synchronization, semen, calving rates, "clean-up" bull costs if not 100 percent AI, and bull maintenance cost reduction. At a

60 percent estimated calving rate, the increased cost per AI calf produced was $43, $42, $41, and $32 for each of the respective synchronization and AI regimes indicated above. The expected increased income over natural service calves was also calculated. This was based on increased maternal value, increased value of breeding stock, increased weight of calves, age advantage of calves, and increased live calves as a result of calving ease and group calving. At the same 60 percent estimated calving rate, the synchronization plus AI advantage per cow over a total natural service program was indicated to be $32, $32, $34, and $36 for each of the respective synchronization and AI regimes indicated above. This analysis also demonstrated that depending on the AI-synchronization regime chosen, labor costs were between 30 and 40 percent of total costs involved. Also, as calving percentage increased, profitability per cow increased.

Other recent comparisons indicate a range in the cost of producing a natural service calf from $29 to $66 and cost of producing an AI calf from $27 to $58 based on various management scenarios.[9, 10, 11]

ABS Global, a leading, AI business in DeForest, Wisconsin, has calculated the cost per calf resulting from natural service sires (Table 17.4).

The estimates in Table 17.4 assume that the new salvage value of the bull will be at least $450. Included in the cost is a 10 percent risk factor to cover the average rate of death and injury. Interest at 15 percent of the purchase price is figured in the maintenance costs. It is assumed that the bull will be used three years and will sire 75 calves. It is also assumed that 1½ cows that would produce additional income could be kept in place of a bull. The service cost per calf will vary with the total number of calves sired, the purchase price

---

[9] "No Bull, No Problem." 1999. Drovers. Vol. 127, No. 4. p. 30.
[10] "The Benefits of AI." 2000. Drovers. Vol. 128, No.2. p. 32.
[11] "Natural Breeding vs. AI." 2000. Drovers. Vol. 128, No. 3. p. 83.

---

**Table 17.4.   Cost per Calf with Natural Service[a]**

| | | | | | | | |
|---|---|---|---|---|---|---|---|
| Bull purchase | $1,000 | $1,500 | $2,000 | $2,500 | $3,000 | $5,000 | $ 8,000 |
| Less salvage | 450 | 450 | 450 | 450 | 450 | 450 | 450 |
| Net cost of bull | $550 | $1,050 | $1,550 | $2,050 | $2,550 | $4,550 | $ 7,550 |
| Bull maintenance[b] (3 yrs.) | 720 | 720 | 720 | 720 | 720 | 720 | 720 |
| Interest on purchase price (15% for 3 yrs.) | 450 | 675 | 900 | 1,125 | 1,350 | 2,250 | 3,600 |
| Risk (10%) | 100 | 150 | 200 | 250 | 300 | 500 | 800 |
| Total cost | $1,820 | $2,595 | $3,370 | $4,145 | $4,920 | $8,020 | $12,670 |
| Cost per calf (75 calves in 3 years) | $24.27 | $34.60 | $44.93 | $55.27 | $65.60 | $106.93 | $168.93 |

[a]Data compiled by American Breeders Service, DeForest, WI.

[b]Maintenance is based on income expected from the beef production of 1½ cows that could be kept in place of a bull.

of the bull, and the years used. Maintenance and depreciation costs must be considered. This table demonstrates that there are several hidden costs involved in keeping a bull on the farm or ranch for breeding.

Information in Table 17.4 allows a herd operator to compare the cost of producing natural service calves when considering the advantages of an AI program. The cost per calf sired for any natural service bull can be estimated on the basis of total calves sired, years used, maintenance and depreciation costs, salvage value, and original price paid for the animal. The average commercial beef producer will use herd bulls costing $750 to $2,500.

Breeders of purebred cattle, and particularly those carrying on a performance-testing program, will usually pay higher than average prices for a bull. However, unless the very top bulls in a feedstock auction are purchased, the level of genetic quality will not approach that available through AI. In turn, such breeders will usually sell calves sired by a superior bull for breeding purposes at well above average prices.

Although there are important costs to consider in using an AI program for beef cows and heifers, it is obvious that the opportunity for genetically improving the economic traits is great, and the return on investment can be high!

## QUESTIONS

1. What are the important advantages of using artificial insemination for beef cattle?

2. What are some of the disadvantages and challenges?

3. What has been the impact of crossbreeding and of the introduction of the "exotic" breeds on the expansion of artificial insemination?

4. On what basis should AI bulls be selected?

5. Why should emphasis be placed on average weaning weight and yearling weight in a cow-calf herd?

6. What steps are necessary to make artificial insemination succeed in a beef herd?

7. What essential equipment should be provided for handling cows to be inseminated?

8. What identification for individual animals would you recommend for the beef herd?

9. How can estrus (heat) in beef cattle best be detected?

10. How does controlled estrus work in beef cattle? What are the advantages?

11. Explain how ovulation is synchronized.

12. What are some of the products used to control the estrous cycle?

13. How does the level of nutrition affect fertility in the beef herd?

14. Why isn't artificial insemination used in more beef herds?

15. What is the attitude of beef registry organizations toward artificial insemination? Is this attitude changing? Explain.

16. Describe the costs involved in producing an AI-sired calf compared to a natural service calf. What hidden costs are involved in keeping a herd bull(s) for breeding purposes?

# U.S. BEEF BREED REGISTRY ORGANIZATIONS

### AMERIFAX (AM)

Amerifax Cattle Association
P.O. Box 149
Hastings, NE 68902
Tel: 402/463-5289
Fax: 402/463-6652
Email: quirk@navix.net

### ANGUS (AN)

American Angus Association
3201 Frederick Blvd.
St. Joseph, MO 64506
Tel: 816/233-3101
Fax: 816/233-9703
Email: angus@angus.org
*Website: http://www.angus.org*

### ANKOLE-WATUSI (AW)

Ankole-Watusi International Registry
22484 W. 239th St.
Spring Hill, KS 66083-9306
Tel: 913/592-4050
Email: watusi@aol.com
*Website: http://www.members.aol.com/
watusi/index.html*

### BEEFALO (BE)

American Beefalo Association
P.O. Box 656
Somerset, KY 42502
Tel: 606/678-5438
Fax: 606/678-5438

American Beefalo World Registry
2225 Old Stage Road
Dillon, MT 59725
Tel: 406/683-6564
Fax: 406/683-6564
Email: info@abwr.org
*Website: http://www.abwr.org*

### BEEFMASTER (BM)

Beefmaster Breeders United
6800 Park Ten Blvd., Suite 290 West
San Antonio, TX 78213
Tel: 210/732-3132
Fax: 210/732-7711
Email: wschronk@beefmasters.org
*Website: http://www.beefmasters.org*

### BELGIAN BLUE (BB)

American Belgian Blue Breeders, Inc.
P.O. Box 35264
Tulsa, OK 74153-0264
Tel: 918/477-3251
Fax: 918/477-3232
*Website: http://www.belgianblue.org*

### BELTED GALLOWAY (BG)

Belted Galloway Society, Inc.
P.O. Box 56
Holly Springs, MS 38635
Tel: 601/252-5744
Fax: 601/252-4386
Email: jhuff@dixie-net.com
*Website: http://www.beltie.org*

### BLONDE D'AQUITAINE (BD)

American Blonde d'Aquitaine
Association
P.O. Box 12341
Kansas City, MO 64116
Tel: 816/421-1305
Fax: 816/421-1991

### BRAFORD (BO)

United Braford Breeders
422 East Main, Suite 218
Nacogdoches, TX 75961
Tel: 409/569-8200
Fax: 409/569-9556
Email: ubb@brafords.org
*Website: http://www.brafords.org*

### BRAHMAN (BR)

American Brahman Breeders
Association
1313 LaConcha Lane
Houston, TX 77054
Tel: 713/795-4444
Fax: 713/795-4450
Email: abba@wt.net
*Website: http://www.brahman.org*

### BRALERS (BL)

American Bralers Association
P.O. Box 75
Burton, TX 77835
Tel: 281/440-5844

### BRANGUS (BN)

International Brangus Breeders
Association
P.O. Box 696020
San Antonio, TX 78269-6020
Tel: 210/696-8231 Ext. 12
Fax: 210/696-8718
Email: jno@int-brangus.org
*Website: http://www.int-brangus.org*

### BRAUNVIEH (BU)

Braunvieh Association of America
P.O. Box 6396
Lincoln, NE 68506

Tel: 402/421-2960
Fax: 402/421-2994
Email: Braunaa@ibm.net
*Website: http://www.braunvieh.org*

Braunvieh Breeders International
P.O. Box 7586
N. Kansas City, MO 64116
Tel: 816/471-1998
Fax: 816/421-1991

### BRITISH WHITE (BW)

British White Cattle Association
of America
P.O. Box 281
Bells, TX 75414-0281
Tel: 903/965-7718
Fax: 903/965-5452
Email: meh@texoma.net
*Website: http://www.britishwhite.org*

### CHAROLAIS (CH)

American International Charolais
Association
P.O. Box 20247
Kansas City, MO 64195
Tel: 816/464-5977
Fax: 816/464-5759
Email: chjoun@sound.net
*Website: http://www.charolaisusa.com*

### CHIANINA (CA)

American Chianina Association
P.O. Box 890
1708 N. Prairie View Road
Platte City, MO 64079
Tel: 816/431-2808
Fax: 816/431-5381
Email: aca@sound.net
*Website: http://www.chicattle.org*

### CORRIENTE (MC)

North American Corriente Association
P.O. Box 12359
N. Kansas City, MO 64116
Tel: 816/421-1992
Fax: 816/421-1991
Email: http://jspawn321@aol.com

### GELBVIEH (GV)

American Gelbvieh Association
10900 Dover St.
Westminister, CO 80021
Tel: 303/465-2333
Fax: 303/465-2339
Email: aga@www.gelbvieh.org
*Website: http://www.gelbvieh.org*

## HEREFORD (HH, HP)

American Hereford Association
P.O. Box 014059
Kansas City, MO 64101-4059
Tel: 816/842-3757
Fax: 816/842-6931
Email: jrick@hereford.org
*Website: http://www.hereford.org*

## LIMOUSIN (LM)

North American Limousin Foundation
7383 S. Alton Way
Suite 100, Box 4467
Englewood, CO 80112
Tel: 303/220-1693
Fax: 303/220-1884
Email: jedwards@nalf.org
*Website: http://www.nalf.org*

## MAINE-ANJOU (MA)

American Maine-Anjou Association
204 Marshall Rd.
P.O. Box 1100
Platte City, MO 64079-1100
Tel: 816/431-9950
Fax: 831/431-9951
Email: anjou1@mindspring.com
*Website: http://www.maine-anjou.org*

## MARCHIGIANA (MR)

American International Marchigiana
Society
Marky Cattle Association
Box 198
Walton, KS 67151-0198
Tel: 316/837-3303
Fax: 316/283-8379
Email: marky@southwind.net
*Website: http://www.marchigiana.org*

## PINZGAUER (PZ)

American Pinzgauer Association
21555 St. Rt. 698
Jenera, OH 45841
Tel: 800/914-9883
Fax: 419/326-5501
Email: Apinzgauer@aol.com
*Website: http://www.afn.org/~greatcow/*

## RED ANGUS (AR)

Red Angus Association of America, Inc.
4201 North Interstate 35
Denton, TX 76207-7443
Tel: 940/387-3502

Fax: 940/383-4036
Email: info@redangus1.org
*Website: http://www.redangus1.org*

## RED BRANGUS (RB)

American Red Brangus
3995 E. 290
Dripping Springs, TX 78620
Tel: 512/858-7285
Fax: 512/858-7084
Email: arba@texas.net
*Website: http://www.Brangusassc.com*

## SALERS (SA)

American Salers Association
7383 S. Alton Way
Suite 103
Englewood, CO 80112
Tel: 303/770-9292
Fax: 303/770-9302
Email: salersusa.org
*Website: http://www.salersusa.org*

## SANTA GERTRUDIS (SG)

Santa Gertrudis Breeders International
P.O. Box 1257
Kingsville, TX 78364
Tel: 361/592-9357
Fax: 361/592-8572
Email: truegert@aol.com

## SCOTCH HIGHLAND (SH)

American Highland Cattle Association
#200 Livestock Exchange Bldg.
4701 Marion Street
Denver, CO 80216
Tel: 303/292-9102
Fax: 303/292-9171
Email: ahca@envisionet.net
*Website: http://www.highlandcattle.org*

## SENEPOL (SE)

Senepol Cattle Breeders Association
P.O. Box 808
Statham, GA 30666-0808
Tel:800/736-3765
Fax: 770/725-5281
Email: lcoley@sales-synergy.com
*Website: http://www.senepolcattle.com*

## SHORTHORN (SS) (SP) (IS)

American Shorthorn Association
8288 Hascall St.
Omaha, NE 68124

Tel: 402/393-7200
Fax: 402/393-7203
Email: hunsley@beefshorthornusa.com
*Website: http://www.beefshorthornusa.
com*

## SIMMENTAL (SM)

American Simmental Association
1 Simmental Way
Bozeman, MT 59715
Tel: 406/587-4531
Fax: 406/587-9301
Email: simmental@simmental.org
*Website: http://www.simmental.org*

## SOUTH DEVON (DS)

North American South Devon Association
2514 Avenue S
Santa Fe, TX 77510
Tel: 409/927-4445
Fax: 409/927-4445
Email: southdevoninfo@aol.com
*Website: http://www.southdevon.com*

## TARENTAISE (TA)

American Tarentaise Association
Box 34705
Kansas City, MO 64116
Tel: 816/421-1993
Fax: 816/421-1991
Email: jspawn321@aol.com

## TEXAS LONGHORN (TL)

Texas Longhorn Breeders Association
of America
2315 N. Main St., Suite 402
P.O. Box 4430
Fort Worth, TX 76164
Tel: 817/625-6241
Fax: 817/625-1388
Email: tlbaa@tlbaa.org
*Website: http://www.tlbaa.org*

## WAGYU (KB)

American Wagyu Association
P.O. Box 4071
Bryan, TX 77805
Tel: 409/260-0300
Fax: 409/846-4945

*For information on other breeds refer to
the following website: http://www.ansi.
okstate.edu/breeds/cattle/*

# REFERENCES

Boyd, L. J. 1992. AI 1992. Hindsight and foresight. Proc. 14th Tech. Conf. on Artificial Insemination and Reproduction. NAAB. p. 6.

Day, M. 2001. Use of progesterone to induce and synchronize estrus: Application of the CIDR. NAAB Symposium on Improving Reproductive Performance at 33$^{rd}$ Res. Symp. and Ann. Mtg. Beef Improvement Federation. San Antonio, TX. pp. 13–25.

Geary, T. 1999. Heat detection systems and estrus management. Proc. 31$^{st}$ Res. Symp. and Ann. Mtg. Beef Improvement Federation. p. 24.

Guidelines for Uniform Beef Improvement Programs (6th Ed.). 1990. Beef Improvement Federation, OSU, Stillwater, OK.

Hafez, E. S. E. (Ed.). 1987. Reproduction in Farm Animals (5th Ed.). Lea & Febiger, Philadelphia.

Huffine. A. et al. 1998. Artificial Insemination Handbook. NAAB. pp. 1–32.

Neumann, A. L., and K. S. Lusby. 1986. Beef Cattle (8th Ed.). John Wiley & Sons, Inc., New York. (Ch. 2.)

NRC Nutrient Requirements of Beef Cattle (6th Revised Ed.). 1984. National Academy Press, Washington, DC. p. 45.

Pace, M. M. 1985. What makes AI and synchronization more profitable? Proc. Ann. Conf. on Artificial Insemination and Embryo Transfer in Beef Cattle. NAAB. p. 28.

Patterson, D. J. et al. 2001. Emerging protocols to synchronize estrus in replacement beef heifers and postpartum cows. NAAB Symposium on Improving Reproductive Performance at 33$^{rd}$ Res. Symp. and Ann. Mtg. Beef Improvement Federation. San Antonio, TX. pp. 26–51.

Perry, E. J. (Ed.). 1968. Artificial Insemination of Farm Animals (4th Ed.). Rutgers Univ. Press, New Brunswick, NJ.

Proc. Ann. Conf. on Artificial Insemination and Embryo Transfer in Beef Cattle. 1966 to 1986. National Association of Animal Breeders, Inc., P.O. Box 1033, Columbia, MO 65205.

Proc. 7th and 8th Tech. Conf. on Artificial Insemination and Reproduction. 1978 and 1980. National Association of Animal Breeders, Inc., P.O. Box 1033, Columbia, MO 65205.

Stevenson, J. S. 1999. Estrus synchronization and induction protocols. Proc. 31$^{st}$ Res. Symp. and Ann. Mtg. Beef Improvement Federation. p. 14.

Thatcher, W. W. et al. 2001. Current concepts for estrus synchronization and timed insemination. Proc. Ann. Conf. and Canine Symp. Soc. for Theriogenology/ACT, Vancouver, BC. p. 129

Wiltbank, M. C. 1998. Update on synchronization of ovulation and estrus. Proc. 17$^{th}$ Tech. Conf. on Artificial Insemination and Reproduction. NAAB. p. 65.

# EXERCISE 18

# Direct Herd Service and Herdsman-Inseminator Training

## OBJECT

To become familiar with the importance of direct herd service, or "do-it-yourself" AI, and the necessity for adequate herdsman-inseminator training courses.

## DISCUSSION

Widespread use of cryogenic refrigerators for storing frozen semen on the farm, a decline in number of dairy herds, and increasing competition from other industries to attract AI technicians from sparsely populated cow areas, have resulted in the selling of semen directly to herd operators. Called "direct herd service," or "do-it-yourself" AI, this practice has been growing steadily for many years. Its main advantage is that it does not require organizations to maintain a large AI technician force. Merchandising becomes less complicated with semen sold on a straw, dose, or unit basis.

Of the 7.5 million dairy cows estimated to be artificially inseminated annually in the United States, nearly 70 percent are serviced with semen sold directly to herd owners. However, this figure can be greatly influenced by region of the country and herd size.[1] Since beef artificial insemination is largely seasonal, it is practical for a large portion—perhaps some 90 percent—to be inseminated by the herd operators or their employees.

At the start, the development of "do-it-yourself" (DIY) programs was looked upon with consternation; however, the passing of time has indicated that (1) with adequate training and supervision by the semen-selling business, herd operators or their trained employees can, in most cases, obtain satisfactory conception rates; (2) adequate inseminator training courses are an integral part of DIY programs; (3) with larger herds, there is the necessity for having the AI inseminator close at hand, as many cows are inseminated on given days; and (4) some herds in sparsely populated cow areas would not have AI service except by direct semen sales.

## Why Herd Owners Adopt Direct Service

An early survey of 62 Michigan dairy operators with 4,596 milking cows indicates the typical reasons dairy operators choose direct service, or the "do-it-yourself" AI plan.[2]

It is noted that 42 percent of these dairy operators gave reasons directly relating to the AI technician for changing to direct service; in 1 of 26 of these cases, a technician was not available. Twenty-nine percent found direct service more convenient, 16 percent believed it to be

---

[1] B. L. Erven and D. Arbaugh. 1978. Artificial Insemination on U.S. Dairy Farms. Report of a Study Conducted in Cooperation with NAAB (ESO 1379). Dept. Agric. Economics and Rural Sociology, Ohio State Univ., Columbus.

[2] L. J. Boyd, et al. 1971. Survey of Michigan Dairymen on Direct Service Artificial Insemination. Paper D-156. Dairy Dept., Michigan State Univ., East Lansing.

**Main Reasons Why 62 Dairy Operators Started Direct Service Artificial Insemination**

| Reason | Number | Percent of All |
|---|---|---|
| A. Technician | | |
|   1. Lost technician | 10 | |
|   2. Dissatisfied with technician or changes in technician | 7 | |
|   3. Did not know when technician would come | 4 | |
|   4. Served as former technician | 3 | |
|   5. Breeds cows at two other farms | 1 | |
|   6. No technicians available | 1 | |
|     Total | 26 | 42 |
| B. Cost—Cheaper | 10 | |
|     Total | 10 | 16 |
| C. Conception Rate | | |
|   1. Better conception rate | 4 | |
|   2. Better timing of insemination | 4 | |
|     Total | 8 | 13 |
| D. Convenience to Dairy Operators or Breeders | | |
|   1. Can breed cows when they want to breed them, can breed at milking time, can breed more easily in loose housing, and can breed in less time than when holding cows for technician | 7 | |
|   2. Did not want to keep a bull | 2 | |
|   3. Store and use semen from own bull | 4 | |
|   4. Have semen from desired bulls when wanted | 3 | |
|   5. Have wider selection of bulls than technician has | 2 | |
|     Total | 18 | 29 |
|     Grand Total | 62 | 100 |

cheaper, and 13 percent claimed better conception rate and better timing of insemination.

The average number of services per conception for these dairy operators was 1.6 and ranged from 112 to 118 services per herd as grouped to size.

This same study found that the cost of direct service was not necessarily cheaper than the cost of service provided by the technician.

It is quite evident that factors other than technician cost influence the adoption of direct service—except for large herds, which are increasing in number. Herd owners should weigh all costs before they decide on a change from a professional technician to direct service. Another factor to be considered is whether or not herd owners can use their time better in managing their herds and farms than in inseminating cows.

In heavily populated cow areas, the cooperative AI organizations in particular maintain a strong corps of trained AI technicians and render a complete breeding service. This no doubt will continue to be the case in areas where the cattle population will support this service. At the same time, direct service will continue to be an important part of cattle improvement programs in which AI is used.

Figures 18.1, 18.2, and 18.3 depict various inseminator training scenes.

## Need for Herdsman-Inseminator Training

Herdsman-inseminators are individuals who inseminate cattle they own or those of their employers. Unlike full-time, or "professional," AI

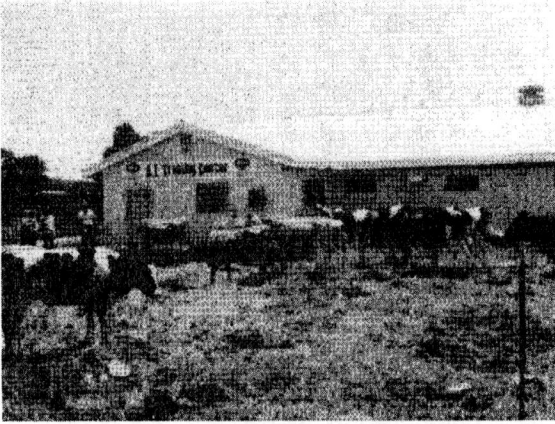

**Figure 18.1.** An AI training center and cows used for practice. (Courtesy, MABC/Select Sires, East Lansing, MI)

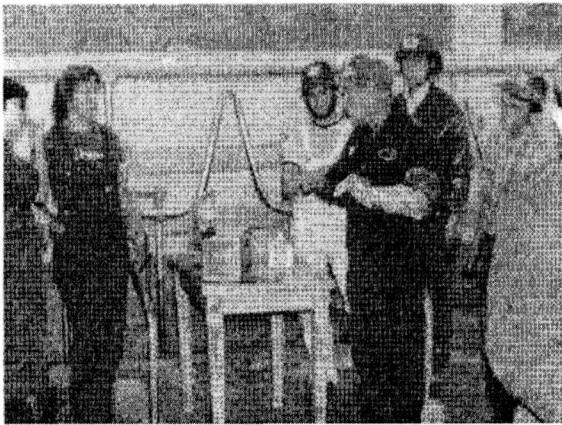

**Figure 18.2.** An instructor explains insemination techniques to a group of direct herd students. (Courtesy, MABC/Select Sires, East Lansing, MI)

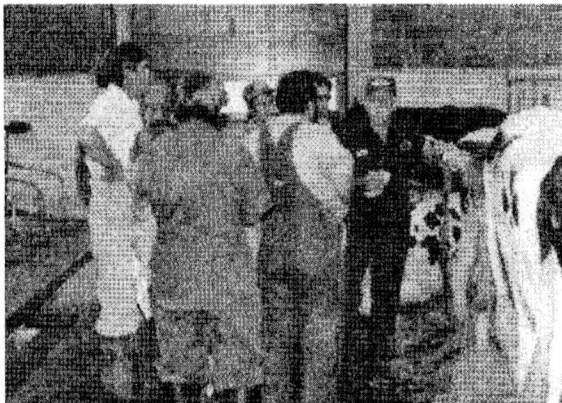

**Figure 18.3.** An instructor demonstrates the recto-vaginal insemination technique. (Courtesy, MABC/Select Sires, East Lansing, MI)

technicians, they do little work outside the herds they or their employers own. They may be individuals who inseminate beef cattle in their own herd or in someone else's herd during a period of six to eight weeks in the spring months. Or they may be dairy operators or dairy herd managers who, for various reasons, purchase frozen semen and inseminate the cattle under their control. The importance of adequate training and supervision to obtain maximum results in such cases cannot be taken lightly.

## Where May Training Be Obtained?

Usually the training of AI technicians is by means of a "short course." Short courses may be from one to two weeks in length; however, herdsman-inseminator training courses are from two to five days. Even one-day "demonstration schools" are held but are not recommended for a total management concept. All short courses are designed to teach the fundamentals of insemination of the cow; proper semen handling and thawing techniques; hygienic measures and reproductive management; record keeping; and, in cases of individuals planning to become full-time technicians, company policies. Sources of training include the following:

**AI Organizations—** Most AI organizations conduct training courses or schools for both insemination technicians and herdsman-inseminators. Such training courses are usually, but not exclusively, designed to provide the necessary technicians that an organization needs for its operations. In some cases, AI organizations hold technician training schools in collaboration with agricultural colleges.

**Agricultural Colleges—** Some agricultural colleges sponsor AI training short courses. In the earlier days of AI, most of the preliminary training for AI technicians came about in this way.

**Private Schools**— With the growing use of artificial insemination in beef herds and the steady development of direct herd AI programs, the demand for training herdsman-inseminators has remained high. The result has been the establishment of AI training schools by private individuals.

## Courses for College Credit

Some colleges and universities in the United States, through their animal or dairy science departments, offer extended training in animal reproduction and artificial insemination. Such courses may be taught over an entire college semester or, in some cases, may include supporting subjects for two school years. College students who expect to enter the field of livestock improvement, which involves AI, will find this more extensive training to be of value.

## Objectives of Short Course Training

The first objective of training schools, whether for professional technician-inseminators, Figure 18.4, or herdsman-inseminators, is to help trainees become proficient in the knowledge and skills necessary to inseminate cows and obtain adequate conception rates. It is also necessary that trainees acquire a knowledge of the female reproductive organs and their general functions. Important, too, is training in the essentials of animal hygiene and the sanitary practices that every person who inseminates farm animals should observe. If success is to result, proper care and handling of semen in the field must be learned and observed. Trainees must also become familiar with the necessary breeding and calving records to be kept. In the case of registered animals, there are special requirements in records that must be met.

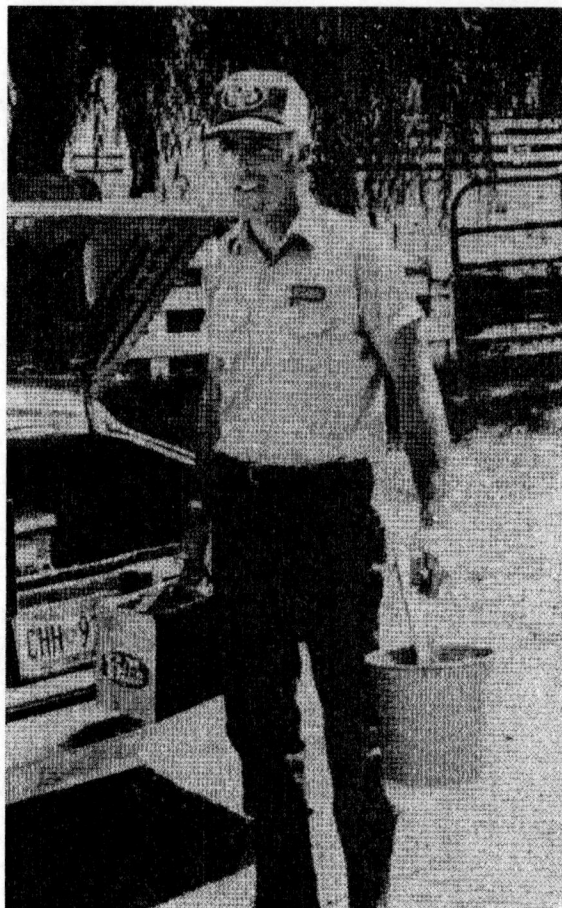

**Figure 18.4.** A professional AI technician prepares to inseminate cows on a Mifflin County, PA, farm. Note his neat appearance, AI kit for equipment, boots, and bucket of water with disinfectant for cleaning boots when work at this farm is completed. An $LN_2$ refrigerator and all equipment and supplies are carried in the trunk of the car. (Courtesy, Sire Power, Inc., Tunkhannock, PA)

## Scope of Training Varies

An early survey of schools for training inseminators, as made by the NAAB, indicated considerable variation in the scope of training provided. This situation was to be expected because there had been no widespread attempt to establish uniform standards and generally emphasize the importance of proper training in this field. Variations existed between schools sponsored by AI organizations, colleges, and private individuals with respect to the time spent on academic phases, the amount of work with live cows, the size and caliber of instructional staff, and the facilities available. Most of the schools surveyed were concentrating efforts on teaching the fundamental information and providing varying amounts of time for practice insemination on live cows. Assistance to trainees after they have completed a training course and gone forth to practice varies greatly. The AI organizations adequately supervise the persons they hire and usually provide a training period with an experienced technician. Most of the schools conducted by private individuals or colleges are glad to render assistance if a trainee runs into difficulties.

In choosing a short course for training, one should determine how much time will be spent working on live cows. Each trainee should have several cows to use exclusively. Several students cannot satisfactorily use the same practice cow, due to the straining and contractions of the cow's rectum following repeated insertions of the palpating hand.

Trainees are urged to select training courses in which the individuals or organizations conducting the school have established reputations for honesty and dependability. Recognizing the need for emphasis on standards for inseminator training, the NAAB, in 1966, established a committee to study the training programs of AI training schools and make recommendations that may be helpful to the industry. From this study, the committee drafted "Recommended Minimum Standards for Training of Artificial Inseminating Technicians and Herdsman-Inseminators," which has been updated to "Recommended Minimum Standards for Artificial Insemination Training." The current recommended minimums follow:

Twelve hours of classroom instruction in
  Anatomy of the cow
  Demonstration of proper insemination
    techniques
  Practice insemination using reproductive organs
  Proper use and maintenance of inseminating
    equipment and semen storage units
  Proper thawing and handling of frozen semen
  Heat detection, signs of heat, methods, and aids
  Cattle identification and herd records

Six hours of live cow insemination practice
  A minimum of three separate sessions
  Two cows per student per course, with each
    having access to a minimum of 10 practice
    cows
  A maximum of eight students per instructor

Cow availability and school size are factors in determining the total days required for AI training. When seeking AI training, be cautious in considering a one-day school that offers a total management concept.

AI training school tuition may vary between sponsoring organizations. Quite often the cost of training will be discounted with equipment or semen purchases. You should inquire directly about training program packages.

## Recommendations

**Field Experience—** It is recommended that trainees spend time riding with experienced technicians to observe field activities firsthand.

**Examinations—** Examinations should involve a test of subject matter and manual skill as an inseminator.

Where state laws require licensing of AI technicians, the course of instruction and training should be adequate to enable students to meet such requirements.

Successful technician-inseminators or herdsman-inseminators must continue to add to their knowledge and skill by study, observation, and practice. Technicians who are not challenged by the opportunity for livestock improvement and are unwilling to accept the responsibilities of their role in working with valuable animals are not likely to find satisfaction in this field. Technicians must continually grow with the job. In so doing, they will command satisfactory incomes and find pleasure in watching the herds under their care make genetic progress.

# QUESTIONS

1. What are the advantages of the "do-it-yourself," or direct herd service, AI program? What are some disadvantages?

2. What factors may influence the cost per cow in calf from direct herd service?

3. Why do some dairy operators prefer the direct herd service program?

4. Why does beef artificial insemination depend heavily on direct herd service?

5. What are considered the most important factors in selecting an AI training course?

6. What training program should be followed if one wishes to become a full-time or a career AI technician?

# REFERENCE

Recommended Minimum Standards for Artificial Insemination Training, National Association of Animal Breeders, Inc., Columbia, MO.

# EXERCISE 19

# Pregnancy Determination in the Cow

## OBJECT

To become familiar with the principles of pregnancy diagnosis in the cow.

## DISCUSSION

Pregnancy diagnosis in the cow is an important part of herd reproductive management. An early determination of pregnancy after insemination is necessary to reduce losses in production time in those animals that did not conceive or did not maintain a pregnancy. By decreasing the average number of days cows are open, the herd calving interval is shortened, which results in higher profitability. Although an animal not returning to estrus after insemination is often assumed to be pregnant, using only external signs as a basis for determining pregnancy is not totally reliable. In addition, there is a small percentage of cows that return to estrus at least once after they have conceived. The AI technician or herdsman-inseminator should be knowledgeable about methods available to help determine pregnancy. This exercise focuses on the clinical determination of pregnancy through rectal palpation. Also, other methods, such as the use of ultrasound and various assays, will be described briefly.

The ability to determine pregnancy through palpation technique is essential for the experienced inseminator in checking cows that may be in heat months after being inseminated, to find out whether they are open or in-calf, before making a repeat insemination.

Also, cows that have an unknown breeding history that the inseminator is requested to inseminate should be checked before breeding. The AI technician or herdsman-inseminator, however, is certainly not licensed to practice veterinary medicine. Cases of doubtful pregnancy or cows that need examination or treatment for subfertility should be referred to a competent veterinarian.

Before a rectal examination of the cow is made to determine pregnancy, first it is important to have a working knowledge of the anatomy and functions of the reproductive tract (see Figure 19.1 and refer to Exercise 4 for more details) and an understanding of events that occur during early pregnancy. Complete breeding records and a reproductive

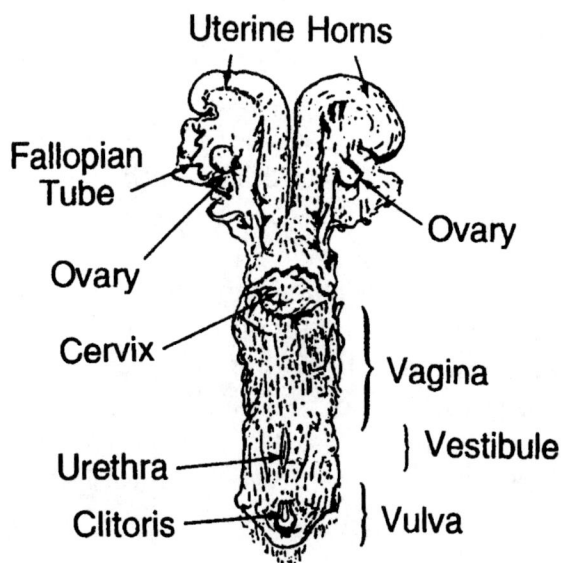

**Figure 19.1.** Reproductive organs in the cow. (Modified from Louisiana Agr. Exp. Sta. Bull. 51)

199

history of the cow are also helpful for an accurate pregnancy examination.

The fertilized cow egg undergoes cellular divisions and enters the uterus 3 to 4 days after ovulation, when it contains 8 to 16 cells. Secretions from the uterine glands nourish the embryo during this early period. The embryo continues to grow rapidly in the uterine horn corresponding to the side on which it was ovulated. The embryo then develops distinct layers of cells that constitute the beginnings of the fetal organs and body parts, as well as the extra-embryonic membranes that eventually attach to the uterine wall to form the placenta. The extra-embryonic membranes elongate and expand into the non-pregnant uterine horn by day 20, when initial stages of implantation begin. By about day 45, attachment is complete and fetal nourishment commences at specific placental sites (placentomes).

## Indications of Pregnancy

Usually the first sign of pregnancy is a cow's failure to return to heat. This is a reliable indication in most healthy cows in herds with a good estrus detection program; however, lack of estrus may mean little in cases of early embryonic death, abortion, pathological conditions that result in pyometra (pus in the uterus), or a persistent *corpus luteum*. It is estimated that about 5 to 10 percent of all cows will show evidence of one heat even though they are pregnant and that about 15 percent of cows not showing heat are not pregnant upon palpation 60 days after insemination. It should be noted here that the presence or absence of small amounts of blood on the cow's tail or rear quarters one or two days after the heat period is not an indicator of whether or not conception has occurred. This metestrus bleeding, which is caused by leakage of small uterine blood vessels, is due to a rapid decline in estrogen level after heat, and it occurs normally

in over 80 percent of heifers and about 40 to 60 percent of cows. Although it is sometimes erroneously believed to be associated with non-pregnancy, metestrus bleeding is actually independent of breeding and conception.

Other outward indications of pregnancy may be observed later in gestation, but they are not very useful for an early pregnancy diagnosis. For example, heifers four to five months pregnant sometimes exhibit swelling, or "springing," of the udder. In older cows, such udder growth is usually not evident until late in pregnancy. Also, the calf can be identified by bumping the flank of the cow (ballottement), but not until around the seventh or eighth month of pregnancy. At that time, the calf can be felt when the fist is intermittently pushed deep into the cow's abdomen at the flank. The fetus will feel like a hard object floating in the abdomen. This ancient method is easy to perform but has little or no practical value in artificial insemination.

Another indicator is the formation of a uterine seal, or thick mucus plug, in the cervix, which can be detected by aid of a speculum and a light and also by rectal palpation. This is of some value in diagnosing, but it is not highly reliable. The cervix always contains some mucus, often of varying viscosity. Some non-pregnant cows show a fairly heavy mucus plug at times, and some pregnant cows show only a small plug.

The most accurate and rapid clinical method to diagnose pregnancy in the cow is by rectal palpation of the reproductive tract (Figure 19.2).

## Rectal Palpation of the Reproductive System

The diagnosis of pregnancy in cattle is generally made from about 35 to 50 days following breeding by palpation of the amniotic vesicle and slip of the fetal membranes, or

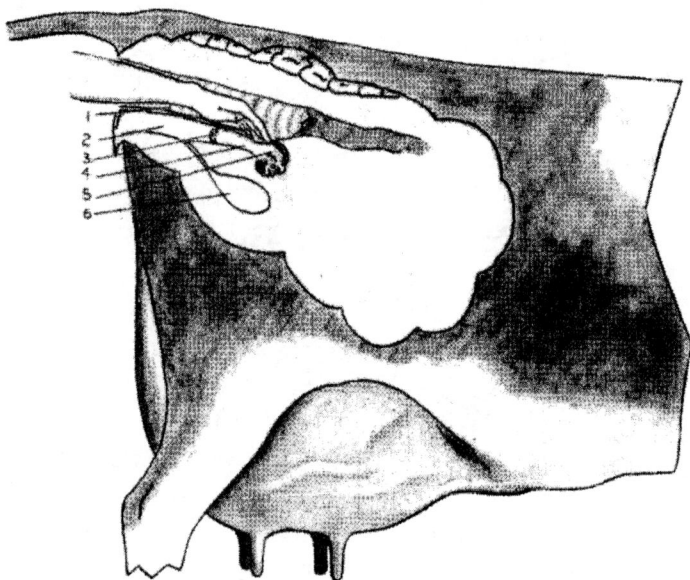

**Figure 19.2.** Rectal palpation of the cow reproductive tract. Non-pregnant ("open") cow shown. (1) rectum, or gut; (2) vagina; (3) *os uteri*, or external cervical opening; (4) cervix and body of uterus; (5) horn of uterus showing right ovary and oviduct; (6) urinary bladder.

from about 80 to 100 days following service by palpation of the fetus, placentomes, or vibration of the middle uterine artery. Detecting any *one* of these signs is considered to be a positive indicator of pregnancy. The novice palpator, however, may want to feel for more than one of these signs to be certain of the diagnosis. Other indicators that suggest a cow or heifer is pregnant are an increase in the size of the uterus, notably the pregnant (gravid) horn; a thinning of the uterine wall and an accumulation of fetal fluids that give the feeling of fluctuation when palpated; the position of the uterus in the pelvic and/or abdominal cavity, which changes as the uterus grows to accommodate a developing fetus; the larger size and persistence of the *corpus luteum;* and a pale-appearing, dry vaginal mucosa. These signs alone, though, should not be relied on to determine pregnancy, because they may also be associated with conditions other than pregnancy.

Dairy operators who strive for a 12- to 13-month calving interval want to know as soon as possible the "story" on the cow heading for a long, dry period or an extended lactation at a low level of production. The beef producer

may use the earlier pregnancy diagnosis (35 to 50 days) for cows inseminated the first time before they are turned out to grass. Since most beef producers try to get all eligible cows (those that come into heat during the AI breeding period) inseminated in a short period, many cows cannot be checked for pregnancy until "round-up time" in the fall. This will usually involve cows 90 to 150 days in calf or open. The rancher often sends cows "not in calf" to market rather than carry them over. In this connection, an accurate pregnancy diagnosis is of great value and does much to improve the calving percentage in the herd.

## PROCEDURE

Experience is necessary to become proficient in pregnancy diagnosis by rectal palpation. It should be realized that there are differences in the genitalia of different animals, not only in non-pregnant animals but also in pregnant animals at the same stage of pregnancy. The ease with which the uterus can be palpated depends a great deal upon the age, condition, size, and breed of the cow. Practical

201

experience is therefore absolutely necessary for any degree of accuracy in diagnosis.

It is also important to understand that rectal examinations for pregnancy must be made with great care to avoid traumatizing the rectum of the cow or the developing fetus. It has been speculated that routine early palpation (at 30 to 45 days) increases the chances of embryonic or fetal death occurring. However, the extent to which early palpation might be a factor in causing death is difficult to measure because the period involved is part of that in which the highest incidence of natural embryonic or fetal death occurs. In any case, the palpator needs to be gentle and exercise care when palpating.

The animal to be examined should be identified and well restrained. Usually the palpator can use one hand (the right) to hold up the cow's tail and the left hand to explore.

The palpator should observe appropriate sanitary precautions and wear protective clothing, boots, and a plastic AI sleeve or shoulder-length rubber glove for examination. All jewelry should be removed from the palpating arm and hand. A bucket of warm water and soap should be available for use in lubricating the anal region of the cow and the gloved hand and arm to be used to examine the cow. The gloved palpation hand is lubricated and inserted into the rectum. Straining by the cow, with contraction of the walls of the rectum, nearly always occurs at this stage. It is best to permit this spasm to pass off before proceeding further and clearing the rectum of feces. (Refer to Exercise 16 for recommended procedures for entering the rectum, removing fecal material, and working through rectal contractions.) The uterus in heifers is normally located in the pelvic cavity when non-pregnant and up to about the third or fourth month of gestation. The uterus in older cows, however, typically lies on or over the pelvic brim when non-pregnant and is displaced into the abdominal cavity soon after conception in some cows or by the second or third month of ges-

tation in others. In heifers or cows in early gestation, a diagnosis for pregnancy can usually be made by palpating the entire length of the uterine horns within the pelvic cavity. However, as the pregnant uterus is displaced into the abdominal cavity over time, it becomes necessary to retract it back into the pelvic cavity for an examination. This can be done, particularly in older cows, up to about the third month of gestation. As in artificial insemination, the cervix is an important internal landmark. When the rectum is emptied, the cervix may be easily located by sweeping the fingers laterally across the floor of the pelvis. As indicated in Exercise 16, the cervix has a hard, gristly feel. It is a round, cylindrical organ some 3 to 4 inches long and about 1 to 1½ inches in diameter. With a good understanding of reproductive anatomy, the palpator can start at the cervix and systematically locate the remainder of reproductive tract structures by feel and examine them for positive indications of pregnancy.

In heifers, the whole of the cervix, uterine horns, and ovaries can be covered by the palm of the hand, about 9 to 10 inches within the rectum. There is often a tendency for beginners to put the hand too far forward. However, in mature animals that have had one or more calves, the horns of the uterus are carried forward and are often out of reach, yet the ovaries can usually still be reached for palpation early in pregnancy. If it is necessary to retract the uterus into the pelvic canal for examination, this can be accomplished by (1) grasping the cervix and pulling it posteriorly, then hooking the intercornual ligament (located at the junction of the uterine horns) with a finger and gently retracting the uterus posteriorly into the pelvic canal, or (2) extending the hand over the pelvic brim, reaching down and cupping the uterus with the palm of the hand, then retracting it up over the brim and posteriorly into the pelvic canal.

## Examination 28 to 50 Days After Breeding

Practice and the development of sensory skills are essential in making an accurate pregnancy diagnosis of the cow 28 to 50 days after breeding. The palpator's knowledge regarding the early development of the embryonic structures and changes in the reproductive tract (ovaries, cervix, and uterine horns) and his or her ability to translate the findings the fingers reveal are matters of concentration and skill. Practicing on cows, when the breeding date is known, can do much to improve skill and confidence. A reasonable amount of speed is desirable in making any pregnancy diagnosis in cattle. If the time of the examination is prolonged, straining occurs, and reliable diagnosis is impossible.

With the palm of the hand downward and proceeding gently, the cervix and dorsal portions of the curled horns of the non-pregnant or early-pregnant uterus can be easily palpated (Figure 19.3). Usually, the entire uterus can be picked up and gently held. By cautiously lifting the hand upward and slightly backward, the horns of the uterus can be un-curled so that each horn can be gently palpated between the thumb and forefinger. The entire length of the horn should be palpated.

Palpation is made for the presence of the amniotic vesicle, which will be felt in the gravid horn. As the thumb and fingers move gently and slowly back and forth along the uterine horn, the vesicle slips between them. The amniotic vesicle is a small spherical structure that is fairly turgid up to six or seven weeks of gestation.[1] Following this period it gradually loses its turgidity until the characteristic "slippery feel" is absent. For this reason, palpation of the amniotic vesicle is most effective from 35 to 50 days of gestation. Usually the amniotic vesicle will be located in the uterine horn on the same side as the ovary containing a corpus luteum; however, in a few cases, the *corpus luteum* of pregnancy is found in the ovary opposite the horn containing the fetus.

The experienced palpator can usually determine the approximate number of days pregnant between 28 and 50 by the feel and size of

---

[1] W. Wisnicky and L. E. Casida. 1948. A manual method for diagnosis of pregnancy in cattle. J. Am. Vet. Med. Assoc. 113:451.

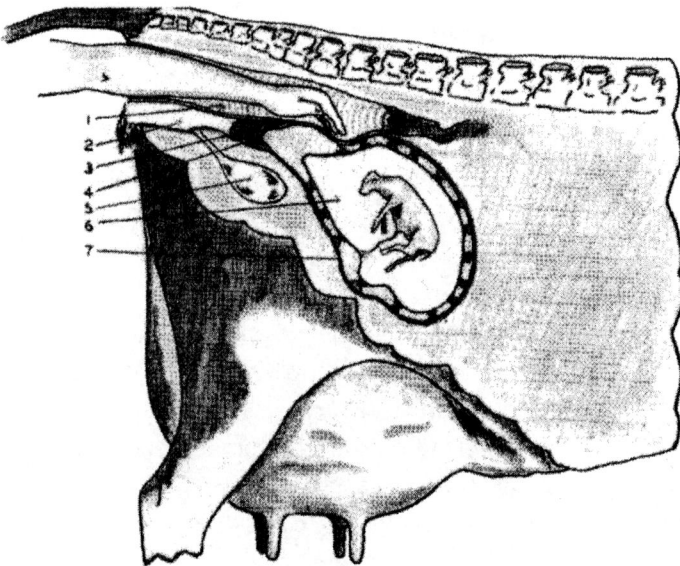

**Figure 19.3.** Rectal palpation of the cow reproductive tract. Pregnant cow shown. (1) rectum (hand and forearm in place); (2) vagina; (3) cervix and cervical plug; (4) cervical canal and body of uterus distended forward; (5) urinary bladder; (6) chorioallantoic sac containing fetus (fetus may be gently palpated by extending hand over the uterus); (7) wall of uterus showing placentomes.

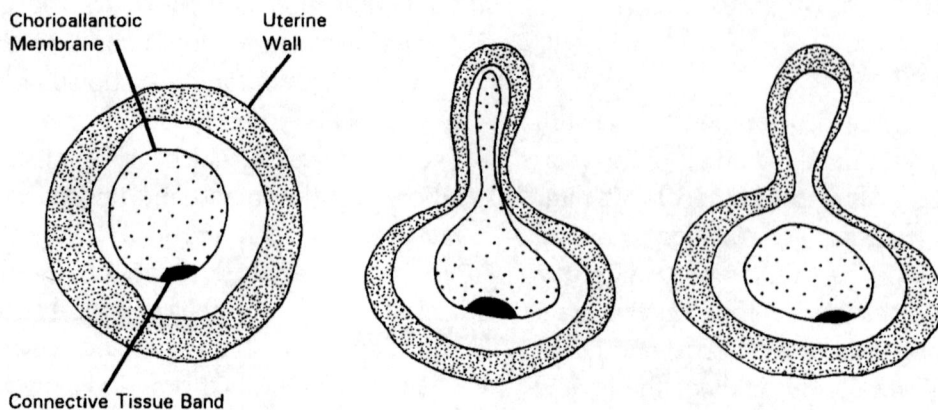

**Figure 19.4.** Schematic drawing of cross-sections of uterine horn of pregnant cow, illustrating "slip of fetal membranes." *Left:* Horn before palpation. *Center:* When compressing the horn by palpation, you can feel the chorioallantoic membrane between your thumb and fingers. *Right:* The chorioallantoic membrane slips back to normal position before the uterine wall escapes between palpating thumb and fingers. In early pregnancy the entire horn is compressed to include the characteristic connective tissue band that contains blood vessels, and is easily distinguished. (From P. L. Senger and J. J. Reeves. Anim. Sci. 454 Manual. Washington State Univ., Pullman. p. 48)

the amniotic vesicle. This can be helpful in determining whether a cow settled to the last or an earlier service or whether or not early embryonic death (fetal absorption) occurred.

In the cow that is pregnant four to five weeks, the fetal membranes (chorioallantoic membrane) can be felt as a separate structure within the uterine horn. These feel much like a shirt or a blouse under the sleeve of a coat. The fetal membranes can be detected by compressing the gravid uterine horn (usually at its widest part) between thumb and fingers before the uterine wall escapes between them. This is known as the "fetal membrane slip" (Figure 19.4). This technique may also be performed later in gestation. It is particularly helpful in distinguishing between pregnancy and other conditions that may cause an increase in the size of the uterine horn(s).

## Pregnancy Determination After 75 to 90 Days

At 21 days following insemination, if the cow is pregnant and healthy, there should be present in one of the ovaries a fully developed *corpus luteum,* and the corresponding uter-

ine horn, or cornu, may be slightly enlarged. If the cow has not become pregnant, the *corpus luteum* will not be present, and a maturing follicle will be forming, usually in the opposite ovary. The palpation of a *corpus luteum* is of greater value when considered with heat dates, etc., in cows that are examined at occasional intervals.

The palpation of the uterine arteries with their characteristic pulse (fremitus) in pregnancy is valuable also. In most cases, the uterine arteries are easily discerned. One middle uterine artery supplies each horn and is the main blood supply to the uterus.

With the onset of pregnancy, the middle uterine arteries increase in volume and the pulsations become more vibratory. This is particularly true for the artery supplying the pregnant horn. In a non-pregnant cow, a uterine artery is about 3 to 5 mm in diameter and has a clearly defined pulse. In the pregnant cow, however, it grows rapidly and finally attains a diameter of over 1½ cm near term. As the artery increases in size, its walls become thinner, and instead of a pulse, it has a characteristic "whirring," or fremitus, that is felt on palpation. There is a heightened or more forceful pressure of blood flow. The uterine artery leaves the caudal end

204

of the posterior aorta or one of the iliacs and passes ventrally "not far from the anterior-median line of the ilium," according to Williams.[2] It is suspended within the broad ligament, which permits it to be readily discerned in the area near the shaft of the ilium. The increase in size of the main artery supplying the pregnant horn can be detected at 60 to 75 days in heifers or at 90 days in older cows. Examination of pregnant cows at various stages of gestation and also of non-pregnant cows will help distinguish the difference in the feel of the uterine artery under various conditions.

The uterus of the pregnant cow undergoes continual enlargement as the pregnancy progresses. Between the second and third month, the change is marked, although not clearly defined. But by the end of the third month, there should be no doubt of the diagnosis. By the fourth month, bulging at the point of the horn in which the fetus is suspended easily can be made out. The rest of the horn is still firm, and there is little difficulty in differentiating between pregnant and non-pregnant horns. The enlargement of the uterine arteries also begins to be felt distinctly at this time. Early in the fourth month, the presence of fluids surrounding the fetus becomes evident, and later the fetus itself can be felt by palpating the uterus from the front and making the fetus rebound back onto the fingertips. By the end of the fourth month, the pregnant horn has enlarged enormously and is lying over the pelvic brim within the abdomen. This has the effect of pulling the cervix forward. The point where it crosses the pelvic brim can easily be determined. The pregnant horn is usually lying slightly to the right of the midline, and the uterine arteries can easily be located (refer to Figure 19.3).

In the early part of the fourth month, placentomes can readily be palpated, and later, parts of the fetus itself can be distinguished. The

placentomes are structures formed by the fusion of uterine caruncles and fetal cotyledons. They are sites where oxygen and nutrients pass from maternal to fetal circulation and waste products pass from fetal to maternal circulation. There is, however, no direct contact between maternal and fetal blood. In the pregnant cow, 70 to 120 placentomes develop around the fetus. They are rounded prominences that can be palpated beginning at around 90 days of gestation, when they are about ½ to 1 cm in diameter. The placentomes enlarge greatly as pregnancy advances, reaching 8 to 12 cm in diameter near term. By the end of the sixth month, the fetus is lying in the right flank, near or on the abdominal floor, and may be palpable through the flank.

When the fetus drops beyond the reach of the operator's hand, diagnosis can be confirmed based on slip of the fetal membranes, palpation of placentomes, and size and fremitus of the middle uterine artery.

## Pregnancy Diagnosis—The Cow: Characteristic Changes in the Reproductive Tract as Pregnancy Progresses

| Status | Characteristics of Reproductive Tract |
|---|---|
| Non-pregnant | Tract lies between rectum and pelvis; uterine horns generally equal in size and may be curled; prominent ovarian structures include *corpus luteum* of the cycle and developing follicle(s); vaginal mucus thin; no cervical plug. |
| Pregnant (Stage of Gestation) | |
| *1 month* | *Corpus luteum* present in one ovary; one horn of uterus slightly enlarged; amniotic vesicle may be palpable; little change in uterine arteries; vaginal mucus thick and stringy; placenta not attached. |

[2] W. L. Williams. 1943. Diseases of the Genital Organs of Domestic Animals (3rd Ed.). Coll. of Veterinary Medicine, Cornell Univ., Ithaca, NY.

| | |
|---|---|
| *2 months* | Pregnant horn enlarged; *corpus luteum* present (large); fetal membranes may be "slipped"; middle uterine artery of gravid horn has slightly stronger pulsations; amniotic vesicle about size of small hen's egg; vaginal mucus thick; plug in os uteri (cervix). |
| *3 months* | Uterus enlarged and begins to drop into abdominal cavity; middle uterine artery enlarged and pulsating stronger than artery of non-pregnant side; small placentomes can be felt through uterine wall; fetus 5 to 6 inches long. |
| *4 months* | Uterus extended well over pelvic area; pregnant horn easily palpated; fetus may be bounced against fingertips; strong pulsations in middle uterine artery; placentomes about size of a quarter; fetus 8 to 12 inches long and 2 to 4 pounds. |
| *5 months* | Cervix located near brim of pelvis and is taut; uterus dropped well over pelvis; placentomes large and palpable; middle uterine artery about 3/8 inch in diameter, with strong pulsations; fetus still palpable, 12 to 17 inches long, and 6 to 10 pounds. |
| *6 months* | Fetus descends to abdominal floor and may be out of reach of hand, but enlarged uterus and prominent placentomes can be felt; uterine arteries larger; pulsations very strong; fetus 15 to 24 inches long and 11 to 22 pounds. |
| *7 months* | Fetus out of reach; placentomes large and palpable; middle uterine artery about ½ inch in diameter; pulsations can be felt throughout tissues; fetus 22 to 30 inches long and 17 to 40 pounds; hairs beginning to form on extremities, back, and end of tail. |
| *8 months* | Fetus ascends and is again palpable; head, legs, and tail can be felt; fetus is 24 to 34 inches long and may weigh up to 70 pounds (Holstein); arterial pulsations very strong on both pregnant and non-pregnant side; mammary glands enlarged—"springing"; some swelling of labia of vulva may be apparent. |
| *9 months* | Fetus obvious (covered with hair, teeth forming, hoofs distinctly formed); labia of vulva swollen and often there is a mucus discharge; mammary glands enlarged and edematous; fetus developed and may weigh 80 to over 100 pounds (Holstein). |
| *9 months to parturition* | Sacral ligaments relax; tail head elevates; area around tail head becomes sunken as parturition nears; cervix relaxes; mucus plug liquefies; mammary system becomes engorged; vulva is swollen and relaxed. |

Through practice and experience, one learns to diagnose pregnancy by rectal palpation. The student or herd operator who examines the reproductive organs in cows by rectal palpation at every opportunity and correlates the findings with breeding records soon has "educated fingertips." Such knowledge and skill are of great value to the inseminator and the herd operator alike. Checking for pregnancy by palpation can save much time and avoid delay in treating or deciding to dispose of cows not in calf.

Rectal palpation is considered the most practical and rapid diagnosis for pregnancy at the present time. If the examiner is competent, rectal palpation can be performed early in gestation, and the result known immediately.

## Other Methods of Pregnancy Determination

**Ultrasound—** In recent years, the use of sound waves for the examination of internal organs and tissues in live animals has steadily increased. Ultrasonic techniques have the advantage of providing detailed morphological information without invading or disturbing the tissues of interest. Transrectal ultrasonic imaging is a clinical method used for determining pregnancy and for examining reproductive tract structures in cattle and other domestic species. This technique utilizes high-frequency sound waves produced by a specialized transducer that is manipulated within the rectum to examine the tissues of interest. Entry into the cow's rectum, removal of fecal material, avoidance of trauma, and sanitary precautions are the same as for rectal palpation. However, a coupling medium also is used in this procedure to act as a lubricant and to eliminate any air spaces between the transducer and the rectal wall.

The transducer acts as a sender of the sound waves and a receiver of the returning echoes, which vary with the tissue consistency. The proportion of sound waves received back from the tissue is processed as electronic signals and displayed as an echo image on an ultrasound viewing screen. Most of the ultrasound units used today are called "B-mode (brightness modality) real-time scanners."[3] With this equip-

ment the processed image appears on the screen as a two-dimensional display of dots, whose brightness is related to the strength of the reflected echoes that return to the transducer. "Real time" refers to the capability of the scanner to capture a moving image, such as fetal heart contractions, ovulations, etc. Different transducers of varying frequencies are available that can be selected to best suit the size and location of tissues to be examined. Under optimal conditions, the bovine fetus can be detected with accuracy by ultrasound techniques beginning about day 18 of gestation. Under typical field conditions, however, 25 to 30 days post-breeding is normal.

The use of ultrasound for examining the cow reproductive tract is increasing among veterinarians, embryo transfer practitioners, and large herd operators. As a reproductive management tool, transrectal ultrasound has much value in determining early on, and with greater certainty, which cows are pregnant and which cows are not pregnant. This allows open cows to be scheduled promptly for re-breeding. Other applications include examination of ovarian structures 30 to 60 days after calving, determination of twins 40 to 55 days post-breeding (Figure 19.5), and fetal sexing at 60 to 80 days

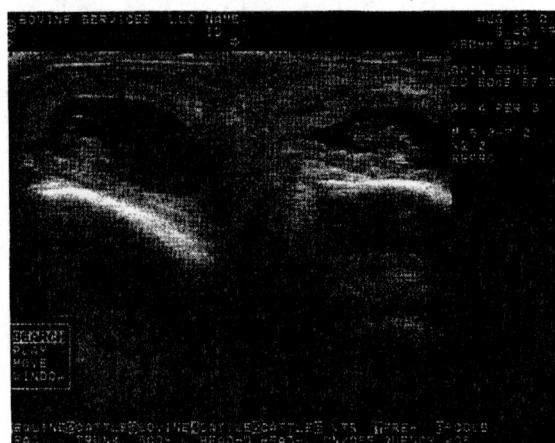

**Figure 19.5.** Ultrasound image of twin bovine fetuses at 39 days. (Courtesy, Jill Colloton, DVM; Bovine Services, LLC., Edgar, WI)

---

[3] P. G. Griffin and O. J. Ginther. 1992. Research applications of ultrasonic imaging in reproductive biology. J. Anim. Sci. 70:953.

of gestation.[4] However, it is probably not practical for the average AI technician or herdsman-inseminator. Ultrasonic imaging requires specialized equipment and training. It is obvious that ultrasound has been very useful as a research tool. The information obtained from this technique has decidedly enhanced our knowledge of reproductive physiology. As equipment costs decline, use of this method will grow in the future.

**Pregnancy Specific Protein B**— Pregnancy Specific Protein B (PSPB) is a substance that is unique to pregnancy and can be detected in the cow's blood early in gestation (day 24 or earlier).[5, 6] It has been demonstrated that this substance is produced by chorionic cells of the cow's placenta.[7] The discovery of PSPB led to the first serological method for determining pregnancy in the cow. This is a very specific laboratory test method that measures the level of PSPB in the cow's blood serum by using radioimmunoassay techniques. Currently, PSPB is being used experimentally. It is quite possible that a reliable on-farm test for PSPB will be developed so that the producer or veterinarian can accurately confirm pregnancy by checking a sample of a cow's blood or blood serum with a simple kit.

**Milk Progesterone**—Progesterone is a hormone produced by the *corpus luteum* (CL) of the ovary during the *estrous* cycle (refer to

Exercise 4). Progesterone levels in the blood are lowest at the time of estrus and highest during the middle of the cycle (about days 6 to 18). In the non-pregnant animal the CL regresses and progesterone levels decline about 2 to 3 days before the next estrus. However, in the pregnant female, the *corpus luteum* is maintained and progesterone is secreted throughout gestation.

In the early 1970's, English and American researchers established that progesterone levels in milk were higher than circulating levels and reflected the variations in blood progesterone levels during the estrous cycle and pregnancy.[8, 9] New York investigators also found that the progesterone content of milk from pregnant cows 19 to 25 days after insemination was about three times greater than that of milk from non-pregnant cows. Obtaining milk samples to measure the progesterone level as a diagnostic method for determining the reproductive status (open or pregnant) of the cow is easier and more convenient than obtaining blood samples. Therefore, various assays for milk progesterone have been developed for use in herd reproductive management.

Normally, a sample of milk collected 19 to 21 days after insemination is tested. Preferably a post-milk sample is collected. The sample is about the same volume as that used for routine butterfat testing. The milk can be frozen until an assay is made, or it may be treated with preservatives to prevent spoilage.

Initially, commercial milk-testing laboratories developed programs to receive and test milk samples for progesterone level. Typically, these utilize automated radioimmunoassay procedures in which the extracted proges-

[4] P. M. Fricke. 1998. Reproductive management of dairy cows using ultrasound. Proc. Dairy Days. U. Of Wisconsin.

[5] J. E. Butler, et al. 1982. Detection and partial characterization of two bovine pregnancy specific proteins. Biol. Reprod. 26:925.

[6] R. G. Sasser, et al. 1986. Detection of pregnancy by radioimmunoassay of a novel pregnancy specific protein in serum of cows and a profile of serum concentrations during gestation. Biol. Reprod. 35:936.

[7] W. P. Eckblad, et al. 1985. Localization of Pregnancy Specific Protein B (PSPB) in bovine placental cells using a glucose oxidase—anti-glucose oxidase immunohistochemical stain. Proc. West Sect. Am. Soc. Anim. Sci. 36:396.

[8] J. M. Booth. 1979. Milk progesterone testing: Application to herd management. J. Dairy Sci. 62:1829.

[9] J. Schiavo, et al. 1975. Milk progesterone in post partum and pregnant cows as a monitor of reproductive status. J. Dairy Sci. 58:1713.

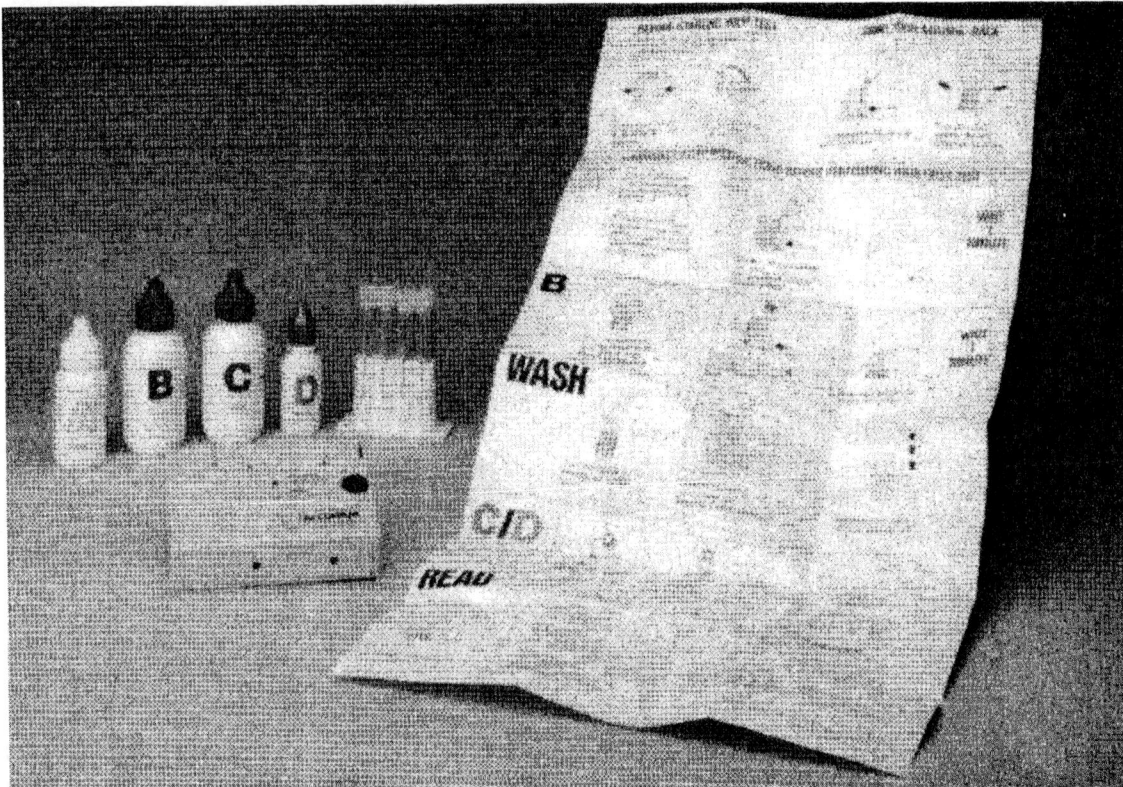

**Figure 19.6.** An on-farm milk progesterone assay kit includes reagents, sample tubes, and instruction sheet. (Courtesy, R. L. Nebel, Virginia Polytechnic Inst. and State Univ., Blacksburg, VA)

terone is compared to known standards to determine milk progesterone concentration. Test results often reach the producer in about two to three days. The sophisticated equipment used in radioimmunoassay procedures is expensive and can limit expansion of this technology to local areas.

Because of the logistics and the time involved with sending samples to a laboratory and waiting for test results, the practicality of centralized milk progesterone testing has been questioned. Consequently, milk progesterone assay kits have been developed for use on the farm by the producer or herd veterinarian. These on-farm test kits measure the progesterone level in milk with a color reaction or substrate change (Figure 19.6). The test kits are not complicated to use, and the results are known immediately.

Actually, milk progesterone testing is more accurate for determining non-pregnancy than pregnancy.[10] If the test indicates a low progesterone level 19 to 21 days after insemination, usually the cow did not conceive to that service and she should be monitored for approaching signs of estrus. Research indicates that the accuracy of predicting open cows is about 95 to 100 percent for low milk progesterone levels 21 to 24 days after insemination. If the test indicates high progesterone levels 19 to 21 days post-insemination, it is likely that the cow is pregnant, but it is not a certainty. The cow should be monitored for estrus, and pregnancy should be confirmed later by ultrasound or rectal palpation. The accuracy of predicting pregnant cows is about 75 to 80 percent for high progesterone levels 21 to 24 days after insemination.

---

[10] R. L. Nebel. 1991. Practical uses of on farm milk progesterone tests. The Virginia Dairyman 55 (September):12.

209

This is because the concentration of progesterone measured reflects only the function of the *corpus luteum,* not necessarily the presence of an embryo or a fetus. Factors that can contribute to decreased accuracy in pregnancy determination by high milk progesterone level include cows with longer than normal estrous cycles, cows initially inseminated at the wrong time, early embryonic death, and certain pathological conditions. On-farm milk progesterone testing is a reproductive management aid that can be used by the producer or veterinarian mainly to determine non-pregnancy or to confirm estrus.

The standard method of palpating the reproductive tract has long been definitive in determining the reproductive status of cows. However, the other methods that have been described can substantially augment the capability of the producer or veterinarian to improve herd reproductive efficiency.

## QUESTIONS

1. What are some of the external signs of pregnancy in the cow? List the positive indicators of pregnancy in the cow.

2. What are the advantages of having all cows in a herd diagnosed for pregnancy from 30 to 40 days following breeding?

3. What are the changes in the cervix, the ovaries, the uterine horns, and the uterine arteries in the pregnant cow?

4. What may cause a pregnant cow to come into heat?

5. What does the term "persistent *corpus luteum*" mean?

6. Explain metestrus bleeding.

7. What are some of the causes of a cow failing to come into heat and failing to develop growing follicles in the ovary?

8. If you were an inseminator and discovered a cow supposedly six months pregnant with pus in the uterus, what would be your advice to the herd owner?

9. Describe the potential applications of ultrasound in bovine reproduction.

10. What is the cellular source of PSPB?

11. Explain how milk progesterone assays can be utilized in herd reproductive management.

# EXERCISE 20

# Reproductive Efficiency—Breeding Problems—Conception Rates

## OBJECT

To become familiar with factors that affect reproductive efficiency in cattle and considerations for improving breeding efficiency.

## DISCUSSION

The efficiency of reproduction in dairy and beef cows is one of the most important factors in determining total production and profitability in the herd. Twenty to 30 percent of all dairy cows are replaced annually. It has been estimated that about 10 percent of all dairy cows require four or more services before they conceive, and 3 to 5 percent of all cows bred do not reproduce at all. To remain profitable, dairy cows must reproduce, and for greatest efficiency, they should calve every 12 to 13 months. Likewise, beef cows should calve every 12 months to produce profitable calf crops. Generally, reproduction problems in cows are related to inefficient management factors, infertility due to various causes, and disease conditions. It is of great economic importance to the dairy and beef producer and the AI business that reproductive efficiency be maintained and that any breeding irregularities be recognized and corrected immediately.

There are numerous factors that intervene between service (insemination) and parturition to prevent a normal pregnancy. Fertility varies among individual animals and consequently also for herds. Probably the best measure of fertility in a herd is the calving rate (percentage of live, normal calves born). However, it also has been customary to measure fertility on the basis of services per conception. In a healthy herd in which fertile bulls are used, an average of about 1.6 to 2.0 services are required per conception. The number of services per conception is useful for analyzing costs and in comparing the fertility of individual cows. The conception rate utilizing AI, on the average, is quite similar to that obtained through natural service in well-managed herds.

Dairy cattle reproduction specialists are now emphasizing pregnancy rates per unit of time (i.e., 21-day periods) or the effective pregnancy rate as a more meaningful measure of herd reproductive success. A 21-day pregnancy rate gives an accurate assessment of the fertility of eligible cows in the previous 21-day period and, compared to other historical measures of efficiency, it allows for more timely intervention to address contributing problems. It takes into account both conception rate (percentage pregnant in the herd after one breeding) and AI service rate (percentage of eligible cows that are bred during the 21-day period). AI service rate is largely an indicator of estrus detection efficiency. The 21-day pregnancy rate is determined by dividing the number of females that become pregnant during this time period by the number of females that were eligible for breeding during the time period. 21-day pregnancy rates are lower than the conception rate per AI. Pregnancy rates of 15 to 20 percent would be considered average to good for today's large dairy operations, while pregnancy rates of 25 to 30 percent would be considered excellent.

Another measure of fertility is the non-return rate that is frequently calculated from insemination records by various AI organizations. Non-return rate is the percentage of cows that are not subsequently rebred within a defined period (usually 60 to 90 days) following an insemination. Non-return rate is used primarily to evaluate the fertility of the semen produced by the AI organization. This fertility information is useful in developing and improving semen processing and handling techniques, evaluating inseminator performance, and communicating the relative fertility of sires to producers for use in their breeding decisions.[1] On the average, about 70 percent of cows inseminated fail to return for service after first service, on a 60- to 90-day non-return basis. Important factors that influence the non-return rate include the inherent fertility of the semen used; semen collection, processing, and storage procedures; insemination technique; cows, herd management, and record keeping.[2]

---

[1] H. Rycroft and B. Bean. 1992. Factors influencing non-return data. Proc. 14th Tech. Conf. on Artificial Insemination and Reproduction. NAAB. p. 43.
[2] Ibid.

However, non-return rate is not a *direct* measure of fertility. Even though cows may be considered as not returning for service after insemination, they could have died, been sold, or been re-inseminated by a different AI organization. Consequently, compared to actual conception rate data (i.e., data based on palpation or other measures), the non-return rate may overestimate the actual fertility. Various accounts indicate the non-return rate can overestimate actual fertility by about 5 to 15 percent. However, when applied to a large number of services in similar herds, the non-return information provides a reliable and useful early estimate of the fertility of the semen produced by an organization.

Various measures of reproductive efficiency and management goals are listed in Table 20.1.

## Management Factors

There are numerous management factors that have an impact on fertility. For AI success, fertile semen must be deposited in the correct location of the healthy cow's or heifer's reproductive tract at the right stage of

**Table 20.1.** Measures of Reproductive Efficiency and Management Goals[a]

| Trait | Definition | Dairy | Beef |
|---|---|---|---|
| First calving | Age (months) | < 24 | 27 |
| Days open | Days calving to conception | < 100 | — |
| First-service conception rate (%) | No. pregnant first service ÷ No. bred first service × 100 | 55 | 65 |
| Calving interval (days) | Days between successive calving ÷ Total cows | < 390 | 360 |
| Services per conception | No. of services in all cows ÷ Total conceptions | < 2.0 | — |
| Total pregnancy rate (%) | No. of cows pregnant ÷ Total cows in herd × 100 | 95 | 95 |
| Calving rate (%) | No. of calves born ÷ Total cows in herd × 100 | 90 | 90 |
| Net calf crop (%) | Total calves weaned ÷ Total cows in herd × 100 | — | > 85 |

[a]Modified from M. R. Jainudeen and E. S. E. Hafez. Cattle and Buffalo. 1987. In: E. S. E. Hafez (Ed.). Reproduction in Farm Animals (5th Ed.). Lea & Febiger, Philadelphia. p. 306.

the estrous cycle. Inefficiency in one or more reproductive management areas can dramatically lower herd fertility.

**Semen fertility** relates to the inherent quality of the bull's semen plus the ability of the respective people in the laboratory and on the farm or ranch to preserve its viability by proper freezing, storage, handling, and thawing. Although individual bulls vary in fertility, AI organizations follow systematic selection and quality control procedures and insure that any substandard samples are discarded. When frozen semen is purchased from a reputable AI organization, the dairy or beef producer can be assured that it has been processed, stored, and handled in a proper manner. All too often, however, low fertility of semen is a result of improper handling of semen after it leaves the AI center. Purchasing semen that has changed hands several times from speculator to speculator should be avoided because mishandling or exposure of semen to damaging temperatures may have occurred. AI technicians and herdsman-inseminators must also follow the recommended semen-thawing procedures to maximize recovery of sperm cells so that the appropriate inseminate quality is obtained. (Refer to Exercise 14.)

**Heat detection efficiency and inseminator skill** are critically important to herd fertility. Failures and errors in detecting estrus continues to be a major management problem in artificial insemination. Missed "heats" are missed opportunities for getting cows bred back soon to meet desired herd calving intervals. Various reports have estimated that up to 50 percent of heats in dairy cattle may not be detected. In addition, many cows are inseminated at the wrong time of the estrous cycle (from about 10 to 30 percent of the cows presented for breeding may not be in heat). This error wastes valuable semen and increases total services per conception. The number of days cows are open can be reduced substantially by improving estrus detection efficiency.

Most cows in estrus can be detected by careful visual observation three to four times a day. Various estrus detection aids may also help improve detection efficiency (see Exercise 16). Adequate reproductive records and proper animal identification are essential for effective heat detection.

The inseminator must have a thorough understanding of the anatomy of the reproductive tract and its relationship to pelvic structures. He or she must be proficient in thawing semen properly, loading the insemination equipment carefully, and depositing semen into the uterus of the cow at the correct time. A major advantage of AI is the reduced potential for the spread of disease. This advantage is made possible by providing semen from disease-free bulls and by using sanitary supplies and techniques in the insemination process. The inseminator, whether a professional technician or a "do it yourself" direct herd customer, must keep insemination equipment clean and sanitary and follow hygienic procedures when introducing the insemination gun or AI tube into the reproductive tract (Exercise 16). Following insemination, the disposable supplies should be collected and disposed of immediately. The inseminator should disinfect his/her boots and the AI kit and should wash his/her hands thoroughly.

**General management** of the herd involves many factors that directly or indirectly affect fertility. The general welfare of cattle is important for maintaining their normal physiological processes. For success, producers must provide cows and heifers with adequate feed and water and with appropriate facilities.

Nutrition plays a key role in reproductive processes. Both nutritional deficiencies and excesses have been shown to impact reproduction. Probably, insufficient energy intake is the greatest nutritional problem seen. Adequate levels of protein, minerals, and vitamins are certainly important. Feeding programs should be designed around the National Research

Council's recommended nutrient requirements for dairy or beef cattle, in conjunction with forage and feed analysis information. Consultation with nutritional experts in formulating specific rations may be beneficial.

A reproductive herd health program[3] in which a veterinarian routinely conducts postpartum examinations of cows and consults with the producer on herd reproductive goals can help identify problems and maximize reproductive efficiency in the herd. Adequate record keeping is essential to this effort. Lifetime records for each cow should include calving dates, heat dates, breeding dates, and exam dates, as well as findings, treatments, and vaccinations. Barn charts and individual cow record forms for dairy and beef cattle are available from most AI organizations.

Improving herd management efficiency can help shorten calving intervals and result in more healthy cows presented for insemination.

## Infertility

Typical causes of infertility in dairy cows have been summarized from various early studies.[4] These sources of reproductive failure are listed in Table 20.2. Theoretically, a calving rate of 60 percent could be obtained considering the total reproductive losses of 40 percent shown in the table. However, data from large-scale field trials using frozen semen have demonstrated actual first-service conception rates to be somewhat lower than this estimate (i.e., 45 to 55 percent). It should be emphasized, though, that higher first-service

---

[3] L. J. Hutchinson. 1984. Reproductive herd health program. In: Ellen R. Jordan (Ed.). Dairy Integrated Reproductive Management. Coop. Ext. Serv., West Virginia Univ. Fact Sheet No. IRM-18.

[4] H. W. Hawk. 1979. Infertility in dairy cattle. In: H. W. Hawk (Ed.). Animal Reproduction. BARC Symp. No. 3. Allanheld, Osmun & Co., Montclair, NJ. p. 19.

**Table 20.2.** Sources of Reproductive Failure in Dairy Cattle[a]

| Cause of Failure | Approximate Percentage of 100 First Services |
|---|---|
| Anatomical abnormalities | 2 |
| Ovulation failure | 2 |
| Lost or ruptured ova | 5 |
| Fertilization failure | 13 |
| Embryonic mortality | 15 |
| Fetal mortality | 3 |
| Total | 40 |

[a] H. W. Hawk. 1979. Infertility in dairy cattle. In: H. W. Hawk (Ed.). Animal Reproduction. BARC Symp. No. 3. Allanheld, Osmun & O., Mantclair, NJ. p. 19.

conception rates are often achieved in individual herds that are well managed and in heifers.

From Table 20.2 it is apparent that in the general dairy cattle population, the greatest losses of potential calves are due to fertilization failure and embryonic mortality. Obviously, efforts to reduce losses in these two areas could have a large impact on reproductive efficiency. Fertilization failure has been associated with semen quality problems/low fertility bulls, insemination timing, and several previous infertile services (repeat breeding). Embryonic mortality has been linked to the fertilization of aged ova (insemination after ovulation) as well as several previous infertile services (repeat breeding). Using semen from reputable AI organizations, maintaining semen viability through proper thawing and handling techniques, and inseminating at the correct time are certainly key components in reducing these losses.

The problem of dealing with "repeat breeder" cows may be more difficult. However, this effort can be facilitated by having good herd records and working with a competent veterinarian. Repeat breeders are those cows requiring three or more services, with true estrus, before conceiving. Dairy herds having an average first-service conception rate of 50 percent might expect about 10 percent of the cows to be repeat breeders.[5] Typically, repeat breeders are subfertile, not sterile. They may suffer from reproductive tract infections and endocrine disturbances that negatively affect (1) sperm storage and transport efficiency or (2) conditions that provide the necessary micro-environment for embryo development. Some improvement in the fertility of repeat breeders has been achieved through hormone therapy. However, culling certain repeat-breeder cows from the herd may be more cost effective over the long term.

## Other factors associated with infertility:

1. Structural abnormalities of the female reproductive tract, such as segmental aplasia (occlusion of portions of the oviducts due to incomplete development) and adhesions of the ovary and adjacent structures, could block the transport of sperm or ova, thereby preventing fertilization. Interestingly, studies have shown that "repeat breeder" cows tend to have more congenital reproductive tract abnormalities than cows of normal fertility. Other abnormalities, such as scarring of the uterus resulting from a previous calving or mechanical injuries, may also contribute to fertility problems.

2. Various studies have demonstrated that higher-producing dairy cows in some herds may experience lower first-service conception rates. Pre-sumably, this effect results from physiological stress related to high milk production. Lucy[6] has discussed a decline in reproductive efficiency in dairy cows since the 1950's/60's. For example, first-service conception rates reported in studies then were 65% compared to 40 to 45% today. In addition, modern dairy cows have longer intervals to first ovulation, higher incidence of anestrous and abnormal luteal phases, lower blood progesterone levels, higher multiple ovulation and twinning rates, and greater embryonic loss. He has surmised that the physiology of the dairy cow has changed over this period. Interestingly though, first-service conception rates in heifers appears unchanged over this period. Physiological adaption to high milk production and management problems associated with larger herd size may be contributing to decreasing reproductive efficiency.

3. Cow age tends to affect fertility. Generally, virgin heifers have higher conception rates than older cows. The reason for this is unclear.

4. High environmental temperatures and humidity, such as experienced in the southern United States during summer months, lower conception rates. In addition to reducing mounting activity, which makes it more difficult to detect cows in estrus, high temperature and humidity stress around the time of breeding can result in fertilization failure or early embryonic death.

[5] M. B. Brunner. 1984. Repeat breeding. In: Ellen R. Jordan (Ed.). Dairy Integrated Reproductive Management. Coop. Ext. Serv., West Virginia Univ. Fact Sheet No. IRM-23.

[6] M. L. Lucy. 2001. Reproductive loss in high producing dairy cattle: where will it end? J Dairy Sci. 84:1277.

5. Post-calving disorders, such as retained placentas, uterine infections (metritis), and cystic ovarian conditions, can decrease subsequent fertility and increase the number of days open.

Normally the cow expels the placenta within 12 hours of calving. However, in cases of abnormal delivery (i.e., difficult calving [dystocia], twins, caesarian sections, abortions, or premature calvings), the probability of retention of the fetal membranes for a longer period is increased. In these cases, various physiological factors result in the lack of complete detachment and expulsion of fetal membranes. Retained placentas result in the delayed involution (return to normal size) of the uterus and chronic inflammation of the reproductive tract. Clean, well-bedded calving areas, proper nutrition, and thrifty body condition help to minimize occurrence of retained placentas. Therapy utilizing hormones or the infusion of antibiotics is aimed at returning the cow's reproductive tract to normal condition as soon as possible. Treatment should be under the supervision of a competent veterinarian.

Metritis is an inflammation of the uterus that may be acute or chronic. A purulent vaginal discharge may be present. Metritis frequently is the result of infection during the period of uterine involution following calving. However, venereally transmitted infection at breeding is also another possible cause. The length of time that inflammation persists and the degree of infection affect the chances for recovery.

Ovarian cysts are follicle-like structures on one or both ovaries that may persist for several days. Follicular cysts are follicles that produce estrogen but do not ovulate. Cows with follicular cysts exhibit recurrent nymphomania over a period of days. Luteal cysts are single structures in one ovary that produce progesterone. Cows with luteal cysts are anestrus (they do not exhibit cycling activity). Both follicular and luteal cystic conditions may be treated by administration of various hormones.

## Infectious Diseases

Reproductive diseases of importance are those that can be spread through sexual contact, particularly in natural service—or even through artificial insemination in the case of an infected bull. However, when using semen from reputable AI organizations that follow comprehensive health-testing protocols, such as the CSS program (refer to Exercise 24), artificial insemination is actually the best defense against reproductive diseases. In a dairy or beef herd that uses bulls in natural service, the likelihood of having venereal disease in the herd is quite high.

**Tuberculosis** is normally a disease of the respiratory tract but may also affect the reproductive organs. It is caused by *Mycobacterium bovis.* Although this disease is largely under control and nearly eradicated in U.S. cattle, there have been past instances in which bulls have infected cows through semen. Tuberculosis testing and eradication programs are regulated by the USDA—Animal and Plant Health Inspection Service (APHIS). Because tuberculosis is a prominent health concern (both to other cattle and to humans), infected cattle that have been identified are slaughtered.

It is incumbent on AI centers to test bulls thoroughly for tuberculosis prior to their admittance and throughout residency during the period of semen production.

**Brucellosis,** or Bang's disease, is caused by the bacterium *Brucella abortus.* Brucellosis organisms invade the placentomes of pregnant cows and interfere with nutrient transfer to the fetus, resulting in abortion after about the fifth month of gestation. In the herd, brucellosis is easily spread through contact with the placenta or fluids from infected cows. Occasionally, a cow does not abort, but the newborn calf is very weak. Infected cows can be brucellosis carriers. There is no cure for brucellosis, and infected animals must be slaughtered. Calfhood vaccination programs are moderately effective in preventing the disease. The human form of brucellosis is called "undulant fever."

The brucellosis testing and eradication program regulated by USDA—APHIS has been successful in efforts to eliminate brucellosis in several areas of the United States. As of September 30, 2001, there were no herds under quarantine for brucellosis.

**Leptospirosis** is caused by spiral-shaped bacteria (spirochetes). There are five serotypes of concern prevalent in the United States (*L. pomona, L. hardjo, L. canicola, L. icterohaemorrhagiae, L. grippotyphosa*) and several other types worldwide. The organisms are found in rivers, ponds, stagnant water, and sewage. Leptospirosis can be spread by cattle ingesting water from contaminated sources. Leptospirosis organisms damage red blood cells and infect the kidneys and udder. From time to time the organisms may be present in the urine. Abortion can occur in cows during about the last three months of gestation. Humans may also be infected and develop flu-like symptoms. Consequently, they should avoid contact with sources of infection (i.e., infected cow's urine, milk, etc.).

In cows, leptospirosis can be prevented with annual vaccinations in "closed herds" or vaccinations more often in leptospirosis problem herds. AI bulls are routinely certified as producing semen free of leptospirosis organisms through routine diagnostic testing. In addition, cryopreservation of semen according to the CSS protocol has been shown to effectively control leptospirosis organisms.[7]

**Trichomoniasis** causes low-grade uterine infections, characterized by temporary infertility. Cows come into estrus irregularly and fail to settle after insemination. Pus containing the protozoan organisms that cause the disease (*Tritrichomonas foetus*, Figure 20.1) accumulates in the uterus and is discharged from the vulva. Abortion occurs during about the first three months of gestation. There is no effective treatment for cows; however, the condition frequently clears up on its own following a period of sexual rest (two to four months).

Trichomoniasis may be prevented by using AI with semen from bulls that are on a routine health-testing and disease-surveillance program.

**Campylobacteriosis (vibriosis)** is caused by the bacterium *Campylobacter fetus* subsp. *venerealis*. Symptoms are similar to trichomoniasis. Irregular estrus periods, low-grade infection, low fertility, and vulvar

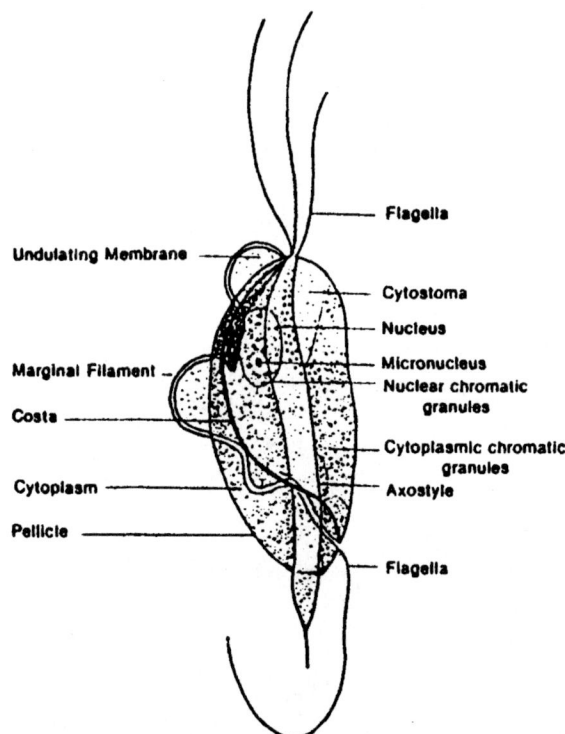

**Figure 20.1.** Protozoan *Tritrichomonas foetus*. (Adapted under the direction of M. E. Ensminger from an original illustration)

[7] S. G. Kim and S. J. Shin. 2000. Glycerol and GTLS effect on leptospira species in bovine semen. Proc. 18th Tech. Conf. on Artificial Insemination and Reproduction. NAAB. p. 63.

discharge typify campylobacteriosis. Abortions may occur between the fourth and seventh month of gestation. After periods of infertility, females develop some immunity and are again able to reproduce. Campylobacteriosis is spread mainly through natural service. It can be prevented by using AI with semen from disease-free bulls. In addition, cryopreservation of semen according to the CSS protocol has been shown to effectively control *Campylobacter fetus* subsp. *venerealis*.[8]

**Bovine viral diarrhea (BVD)** virus can cause abortion during the first three months of gestation or result in weak, stunted calves. It may also result in infertility in the cow. There are several strains of the virus that produce various forms of disease. In one form of the disease, animals become infected *in-utero* but do not develop antibodies to BVD. Infected cows are detected only by virus isolation methods on samples of blood or other body fluids. These "persistently" infected animals will shed virus throughout their life without showing disease symptoms. These animals frequently infect their herdmates.

CSS-approved AI centers are required to test all bulls for persistent BVD infection to insure that the virus will not be transmitted in semen.

There is no effective cure for BVD infection; however, various vaccination strategies may be effective in preventing infection.

## Other Organisms Affecting Reproduction

**Mycoplasmas, ureaplasmas, and *Haemophilus somnus*** have all been associated with infertility and abortion in cattle.[9] These organisms inhabit the mucous membranes of the lower urogenital and upper respiratory tract of cattle and at times are opportunistic pathogens. They have been associated with poor conception, granular vulvitis, vaginitis, endometritis, salpingitis (inflammation of oviducts), and abortion in the cow. All three organisms have also been isolated from unprocessed bull semen.

As diagnostic tests for these organisms are not currently practical for screening AI bulls, effective control is achieved through the treatment of neat semen and semen extender with the combination of gentamicin, tylosin, and Linco-Spectin (see CSS antibiotic combination in Exercise 24) according to methods described by Shin, et al.[8] Double sheathing of the AI gun or insemination tube may also aid in reducing the number of these organisms introduced into the uterus from more contaminated areas of the vulva and vagina (see Exercise 16 for procedure).

***Chlamydia psittaci*** organisms have been isolated from cattle and are associated with epizootic bovine abortion in females, seminal vesiculitis in bulls, and arthritis in calves. Various vaccines are available.

**Bovine Herpes Virus-1 (BHV-1),** more commonly called "IBR virus," causes infectious pustular vulvovaginitis (IPV) in females and balanoposthitis in bulls. IPV in heifers is characterized by pain upon urination and defecation, mucopurulent discharge from the vulva, and white pustules on the wall of the vulva and vagina. Susceptible pregnant females exposed to BHV-1 may abort immediately or after a period of time (weeks to months). Also, studies have indicated that

---

[8] S. J. Shin, et al. 1988. A new antibiotic combination for frozen bovine semen. I. Control of mycoplasmas, ureaplasmas, *Campylobacter fetus* subsp. *venerealis* and *Haemophilus somnus*. Therio. 29:577.

[9] D. H. Lein. 1986. Current role of ureaplasma, mycoplasma, *Haemophilus somnus* in bovine reproductive disorders. Proc. 11th Tech. Conf. on Artificial Insemination and Reproduction. NAAB. p. 27.

[8] Ibid.

BHV-1 may result in temporary infertility following intramuscular vaccination or natural infection. Vaccination strategies for calves and breeding-age females are frequently followed. Generally, AI centers maintain populations of IBR seronegative bulls.

**Blue tongue virus (BTV)** rarely causes clinical disease in cattle. The virus is transmitted by a biting gnat *(Culicoides variipennis)*. Presumably, the virus could cause early embryonic or fetal death in viremic pregnant females. The possibility exists for BLU virus being shed in the semen of viremic bulls. AI centers generally maintain populations of BLU negative bulls in vector-free environments. Also, the semen from BLU seropositive bulls may be safely used when the non-viremic status of the bulls is continuously monitored by diagnostic testing.

Prevention is the best means of controlling disease in the herd, but prompt treatment of any reproductive abnormality will aid in maintaining an efficient breeding program.

## CONCLUSION

Having a good understanding of the many factors that affect herd conception rate is an essential first step for improving reproductive efficiency. Obviously, a complete and accurate record system also helps the producer and the veterinarian identify problem cows and monitor reproductive performance. The producer should work closely with the herd health practitioner in setting herd goals to maximize reproductive efficiency and reduce disease conditions. Improvement in various management areas (particularly estrus detection efficiency and semen handling and insemination procedures) can have a marked impact on reducing reproductive failure in the herd.

## QUESTIONS

1. What are the main factors associated with lowered reproductive performance in dairy and beef herds? What are the economic consequences of lowered fertility?

2. How is fertility usually measured in the herd? Explain.

3. Explain the difference between conception rate and 21-day pregnancy rate.

4. How does a dairy or beef producer know there are reproductive problems in the herd?

5. List several management factors that affect herd fertility in an AI program. Which factors have the greatest impact on fertility?

6. Explain the importance of adequate record keeping as it relates to herd reproductive performance. What specific information should be recorded?

7. Identify sources of infertility, and explain how a dairy or beef producer can have an impact on improving herd fertility.

8. List the reproductive diseases of importance, and explain how they are controlled and/or prevented.

# REFERENCE

Fricke, P. M. 2002. Measuring reproductive levels. Ontario Dairy Farmer. Vol. 16, No. 1, p. 30.

Fricke, P. M. 2002. The equation of reproduction. Proc. 19th Tech. Conf. on Artificial Insemination and Reproduction. NAAB. In-press.

Mohr, P. 2001. A measure that matters. Dairy Today. April. p. 8.

Morrow, D. A. (Ed.). 1986. Current Therapy in Theriogenology. W. B. Saunders Company, Philadelphia. Section V, Bovine, pp. 93-450.

# EXERCISE 21

# Embryo Transfer (ET) and Related Practices

## OBJECT

To become familiar with the technology, advantages, and disadvantages of embryo transfer (ET); to review the progress being made and the biotechnology involved in splitting embryos, cloning, and *in vitro* fertilization.

## DISCUSSION

Most of the emphasis in cattle improvement has been directed toward the genetic influence of the male because of the large number of progeny involved. However, the use of embryo or fertilized ova transfers offers the opportunity for a cow to produce many offspring in a single year, thus increasing her genetic impact. Progress in the commercial application of embryo transfer has been considerable. In 2000, there were 237,181 embryos from 37,680 recoveries in the United States reported by 133 embryo transfer businesses.[1] On a worldwide basis, the International Embryo Transfer Society (IETS) indicates that more than 113,000 cows were flushed, resulting in over 660,000 transferrable bovine embryos in 2000, of which 528,000 were transferred (Table 21.1).

Embryo transfer has been used extensively in purebred beef and dairy herds. In 2001, the Holstein Association USA reported that a total of 17,046 Holsteins (6,202 males and 10,844 females) resulting from embryo transfer were registered.[2]

The technique for treating females hormonally so that more than the usual one egg (ovum) is released from the ovary during the estrous cycle is called "superovulation" (Figure 21.1). Often, a healthy, properly treated, fertile cow will ovulate 5 to 20 eggs. On the average, about 5 or 6 of these will be of acceptable quality for transfer. The eggs can be fertilized by means of artificial insemination, and six to eight days later flushed from the reproductive tract of the cow. Those suitable, while in the early cell division stage, may be transferred to recipient animals that are in the proper stage of estrus.

The earlier technique for recovery of fertilized eggs and their transfer employed surgical procedures; however, present-day techniques involve the successful flushing of the fertilized eggs from the donor cow. Transfer of the recovered fertilized egg(s) into the recipient animal is also commonly done by non-surgical means similar to AI techniques. These developments have done much to accelerate the practice of embryo transfer.

Frozen embryos from sheep, goats, cattle, horses, and several other species have been successfully preserved for many months.[3] As early as 1977, an AI firm—Carnation/Genetics,

---

[1] Personal communication, Don Ellerbee, American Embryo Transfer Assoc. (AETA)

[2] Irma Robertson Holstein Association of America, 1 Holstein Place, Brattleboro, VT 05302-0508. 2002. (Personal communication.)

[3] Transplantation of zygotes. 1976. Proc. 8th International Congr. Animal Reproduction and Artificial Insemination (Krakow, Poland). p. 229.

**Table 21.1.** Overall Activity of *In Vivo*-Derived Bovine Embryos in 2000[a]

| Continents | Flushes | Transferable Embryos | Number of Transferred Embryos | | |
|---|---|---|---|---|---|
| | | | Fresh | Frozen | Total |
| Africa | 1,205 | 7,049 | 3,566 | 3,197 | 6,763 (1.3%) |
| N. America | 50,527 | 287,460 | 102,285 | 122,166 | 222,451 (42.5%) |
| S. America | 9,327 | 56,645 | 45,679 | 38,842 | 84,521 (16.0%) |
| Asia | 12,225 | 89,063 | 15,046 | 43,925 | 58,971 (11.1%) |
| Europe | 22,734 | 125,035 | 47,270 | 58,698 | 105,968 (20.1%) |
| Oceania | 17,040 | 99,068 | 32,410 | 15,456 | 47,866 (9.0%) |
| Total | 113,058 | 664,320 | 246,256 | 282,284 | 528,540 |

[a]Modified from M. Thibier. 2001. Statistics of the ET industry around the world. International Embryo Transfer Newsletter (IETS) 19:4. The percentage of dairy and beef donors varies between countries. In 2000, the percentages were 39% (dairy) and 61% (beef) for the U.S. and 74% (dairy) and 26% (beef) for Canada.[a]

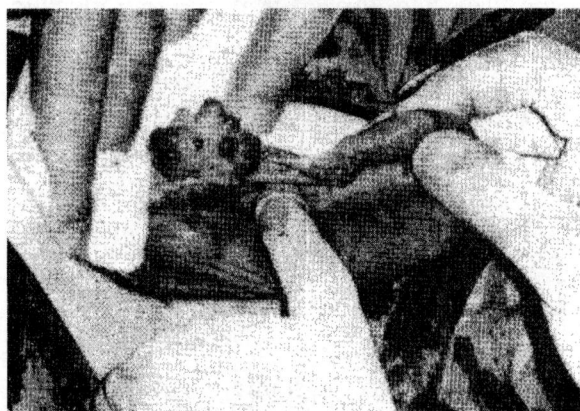

**Figure 21.1.** Exposed horn of the uterus showing an ovary with numerous ovulation points following treatment for superovulation. (Courtesy, former Carnation/Genetics Division, Hughson, CA)

Hughson, California—reported confirmed pregnancies from embryos (obtained nonsurgically) stored for six weeks in liquid nitrogen (−320°F [−196°C]).[4] Modern Ova Trends, an embryo transplant business in Norval, Ontario, Canada, announced the birth of a Holstein heifer on April 20, 1977. The calf resulted from an embryo collected in 1976 that had been frozen at −320°F (−196°C) for several months, then thawed and transferred into a crossbred recipient. This calf is believed to be the first calf born in North America from a frozen-thawed embryo. With the advent of better culture methods and processing procedures, frozen embryos, like frozen semen, have become readily available to cattle breeders.

The number of progeny one cow could produce in a year as a result of superovulation and embryo transfer is probably undetermined; however, Alberta Livestock Transplants, Ltd., Alberta, Canada, reported that the Swiss Simmental cow Big T Furka, owned by Big T Stock Farms, Pennant, Saskatchewan, produced 30 calves in one year from two transplant operations.[5]

---

[4] Ova transfer news from Carnation/Genetics. 1977. Advanced Animal Breeder (November). p. 10.

[5] Better Beef Business. February 1976. p. 47.

## Advantages of Embryo Transfer

1. It increases the genetic impact of a cow by providing a significant number of offspring.

2. It can be an early progeny test for transmission of undesirable genetic traits by females or males.

3. It enables better herd replacements due to female contributions in number of progeny provided.

4. In the case of heifers or young cows, the production of numerous offspring in a short time enables the early measurement of the dam's transmitting ability (see "Multiple Ovulation and ET [MOET]" later in this exercise).

5. It provides an added source of income to a purebred breeder who has superior females, through the sale of both male and female offspring.

6. Frozen embryos from high-producing cows may be shipped for use in other herds (and in other countries), and they provide greater genetic potential for improvement.

7. It may aid reproduction in cows that fail to settle due to adhesions, cystic ovaries, or other abnormalities of the reproductive tract. (*Note:* Due to the expense involved in embryo transfer, the exact cause of infertility in a cow should be determined before this approach is used.)

8. Where desired, twins or identical progeny, as well as animals of predetermined sex, may be obtained by utilizing the necessary biotechnology.

9. The use of embryos from known disease-free females that have been inseminated with semen from disease-free males virtually eliminates the likelihood of spreading infection to the recipient.

## Disadvantages of Embryo Transfer

1. The cost is fairly high and will not pay dividends on offspring unless they are from the most outstanding and meritorious females and males of the breed. A conservative estimate would be $500 to $1,000 and higher per ET calf. Included in the cost are professional fees, drugs, travel expenses, recovery of the fertilized ova, evaluation and storage of the fertilized ova, and the transfer to the recipient animal in the proper stage of estrus. In addition, there is the cost of blood typing the donor and special registration fees for ET offspring.

   Recipient costs amount to some $500 or more per calf and include delayed natural reproduction, the cost of synchronization, and the fact that about 6 to 8 recipient animals need to be kept for each transfer. These costs must be considered for each ET calf obtained. When several transfers are made at the same time, as may apply to large herds, the cost per ET calf is reduced.

2. On the average, one-half of the ET calves will be bulls. Dairy bull calves have a limited market unless from a cow and by a sire that have appeal to the AI industry. Beef breeders usually have strong demand for bulls from their best cow families.

3. The response to hormone treatment is erratic. Some females respond better than others, and some cows become

refractory after repeated injections with protein hormones.

4. Careful selection must be made of cows to be superovulated for embryo transfer. There is a tendency for herd owners to make embryo transfers from "the best cow in the herd" yet not truly in the upper 2 to 5 percent of the breed, and little genetic gain, population-wise, is made. It must be kept in mind that the "payoff" for ET is the sale of breeding stock, not increased milk production or more pounds of beef, which can be obtained more cheaply through the use of production-proven AI sires.

The technology for embryo transfer and associated practices is being improved continually, and more livestock operators are using it. The cost per ET animal probably will be reduced as experience and research further refine the processes.

## Reproductive Technologies

Reproduction in cattle involves the union of male and female gametes (sperm and ova). More technically, however, it is the union and random recombination of the DNA from the male and female pronuclei that determines the genetic make-up of the resulting offspring. The ovum undergoes changes known as meiosis as it matures and is ready for fertilization. These changes are completed and the chromosomal pattern established after ovulation and penetration by the sperm.

Research in fast-developing areas of biotechnology has demonstrated that the DNA molecule in sperm, ova, or body cells can be probed and that the genes associated with certain traits, such as milk production, body characteristics, and disease resistance, can be identified and isolated and individual

cells manipulated to produce a "made-to-order" or genetically modified individual.

Included under the heading of "Reproductive Technologies" are splitting embryos, sexed semen, cloning, *in vitro* fertilization, and embryo transfer. Each of these will be discussed briefly in general terms. Other biotechnologies are being researched continuously, and the reader is encouraged to stay abreast of new developments.

For additional information on developments in genetic engineering and emerging technologies, refer to "Animal Biotechnology: Technology Transfer and Industrial Needs" and other references at the end of this exercise.

## Splitting Embryos

The splitting of embryos by microsurgical means to obtain identical twins or to increase pregnancies per se has been an important part of the ET business. The bisection of morula- to blastocyst-stage embryos results in identical multiple offspring prized by some research workers and cattle breeders.

## Sexing Embryos

Another advantage of the ET technique is that the sex of the expected calf can be predetermined before the fertilized ova are transferred. Canadian workers reported in 1976 that by using biopsy methods and chromosome analysis, they could accurately determine the sex in 14- to 15-day-old embryos.[6] In recent years, these procedures have been applied to earlier-aged embryos. Chromosome analysis or karyotyping of blastocyst-stage embryos now appears to be accurate. Disadvan-

---

[6] D. Mitchell, et al. 1976. Sexing and transfer of bovine embryos. Proc. 8th International Congr. Animal Reproduction and Artificial Insemination (Krakow, Poland). p. 258.

tages are that biopsy methods require removing some cells from the embryo and killing them, and that readable sets of chromosomes are sometimes not obtained. The use of fluorescent-labeled antibodies to specific male antigens and the polymerase chain reaction (PCR) detection of male-specific DNA fragments are two methods of embryo sexing that show promise. Sexing embryos is now more practical but still expensive and generally cannot be done on the farm. This practice will be referred to in the pages to follow. (For sexing procedures, see Section 4.2 of *Embryo Transfer in Dairy Cattle,* cited in the references at the end of this exercise.)

## Sexed Semen

For many years, investigators throughout the world have attempted to separate sperm bearing the Y chromosome (male producing) from those bearing the X chromosome (female producing).[7,8] For a review of the background and status of semen sexing, refer to Amann, 1988; Polge, 1996; and Garner, 2001 (see references). Obviously, for a cattle breeder to be able to choose the sex of a calf before insemination would be of considerable economic importance. Until recently, no method of separating sperm into the X and Y categories had proven to be reliable. However, Johnson and others (see references to Johnson, 1989; Johnson, et al., 1989; Cran, et al., 1995; Lindsey, et al., 2000) successfully separated live X- and Y-bearing sperm of rabbits, boars, bulls, and stallions based on DNA content using flow cytometry techniques. Results from inseminating the "sorted" sperm showed a marked deviation in the sex ratio of offspring, closely matching the predicted proportions of X- and Y-bearing sperm that were determined from a sample of the semen that was inseminated. This method is very slow for the commercial laboratory with relatively low yield, and there appears to be some reduction in fertility of the sexed semen. Nevertheless, this technology has been commercialized in the United Kingdom and bovine sexed semen is being sold there. AI centers in the United States are conducting field trials hoping to make this technology available in the U.S. market in the near future.

Sexed semen, if available with a normal degree of fertility and with the ability to produce a significant change in the sex ratio, would be less expensive and much more convenient than sexing embryos.

The benefits the cattle-breeding industry could derive from successful sexing techniques of bovine embryos and semen would be immense. The desire for a bull calf out of an outstanding cow might possibly be fulfilled on order.

## Cloning

The term "clone" refers to a group of genetically identical cells descended from a single ancestor. In animal reproduction, cloning indicates offspring that have exactly the same genetic make-up as the progenitor. With the growing knowledge regarding the role of the cell nucleic acids DNA and RNA, genetic engineering is steadily expanding in both plants and animals.

Cloning in farm animals gives rise to a greatly increased number of offspring with the same genetic composition. An example, occurring occasionally under natural conditions, is identical twin calves. They originate from a single fertilized ovum that divides in the embryonic stage to form two identical animals. Cloning, in practice, involves the manipulation of embryonic cells to create an

---

[7] Sex Ratio at Birth—Prospects for Control. 1971. Symp., American Society of Animal Science, Champaign, IL.
[8] B. C. Bhattacharya. 1975. Sex selection—How soon? Farm Journal (January). p. 8.

individual with the same genetic make-up as the donor. Essentially, cloning is successful because all of the body cells of an animal have the same basic genetic information in their nuclei. Theoretically, any body cell nucleus could provide the "blueprint" (genetic instructions) for a copy of the adult animal and be used in cloning. However, at some point during embryogenesis, cells differentiate and their developmental fate becomes irreversibly set, acquiring only those characteristics typical for a specific cell type. For example, some cells are destined to be heart muscle, while others will be nerve cells or intestinal cells. It is believed that the differentiated cells vary in their appearance and functions because they express or make use of only certain genes or portions of the total DNA in their nuclei.

Until 1997, conventional wisdom was that cloning required the use of early (undifferentiated) embryonic cells that are totipotent or still have the full potential to develop into an adult animal.[9] Using adult cells, Wilmut and Campbell,[10] researchers at the Roslin Institute in Scotland, created Dolly, the first sheep from (differentiated) udder cells. This was the first time the complete genetic material from an adult mammalian cell was used to develop an identical new individual. Previously, only embryonic cells had been used.

**How Cloning Is Done**— Although there are many variations in the technique between laboratories, the basic procedures are:

1. Collection of cells to be grown. These may be embryonic stem cells or new differentiated cells such as mammary gland cells (Dolly).

2. Cells are grown in culture.

3. Nuclei are extracted from the cultured cells.

4. The nuclei are inserted into an egg cell that had the nucleus removed (nuclear transfer).

5. These cells with their transplanted nuclei can be implanted directly into a recipient female, or

6. A whole donor cell can be fused with an enucleated egg cell.

7. The embryo is broken up into its components after reaching about 16 cells.

8. Resulting cells are fused with other enucleated egg cells.

9. These second-generation cells can then be transferred to recipients.

Another variation is to obtain donor cells and manipulate the genome through targeted gene replacement. Transgenic animals are then created when DNA is inserted into their gene makeup from another source.

**In Summary**— Cloning in cattle may revolutionize herd improvement methods. For example, the owner of a dairy herd could have an unfertilized ovum flushed from a cow of lower merit, the nucleus removed, and a donor's superior cell inserted. The result would be a heifer that is a duplicate genetically of the donor embryo. More importantly, female clonal lines could be developed and performance tested for various production traits by methods used for progeny testing of bulls. After performance testing, embryos could be produced from selected clonal lines by re-cloning procedures, and replacement heifers could be produced with a known potential in production traits for a specific environment.[9]

Cloning, while offering spectacular possibilities in cattle improvement, also presents some

[9] J. J. Sullivan, S. L. Stice, and C. L. Keefer. 1992. Potential application of embryo cloning. Proc. 14th Tech. Conf. on Artificial Insemination and Reproduction. NAAB. p. 30.
[10] Ian Wilmut and Keith Campbell, 1997. Nature, February 27, 1997.

challenges. The techniques for cloning are still being investigated, and improvements are being made. At present, about 20 to 25 percent of the transfers of nuclear material from the donor to the recipient are successful. The actual calving rate has been reported to be somewhat less.[11] The cost is quite high, and there have been concerns about a higher than normal percentage of large calves at birth.[12] Also, cloned offspring will all be of the same sex.

Another aspect of cloning is that if one uses the genes from older generations of cattle over an extended period of time, there is a loss in the improved production potential in succeeding generations, compared to genetic gains continually achieved through young sire-proving programs.

Cloning as a tool in animal breeding will likely help develop female cloned lines to increase production and disease resistance. Likely the most significant impact will be to produce transgenic animals to produce pharmaceuticals, including human vaccines and blood plasmas, nutraceuticals (a group of products made up of dietary supplements and medically beneficial foods), and xenotransplantation (a process to produce organs for transplant into humans). Cloning simplifies the production of transgenic animals from the body cells of a single donor.

Cloning in cattle is being investigated by laboratories in the United States, Canada, and several other countries with the intent of developing a commercial enterprise. As time passes, the story of cloning will continue to unfold. The reader is urged to study the references at the end of this exercise and to follow current reports.

---

[11] J. J. Sullivan, et al. 1992. Update on commercialization of bovine embryos cloning. Proc. 11th Ann. Conv. American Embryo Transfer Assoc. (AETA) (Atlanta). p. 28.
[12] G. E. Seidel. 1992. Overview of cloning mammals by nuclear transplantation. Proc. of Symp. on Cloning Mammals by Nuclear Transplantation (Ft. Collins, CO). p. 1.

## In Vitro Fertilization

The term "*in vitro*" refers to outside the live body. *In vitro* fertilization is carried out by placing eggs (oocytes) and sperm in culture dishes or test tubes so that, under suitable conditions, fertilization can take place.

*In vitro* fertilization in cattle is a complex process and to date is used mostly in research work; however, it has the potential for commercial production of genetically superior embryos. It is more expensive and complicated than embryo transfer. Chief uses of *in vitro* fertilization in cattle at this time are (1) to remedy infertility, such as blocked Fallopian tubes, failure of fertile ova to be released, or infections of the oviducts that prevent pregnancy; (2) to obtain calves from valuable cows that have been badly injured or are sick and not likely to survive (eggs or oocytes from such animals, even up to a few hours after death, often are viable and capable of fertilization); and (3) to serve as a research tool in investigating gamete maturation, interaction, and fertility.

Oocytes for *in vitro* fertilization may be obtained from the oviducts. Large pre-ovulatory oocytes also can be obtained surgically. Another method is to use the more mature oocytes obtained from the ovaries of slaughtered cows. Ultrasound technology has enhanced the ability to recover oocytes from live animals.

The collected mature oocytes are co-cultured with capacitated sperm and allowed to incubate at body temperature of the cow for 6 to 24 hours. If fertilized, oocytes will be in the two-cell stage in about 12 to 24 hours. However, they need to develop to the morula or blastocyst stage before being transferred to the uterus of the recipient animal. In order to bring the fertilized oocytes to the proper stage of development, several methods may be used. These include (1) transferring the oocytes to the oviduct of a cow by surgical means and (2) culturing the embryos for several days in a media containing oviduct cells. Even this method

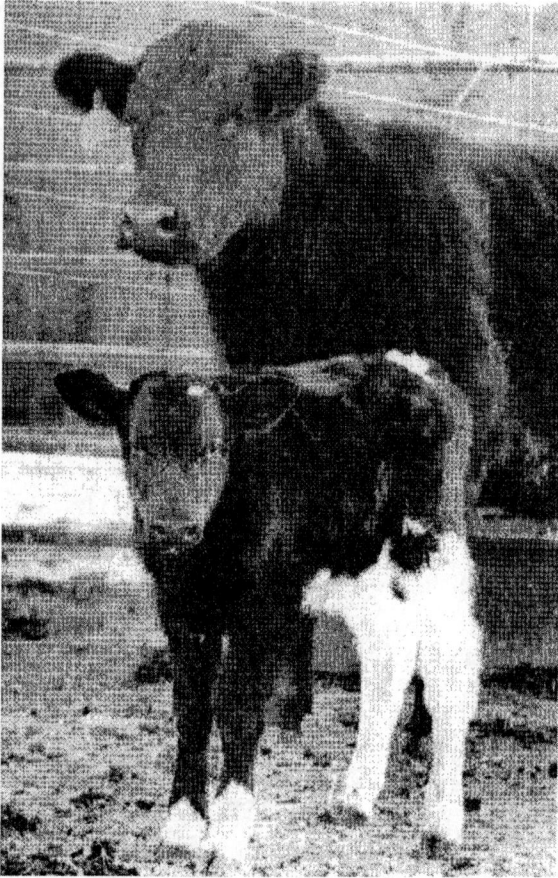

**Figure 21.2.** Missouri's first "test tube" calf, born December 26, 1989, is pictured with its surrogate mother at the University of Missouri, Columbia, MO.

implanted in a surrogate cow. The resulting calf, carried full term and normal in all respects, is shown in Figure 21.2.

It is to be expected that as techniques improve and experience is gained, there will be greater use made of *in vitro* fertilization and it could be a better method for obtaining embryos than superovulation and embryo recovery. This technique is in wide use to address infertility problems in humans.

## Multiple Ovulation and ET (MOET)

The term "MOET" was first used in other countries by researchers and breed recording organizations. The use of multiple ovulation and embryo transfer, along with other aspects of reproductive technologies, may substantially speed up cattle improvement (see discussion on cloning). Basically, MOET requires large nucleus herds or enough cooperating herds ("clusters") to form a working group of 1,000 or more animals. Preferably, all of the animals should be maintained under similar management and environmental conditions to reduce variation.

Although the large number of offspring in a bull's progeny test allows for very accurate selection of sires as parents of the next generation, a bull is relatively old (at least five years) by the time his genetic potential is estimated. The advantage of the MOET approach is in the reduction of the long generation intervals that occur with progeny tests. MOET programs provide a trade-off of increased generational turnover rate versus the lower risk of more accurate progeny tests. In the MOET program the best females, particularly heifers, based on genetic values (production, pedigree, performance of relatives such as full or half sisters), are selected for the project. Older females that meet the selection standards are not to be overlooked. The animals are superovulated and bred by AI to the best bulls available.

has a low rate of success, but it is the method of choice for most applications. Some calves—notably in Wisconsin and Missouri—have been produced by using this method.

As an example, through the research efforts of Dr. John Sikes, Dairy Unit, Department of Animal Science, University of Missouri-Columbia; graduate student Tammie Schalue-Francis; and Cliff Murphy, D.V.M., a "test tube" calf was born December 26, 1989. The method used was to procure an egg (oocyte) from a cow of unknown ancestry at a slaughterhouse. In a petri dish, the egg was matured and then fertilized using semen from a Holstein bull. The media surrounding the egg contained oviduct cells. After seven days of incubation, the young embryo was non-surgically

Heifers may produce embryos at 12 to 15 months of age. The embryos are transferred into high-indexed females, and the resulting progeny compared to each other for the various economic traits. The best of these are bred and superovulated at an early age, and the next generation is on the way. Semen may be sexed, embryos split, and cloning utilized. Selection is largely through females, with 5 to 10 percent of the best ones being retained for succeeding generations. Since the generation interval may be reduced some 50 percent, theoretically the genetic gains are increased accordingly. Most of the selection of animals to carry on is from the female lines. Bulls selected for use will be largely the best AI bulls available; but as time progresses, young bulls (brothers of the best females in the nucleus herd) will be used. Males can be evaluated from full sisters' production records at an earlier age than possible from progeny testing. Even though unproven, many of these young sires will be genetically superior to even the best sires routinely proven by conventional methods. The young sires will be progeny tested, with the poorest going to slaughter, as will also be true of the least productive females.

The net purpose of MOET is to provide a nucleus of highly superior animals that can be used to supply the genetic material for improvement of the cattle population at a faster rate than through the time-consuming progeny test method. However, MOET is expensive, there may be selection errors, females may not respond well to superovulation, and numbers of planned pregnancies may be variable. Whether or not MOET will successfully change the rate of genetic progress is largely an unknown that will be determined over time. Because of the expense, MOET herds have not been established as rapidly as some expected. Several companies involved in cattle improvement in North America have adapted portions of the MOET concept in their standard progeny test programs.

## Health Control Measures Critical in an ET Program

The possibility of introducing disease into a herd by means of embryo transfer should not be ignored. Disease-free embryo donors and recipient animals are vital for a successful and healthy ET program.

The use of frozen embryos has reduced the need for a large number of recipient animals. Some producers, however, find it necessary to obtain recipient animals outside their herds. Such animals may create health problems. The sometimes-expressed idea that almost any animal can serve as a recipient to incubate a developing embryo is misleading. The recipient animal must be free of infectious diseases that may cause death of the fetus and abortion. In addition, the recipient dam should be free of chronic, low-level infections that can be transmitted from the dam to the fetus or newborn calf. These low-level infections do not usually result in abortions or weak calves at birth. The recipient dam obtained from outside sources is usually in the herd only a short time. She may not show clinical signs of disease herself but may transmit viral agents to the calf she is carrying and subsequently introduce a growing chronic disease problem into the breeder's herd. Such disease transmissions have been evidenced by the birth of BVD-infected calves after ET using BVD-contaminated fluids and also by a limited study of BVD-infected young bulls rejected by AI centers showing a higher number of infected calves than those from uninfected bulls in the same centers.[13]

There are many advantages in using recipient heifers from the owner's breeding herd. Paratuberculosis (Johne's disease),

---

[13] T. Howard. 1992. Herd health and ET must be managed together. Hoard's Dairyman (September 25). p. 654.

bovine leukosis, and persistent BVD are sometimes not detected in apparently well-managed herds because the infection is at latent levels. However, introducing new animals or using recipient herds that have frequent replacements greatly increases the chance of exposure to these diseases. Therefore, a complete and efficient testing and vaccination program is necessary. Immunization of recipient animals should be completed at least a month before the embryo transfer is made. It is recommended that in addition to the usual tuberculosis and brucellosis tests, recipient animals also be tested for paratuberculosis (Johne's disease), leukosis (BLV), and persistent BVD (by virus isolation methods). Arrangements for these tests should be made with the herd veterinarian. These tests are not too expensive if made on a herd basis. Freedom from the above diseases is essential if frozen embryos are to be sold outside the herd or in foreign markets. If persistent BVD becomes established in a herd, the virus can be transmitted from dams to calves for several generations. Also, pregnant cows exposed to animals shedding the virus can become infected, and additional infected calves result.

Another important item to consider in the recovery, washing, and freezing of embryos is that bovine blood products, such as bovine fetal serum or bovine serum albumin, are utilized. These products are made up from the pooled blood of fetal calves as a slaughterhouse by-product. Such fluids, while not the only source of BVD virus, have the potential to introduce the virus at the optimum time for fetal infection. The herd veterinarian and the ET company should collaborate in the necessary testing, vaccination, and embryo transfer procedures to guard against transmission of persistent BVD infections. Obviously, if all recipient animals can be provided from the breeder's own herd, the opportunity for the spread of infections is much reduced. If beef heifers are purchased for recipients, it should be

kept in mind that the use of growth-promoting hormones, parasite medication, or recent vaccination will alter the response to estrus control products. The producer, the veterinarian, and the ET company should cooperate to synchronize the program, keeping the above facts in mind. For further information on disease control requirements and procedures, refer to the CSS Minimum Requirements (Exercise 24) and the 3$^{rd}$ Edition of the *Manual of the International Embryo Transfer Society* (1998).

## On-the-Farm Embryo Transfer

As the techniques have improved and experience has been gained, many embryo transfers are made at the cattle breeder's farm. Non-surgical procedures are generally used. The ET operator typically has a well-equipped van or vehicle in which the necessary laboratory work can be carried out. After treatment of the donor animal to bring about superovulation and fertilization of the shed eggs, the eggs are flushed from the uterus at the proper stage and transferred into one or more recipient animals. The recipient animals will have been synchronized with the donor for estrus.

The herd owner supplies the recipient animals as well as the donor. It may require 6 to 8 recipients in order to utilize all of the recovered fertilized eggs and to have the recipients in the proper stage of heat for each transfer made. (See the first paragraph of "Disadvantages of Embryo Transfer" earlier in this exercise.)

## ET Companies—Skilled Technicians

The herd operator who desires to have embryo transfers made should procure professional, experienced, and well-trained personnel to do the job. The success of any ET program is highly dependent upon the ability and skill of the persons carrying out the procedures.

ET firms are available in most livestock areas. Some of these companies, maintain a herd of recipient animals and have cattle-handling facilities, as well as the laboratory equipment necessary to carry out the complete ET procedure at their headquarters. In such instances, the donor animal is moved to the ET firm's headquarters and kept there as long as transfers are to be made or until eggs are collected, frozen, and stored.

Most ET firms carry out the entire procedure at the herd owner's farm with some laboratory facilities such as might be available at a veterinary hospital. Successful ET programs are being carried out by both large and small firms, whose operators are skilled and knowledgeable in all phases of reproduction, embryo transfer, and artificial insemination.

These companies are usually staffed by professional workers who have had training and experience in reproductive physiology, veterinary medicine, and artificial insemination. A veterinarian is usually involved, and wisely so, because of the need to administer drugs in the proper amounts and in the necessary sequence for the successful synchronization of donor and recipient animals. While the charges for professionals in their field vary, the ET business should be selected on the basis of a proven record of successful pregnancies. Skilled operators obtain a 50 to 70 percent pregnancy rate. The bottom line for a producer is the number of ET offspring that can be sold or added to the herd.

## Choose the ET Company Carefully

When choosing an ET company, a herd owner should determine clearly what ET services are required. Should the donor be collected on the farm or sent to the headquarters of an ET business? Should the recipients come from the owner's herd or from the ET firm?

How many embryos should be utilized in the fresh state, and how many should be frozen and stored?

If the cattle-housing facilities of an ET company are to be used, it is a good idea to inspect them before making an agreement for service. A careful check should be made on disease control measures; that is, what health tests are required before an animal is admitted to the premises, and what tests are carried out after admittance? Are quarantine quarters available? Are the premises clean? Does the staff have a positive attitude toward animal health requirements? Health requirements should be such that if embryos are to be exported, they will qualify. As a rule, health tests will include those for all diseases commonly found in cattle, plus any other health tests that are required in the countries of destination.

An agreement should be drawn up specifying the services to be rendered and the responsibilities of all parties. Price for the services should be agreed upon. Charges may be based upon pregnancies diagnosed at 60 to 90 days or upon services rendered regardless of results. Both methods have advantages and disadvantages. If few or no pregnancies are obtained, the second plan can be very expensive.

Embryo transfer is much more difficult than artificial insemination. It cannot be learned in a short course of a few days' duration. Education in reproductive physiology, artificial insemination, and veterinary science, plus technical skill and cattle management know-how gained by experience, are prerequisites for beginning ET operators. Proficiency will come only with time and experience. The herd owner contemplating embryo transfer in the herd should avoid inexperienced or beginning operators unless they will be assisted by trained and skilled personnel.

Many of the ET businesses in the United States, Canada, and overseas are members of at least one of three associations organized to further and guide the ET program. A certification program has been established for ET companies. Certification requires that personnel of the firms be competent in all transfer techniques, regulations, and record keeping. A letter to one or more of these associations will provide a herd owner with a list of businesses or companies that furnish ET services. The address of each follows:

American Embryo Transfer Association (AETA)
P.O. Box 2118
Hastings, NE 68902-2118

International Embryo Transfer Society (IETS)
1111 N. Dunlap Ave.
Savoy, IL 61874

Canadian Embryo Transfer Association (CETA)
P.O. Box 2000
Kemptville, Ontario, Canada K0G 1J0

In selecting an ET business, a herd operator should ask for a list of clients in the area and check with them regarding embryo recovery rates and percentage of pregnancies obtained.

## PROCEDURE

### Selection of the Donor Cow

The cow or heifer selected as a donor for the ET program should be well above the breed and herd average in the potential for the production of milk or meat. She should be of desirable conformation and free from inherited defects. For dairy cows, a high cow index value is the best indicator of good genetic potential. The cow index is a measure of genetic transmitting ability for milk, fat, protein, and dollar income. Since many dairy cattle breeders who use embryo transfer expect to produce animals that will bring a premium price at public or private treaty sales, only a cow that has a high cow index, a high production record herself, a high official classification score, and a popular pedigree with a depth of

good breeding and production should be used as a donor. It is donor cows with the above criteria, bred to high PTA bulls in AI, that produce young sires of interest to AI centers or, in some cases, breeder syndicates.

The donor should be thrifty and free of disease, should be cycling regularly, and should have a history of regular calving.

As a rule, older cows, largely because they have produced well, have had several superior offspring, and have classified high, are chosen as donors; however, dairy producers should not overlook heifers with a high cow index. Older cows fall behind in genetic potential because each generation of cattle is superior as genetic progress is made. The individual who wishes to build genetic potential for production in a herd should emphasize the use of high-ranking AI sires and use embryo transfer to a limited extent.

### Selection of Recipients

Well-grown heifers at least 15 to 16 months old are generally selected as ET recipients. Lower-producing dairy cows, if in sound reproductive condition and 60 days post-partum, may also be used. Providing suitable recipients is the major cost in embryo transfer. It may require from 6 to 8 cows or heifers for use with each donor animal. This is because not all recipients will respond to estrus synchronization drugs and because some may come into heat too early or too late to be suitable for embryo transfer. However, with successful cryopreservation techniques available, the need for many recipients is not as critical, since any extra embryos can be frozen and stored for later use.

There are two ways to provide recipient animals. The first method is to use animals from the owner's herd. This plan, while reducing transmission of disease, is not without considerable expense. Heifers are committed for months, and normal breeding is delayed. If cows are used, milk production is lost, and the recipients are delayed in natural calving. The second method is to obtain recipients from an ET company, usually at a fee of $1,100 to $1,500 per pregnancy. Salvage value of a recipient is recovered by the cattle breeder. While these costs seem high, a cattle breeder with a limited number of animals may not have enough animals available to serve as recipients. Often, it is unwise to purchase recipient heifers from other herds because of the danger of introducing disease and the uncertainty of the reproductive pattern of such animals. The owners of donor animals will have to choose the plan best for them. In any event, the resulting calf produced by embryo transfer must command a high figure if sold, or it must be of unusual value in the herd breeding program.

## Heat Synchronization of Donor and Recipients—Superovulation

To be successful, the timing of the embryo transfer and the estrous cycles of the donor and the recipients should coincide as closely as possible. The donor animal should have two normal heat periods before synchronization of the recipients is begun. It is wise to have a veterinarian check both the donor and the potential recipients to make sure the reproductive tract of each is normal. Hormone treatment is used to synchronize the estrus periods and to produce superovulation. There are several variations in the treatment schedule due to the preference of the ET operator, the drugs available, and the size and breed of the animals. (See Exercise 17 for estrus synchronization.)

The donor superovulation injection program is begun between days 9 and 14 so as to induce the production of more than one egg. Eight injections of 5 mg of FSH (follicle-stimulating hormone) each are given at 12-hour intervals (AM and PM). On days 3 and 4 of the injection schedule, the amount of FSH

is decreased slightly, and an injection of prostaglandin is given. (Some operators use only one prostaglandin injection.) Estrus usually occurs about 36 to 60 hours after the initial injection of prostaglandin. Administering prostaglandin toward the end of the FSH injection period causes the *corpus luteum* to regress. The recipient animals are also administered prostaglandin about 12 to 24 hours before the donor is so treated. This schedule of treatment helps the necessary synchronization of estrus between the donor and the recipients.

The donor animal should be artificially inseminated once or several times. Usually donors are inseminated at 12 hours and again at 24 hours after standing heat is observed. If available, multiple units of semen from a highly fertile bull may be used at each insemination. A plentiful supply of viable semen in the donor's reproductive tract is necessary because ovulation occurs over a period of several hours (even a day or two).

Another plan of superovulation is to replace the FSH injections described above by giving the donor cow a single injection of pregnant mare's serum gonadotropin (PMSG). This hormone is follicle stimulating, similar to FSH, and it also has some luteinizing (LH) action. Both hormones are needed. The injection may be administered any time during the estrous cycle. Treatment of the donor with PMSG followed by prostaglandin is successfully used by some ET workers.

As the time nears for embryo transfer, estrous cycles of the donor and the recipients should be checked every few hours and the observations recorded. The heat cycles of the donor and the recipients to be used should be in close agreement. If prostaglandin is used, the difference in time might vary some 6 to 18 hours; however, the best results in successful embryo transfer are obtained when the donor and the recipients are in heat the same day.

## Collecting the Embryos

Since virtually all embryos are collected by non-surgical means, only this method will be discussed. For background on surgical recovery of embryos, see the references for this exercise.

Flushing the uterus of the donor cow should begin six to eight days post-estrus, because it takes from three to five days for the embryos to descend the oviducts and reach the uterus. Most of the embryos will usually be in the upper horns of the uterus. The anterior part of the uterine horn, particularly on the side with the superovulated ovary, is the area to be flushed. A specially designed catheter, a flushing medium of phosphate-buffered saline, and the appropriate collecting cylinders, beakers, and dishes are necessary for currently used collection methods. For more specific information on flushing media and other media used in embryo transfer, refer to Appendix IV, page 616, of the work by E. S. E. Hafez cited in the references.

An elongated two-way Foley catheter, about 28 inches long, is used (Figure 21.3).

As will be noted, one of the passages of the collection device leads to a small balloon. Inflated, this balloon has a capacity of 10 to 25 ml of air, which occludes the uterine lumen and prevents leakage of the flushing medium. Through the second passage of the catheter, the flushing medium is introduced and recovered. By releasing a tubing clamp, the medium enters the uterus by gravity flow. Alternatively, the medium may be forced into the uterus by a syringe that is also fitted with a clamp. The delivery tube (with clamp) leads to a collection receptacle, which receives the returned flushing medium containing embryos.

In the collection procedure, the steps generally are:

1. A local anesthetic is injected between the vertebrae on the rump of the cow to reduce rectal contractions.

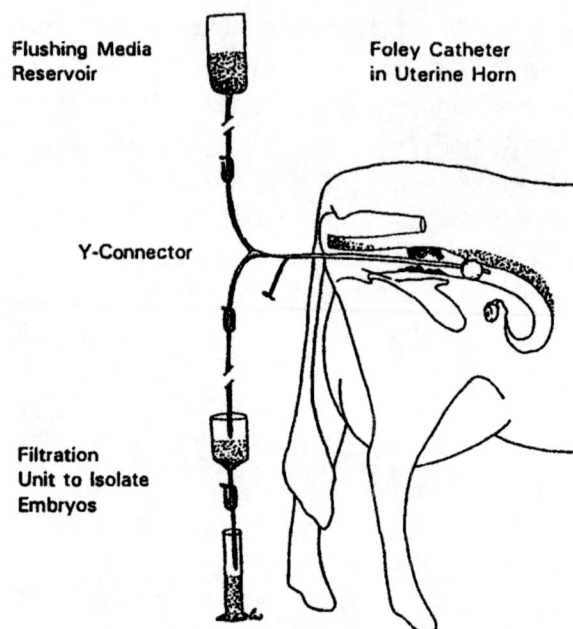

**Figure 21.3.** Non-surgical embryo recovery using a two-way Foley catheter. The uterine horns are flushed with media, and embryos are collected. The catheter balloon occludes the uterine lumen, preventing leakage of the flushing medium.

2. The vulva area of the donor is thoroughly cleansed so as to reduce contamination of the embryos.

3. The catheter, if necessary strengthened by a steel stylet placed inside it to give rigidity, is passed through the cervix in much the same way as an AI tube.

4. When the catheter is in place, the balloon is inflated so that it closes the lumen of the appropriate uterine horn slightly past the bifurcation of the uterine horns. The stylet, if used, is then withdrawn.

5. The medium container is filled with the fluid at body temperature, and with the collecting tube closed, about 15 to 20 ml of fluid are infused to prime the tube. Then, additional medium is infused into the uterine

horn until it becomes rigid as determined by palpation per rectum. The delivery tube clamp is released, and the fluid drained into the collection container (Figure 21.3). The process is repeated several times, with the uterus massaged per rectum. Up to about 500 ml of fluid may be used for each flushing so as to recover as many embryos as possible. Should *corpora lutea* be found on both ovaries, both horns of the uterus should be flushed. Following flushing, the balloon is deflated and the catheter removed. Since there may be some irritation of the cervix by introduction of the catheter, an antiseptic solution should be infused into the uterus.

6. The flushed media (usually collected in glass or plastic cylinders) is allowed to stand for several minutes to let the embryos settle to the bottom. Avoiding agitation, the top portion of the fluid is carefully siphoned off. The bottom portion, which contains the embryos, is separated into smaller amounts and examined under a stereo microscope at a magnification of $10\times$ to $60\times$. As the embryos are located, they are placed in a holding medium and evaluated microscopically for quality. Alternatively, an embryo filter apparatus can be used to "catch" or collect the embryos as the flushed media passes through it. Embryos then are rinsed from the collection grid. This is the current method of choice.

The embryos selected for transfer should be round and full, with an unruptured zona pellucida and the normal development (cell divisions) with respect to the time of recovery. Misshapen ova come in many forms and should be discarded. Likewise, single-cell ova should be discarded, as they are unfertilized. Two-cell ova, if only two days old, are generally fertilized and may be considered normal; however, if the uterus is flushed later than two days following estrus, the two-cell ova should be discarded. The embryos considered normal will generally have from 2 to 64 cells, with the number of cells varying with the time of flushing. Some will have 16 cells or more, with older embryos in the morula and blastocyst stages. Generally, about five to eight of the embryos obtained will be acceptable for transfer.

Many ET practitioners make use of one of the microsurgery stations that have been developed for various embryo-related procedures. An example of a micromanipulator system is shown in Figure 21.4. This system is especially suited for field work. It consists of a zoom stereo microscope with illuminated base (incident and transmitted light), a heating stage, and micromanipulators with micrometer adjustments that provide the

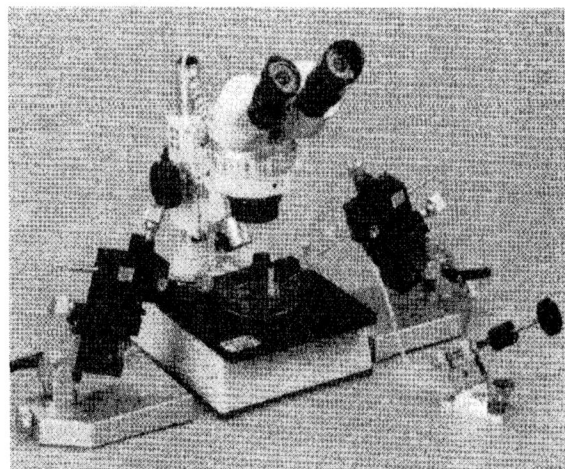

**Figure 21.4.** A micromanipulator system used for microsurgery and other embryo-related procedures. (Courtesy, Minitube of America, Inc., Madison, WI)

necessary working distance to perform the desired microsurgery. The unit may be transported for use by those ET operators who perform their services at the client's facilities.

7. The recovered ova selected for use should be maintained at a temperature of 99°F (37°C) and kept sealed in the collection vessel until transferred. After selection, embryos should be transferred to the recipient animal as soon as possible to insure high viability. Good quality embryos not utilized immediately following collection may be frozen in liquid nitrogen and stored for future use in much the same manner as semen is frozen and stored.

## Making the Transfer

There are two methods of embryo transfer, surgical and non-surgical. The non-surgical method is widely used and conducted as follows:

1. The recipient animal is given a light epidural injection of anesthesia between the vertebrae of the rump to reduce rectal contractions.

2. The embryo to be transferred is drawn into a 0.25-ml insemination straw and then placed into the standard AI gun equipped with a sheath.

3. The insemination gun is carefully worked through the cervix and into the horn of the uterus corresponding to the ovary that has a *corpus luteum*. The embryo should be deposited as deep into the uterine horn as feasible without using force (force can result in trauma and infection). If no *corpora lutea* are found, the recipient should not be used, as a functional *corpus luteum* is necessary for pregnancy.

If twins are desired, an embryo should be placed in both horns of the uterus of the recipient with a *corpus luteum* present.

The surgical method is carried out in this manner:

1. The recipient is prepared for surgery by shaving an area about 6 inches square located some 6 inches in front of the hipbone joint. The area prepared should be on the side where the *corpus luteum* is present (indicating the ovary where ovulation occurred).

2. A local anesthetic is injected at the shaved area.

3. The area is scrubbed with alcohol, and a 2-inch incision is made with a scalpel.

4. The uterus and the ovaries are brought near the opening of the incision by grasping the uterus with the fingers of a surgical-gloved hand.

5. A small incision is made in the exposed uterine horn with a blunt needle.

6. The embryo is drawn into a 0.25-ml straw attached to a small syringe and deposited into the uterus.

7. The incision is closed with a few stitches.

The surgical method has a slightly higher pregnancy rate than the non-surgical method.

The non-surgical method of embryo transfer is faster and less expensive than the surgical method; however, there is greater danger of infections in the reproductive tract, since the uterus is more susceptible when under the influence of progesterone from the *corpus luteum*. But with growing experience and improving technology, the danger is being reduced, and the non-surgical method is the primary technique for transfer.

## Embryo Cryopreservation

The freezing and storage of good quality embryos (cryopreservation) makes it possible for the full advantages of embryo transfer to be realized.

Like all mammalian cells, embryos require a protective agent to minimize the rigors of freezing and thawing. A commonly used cryoprotective solution for freezing embryos consists of modified Dulbeccos phosphate-buffered saline containing bovine serum albumin or heat-treated serum, 10 percent glycerol, and appropriate antibiotics (see page 616 of the work by Hafez cited in the references). Embryos are placed in this solution for about 30 minutes at room temperature so that the glycerol permeates the cells. The embryos, with a small amount of the cryoprotective solution, are put into plastic straws for freezing. Glass ampules are no longer used.

The cooling of embryos must be controlled to avoid the formation of large ice crystals inside the cellular structure. The straws are rapidly cooled from room temperature to about 21°F (−6°C). Then, the embryos in straws are cooled slowly at a rate of about 0.9°F (0.5°C) per minute to about −22°F ( 30°C). After a short holding period at −22°F (−30°C), the embryo units are cooled rapidly by transferring them into liquid nitrogen (−320°F [−196°C]). The cryopreserved embryos may be stored for years if kept immersed in liquid nitrogen. Once embryos thaw, they must be used immediately. They cannot be refrozen and maintain viability.

Embryos in 0.5-ml straws may be thawed for use by transfer to water at a temperature of 70° to 99°F (21° to 37°C). The smaller diameter (0.25-ml) straws can be rapidly warmed in air and transferred to 99°F (37°C) water. After recovery of an embryo from a straw, the glycerol cryoprotectant is removed from the embryo before transfer. This is accomplished by stepwise washing of the embryo in buffered sucrose solutions containing incrementally lower concentrations of glycerol. Typically four to six washings for about six minutes each are used. The last washing solution contains no glycerol.

**One-Step Straw (Direct Transfer) Method**—An increasingly used method of embryo cryopreservation is to place one embryo in a straw (0.25 ml) with a small amount of the cryoprotective solution and to fill the remainder of the straw with buffered sucrose diluent. The two solutions are separated by a small air bubble. When thawed, the cryoprotective solution is dislodged by simply shaking the straw to remove the air bubble and permit the embryo to move into the diluting medium (buffered sucrose solution). The embryo is then transferred into the cow from the same straw in which it was frozen. This Direct Transfer method is utilized as soon as the embryo has been thawed, similarly to the way frozen semen is utilized in AI practice. Since the embryo does not have to be removed from the straw in the Direct Transfer method, technical errors associated with washing the embryo can be eliminated, making this method practical for use under on-farm conditions.

## Regulations Governing Embryo Transfer for Registered Cattle

With the growing use of embryo transfer in cattle beginning several years ago, most cattle registry organizations have adopted regulations to insure the accuracy of parentage and the proper identification of the resulting offspring. Frozen embryo labeling requirements have been approved by the International Embryo Transfer Society. Although these requirements are used as a guide by many breed registry associations, there are variations among organizations. *Every breeder of registered cattle or other livestock who decides to use embryo transfer should contact the respective breed registry organization and*

**Table 21.2.** Other Species E.T. Activity—2000

| Species | Flushes | Transferrable Embryos | Number of Embryos Transferred | | | |
|---------|---------|-----------------------|--------|--------|---------|--------|
| | | | Fresh | Frozen | Storage | Export |
| Sheep | 2,846 | 18,781 | 1,414 | 3,472 | 3,760 | 9,370 |
| Goat | 1,504 | 11,492 | 9,912 | 607 | 1,315 | 687 |
| Cervids | 374 | 1,499 | 743 | 521 | 285 | 252 |
| Equine | 5,398 | 3,139 | 2,755 | 75 | 100 | |
| Swine | 260 | 9,043 | 7,091 | | 5,910 | |
| Totals | 10,382 | 43,954 | 21,915 | 4,675 | 11,370 | 10,309 |

*follow the requirements set forth for the recording of ET animals.*

A copy of frozen embryo labeling requirements recommended by the International Embryo Transfer Society and adopted by the Holstein Association USA, Inc. appears in Appendix E.

## Embryo Transfer—Other Species

Embryo transfer technology is increasingly utilized in species other than bovine. Reporting of this activity is lacking; however, the best estimates for flushes and transferrable embryos in 2000 are presented in Table 21.2. (See Thibier in the references.)

There certainly is embryo transfer potential in species other than bovine.

## Embryo Sales—Exports

The sale of embryos from outstanding cows has become a growing addition to the income of cattle breeders. Frozen embryos are sold domestically and internationally. In 2000, there were 16,821 embryos exported (8,538 beef and 8,283 dairy) from the United States. One of the considerations in the sale of frozen embryos is that they are not a means of spreading cattle diseases. Many diseases are caused by viruses, including BLV (bovine leukemia virus), BVD, IBR, and BLU (blue tongue), etc. However, there is less risk of spreading disease through embryos or semen than through live animals.

In order to protect the integrity of embryo transfer programs in the United States, the American Embryo Transfer Association (AETA) certifies ET companies. It also cooperates with the USDA's Animal and Plant Health Inspection Service (APHIS), the U.S. Animal Health Association (USAHA), and the Foreign Agricultural Service (FAS) by assisting in the development of regulations for the export and import of embryos. The Canadian Embryo Transfer Association (CETA) also works closely with the Canadian Food Inspection Agency. The cattle breed registry organizations, as well as companies and individuals engaged in embryo sales, are guided by these regulations.

The NAAB subsidiary Certified Semen Services, Inc., provides a guide for the production of disease-free semen. The production and handling of frozen embryos, so as to control the transmission of disease and avoid contamination, is an obligation of all concerned. Information on regulations may be obtained from any of the previously mentioned sources.

# QUESTIONS

1. Why do cattle breeders utilize embryo transfer?

2. What are the chief advantages of embryo transfer?

3. What are the disadvantages of embryo transfer for a purebred cattle breeder?

4. What are the requirements for a donor cow (dairy breeds)?

5. How would you provide recipient animals?

6. Why is synchronization of estrus in the donor and the recipients vitally important?

7. How is superovulation brought about?

8. Why is prostaglandin ($PGF_{2\alpha}$) used in most superovulation methods?

9. How are embryos recovered from the donor?

10. What are the advantages of non-surgical vs. surgical embryo transfer?

11. How would you select a company to perform embryo transfer in your herd?

12. If you decide to engage in the practice of embryo transfer as a business, how would you proceed in getting the necessary training and experience?

13. When frozen embryos are sold, what precautions should be followed with respect to the control of disease?

14. What are the requirements for registering purebred dairy cattle resulting from embryo transfer?

# REFERENCES

Amann, R. P. 1988. Treatment of sperm to predetermine sex. Proc. 12th Tech. Conf. on Artificial Insemination and Reproduction. NAAB. p. 127.

Animal biotechnology: Technology transfer and industrial needs (Proc. NCR-150 Symposium). 1992. Anim. Biotech. 3(1):1.

Brackett, Benjamin, George E. Seidel, Jr., and Sarah Seidel (Eds.). 1982. New Technologies in Animal Breeding. Academic Press, New York.

Cran, D. G. et al. 1995. Sex pre-selection in cattle: a field trial. Vet. Rec. 136:495.

Dochi, O., Yamamoto, Y., Saga, H., Yoshiba, N., Kano, N., Maeda, J., Miyata, K., Yamauchi, A., Tominaga, K., Oda, Y., Nakashima, T., and Inohae, S. 1998. Direct transfer of bovine embryos frozen-thawed in the presence of propylene glycol or ethylene glycol under on-farm conditions in an integrated embryo transfer program. Theriogenology. 49(5): 1051–1058.

Foote, R. H. 1999. Development of reproductive biotechnologies in domestic animals from artificial insemination to cloning: a perspective. Cloning. Vol. 1, No. 3. p. 133.

Garner, D. L. 2001. Sex-sorting mammalian sperm: concept to application in animals. J. Androl. Vol. 22, No. 4. p. 519.

Hafez, E. S. E. (Ed.). 1987. Reproduction in Farm Animals (5th Ed.). Lea and Febiger, Philadelphia. (Chs. 25, 27, 28 and Appendix IV.)

Humes, P. E., and R. A. Godke. 1985. Genetic impact of embryo transfer in beef cattle. Proc. Ann. Conf. on Artificial Insemination and Embryo Transfer in Beef Cattle. NAAB. p. 38.

Johnson, L. A. 1989. Progress toward achieving sex preselection in farm animals. J. Anim. Sci. 67 (Suppl. 1):342 (Abstr.).

Johnson, L. A., J. P. Flook, and H. Hawk. 1989. Sex preselection in rabbits: Live births from X and Y sperm separated by DNA and cell sorting. Biol. Reprod. 41:199.

Johnson, L. A. 2000. Sexing mammalian sperm for production of offspring: The state-of-the-art. Animal Reproduction Science 60-61 (2000) p. 93–107.

Leake, Linda L. Sci fi. Repro. Dairy Today. April 2001. p. 16.

Lindsey, A. C. et al. 2000. Hysteroscopic insemination of fresh and frozen un-sexed and sexed equine spermatozoa. In: Proc. 5th Intl. Symp. Equine Embryo Transfer. Saari, Finland.

McCue, P. M., Squires, E. L., Bruemmer, J. E. and Niswender, K. D. 2001. Equine embryo transfer: techniques, trends and anecdotes. SFT Annual Conference Proceedings. p. 229–235.

Polge, E. J. C., 1996. Historical Perspective of AI: Commercial Methods of Producing Sex Specific Semen, IVF Procedures. Proc. 16th Tech. Conf. on Artificial Insemination and Reproduction. NAAB. p. 7.

Schenk, J. L., 2000. Apply Sperm Sexing Technology to the AI Industry. Proc. 18th Tech. Conf. on Artificial Insemination and Reproduction. NAAB. p. 73.

Seidel, George E., Jr., and R. Peter Elsden. 1997. Embryo Transfer in Dairy Cattle. W. D. Hoard & Sons Company, Fort Atkinson, WI.

Stringfellow, D. A., and S. M. Seidel (Eds.). 1990. Manual of the International Embryo Transfer Society. 1990. IETS, Champaign, IL.

Thibier, M. 1992. Statistics of the ET industry around the world. Embryo Transfer Newsletter (IETS) 10:10.

Thompson, J. 1993. Is MOET in your future? Holstein World 90 (March Bonus):26.

Van Wagtendonk-de Leeuw AM, Den Daas JHG, Kruip ThAM, Rall WF. 1995. Comparison of the efficacy of conventional slow freezing and rapid cryopreservation methods for bovine embryos. Cryobiology, 32:157–167.

Current literature as assigned by the instructor.

## WEB SITES

American Embryo Transfer Association
   *http://www.aeta.org*

Canadian Embryo Transfer Association
   *http://www.ceta.ca*

International Embryo Transfer Society
   *http://www.iets.org/*

Cloning
   *http://genomics.phrma.org/*

————————————————— **PART FOUR**

**Sire Selection;**

**Bull Health and Management;**

**AI Organizations;**

**Employment Opportunities**

# EXERCISE 22

# Selection of Sires for AI Use

## OBJECT

To review considerations involved in the selection of dairy and beef bulls for artificial insemination.

## DISCUSSION

Bulls selected for AI should transmit to their offspring the genetic potential for well-above-average milk or meat production. In addition, the progeny must be of desirable conformation, be long wearing, have quiet disposition, and be free of genetic defects. Genetic improvement of cattle through the use of artificial insemination calls for a continual replacement of the lower-production-transmitting bulls by younger, proven bulls with superior genetic merit. The success of this program in dairy cattle is well illustrated in Table 1.1 by the fact that milk production per cow almost quadrupled in the United States in a span of some 60 years. The development of guides for selecting and proving young sires and the heavy use of superior sires through artificial insemination have significantly contributed to these attainments.

Both production-proven, Figure 22.1, and promising young sires are used in AI. The objective is to have a sufficient number of superior-production-proven sires to breed to most of the cows (some 70 to 80 percent). The remainder of the cow population is bred to promising young sires that are being sampled. Since every proven sire was once unproven, it is important to use a combination of young bulls and proven sires.

## PROCEDURE

Sires to be used for artificial insemination are selected on the basis of traits that are economically important to those who will own their offspring. In addition, the AI organization needs to consider the fertility of a bull when semen is frozen and used in many herds, the demand (popularity) for semen, and justification for the bull's purchase price—i.e., will he provide sufficient income to justify his purchase price?

Following are some factors generally considered by AI businesses in selecting bulls:

1. ***Genetic evaluations for production traits***—For a proven sire, genetic evaluations can provide fairly accurate information with regard to his transmitting ability for improved production. For dairy bulls, special attention should be given to PTA's for milk, protein, and fat. For beef, bulls should be selected for high growth while maintaining birth weight or calving ease. Reliability or accuracy should be considered as well. Check the number of daughters that have contributed production records to the bull's evaluation and see if these daughters are evenly distributed in many herds.

    For a young sire, genetic evaluations are not as accurate but still provide useful information. While these evaluations do not include production information from offspring,

**Figure 22.1.** These sires have been very influential in their breed. Not only have they sired many offspring, they have also sired top AI bulls in the next generation. Becoming familiar with the influential sires will assist you in pedigree analysis and in communicating with breeders.

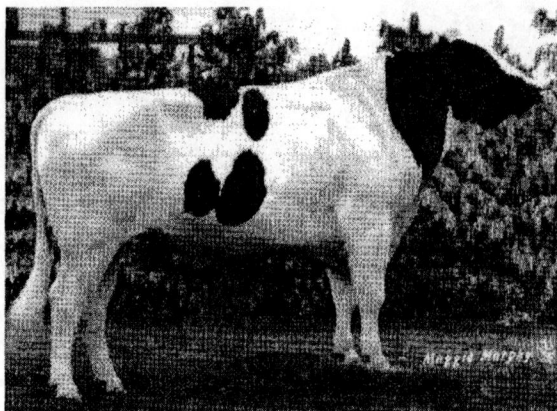

**Figure 22.1A.** Holstein 8H1464 BIS-MAY TRADITION CLEITUS 1879085 (Eastern AI Coop., Ithaca, NY)

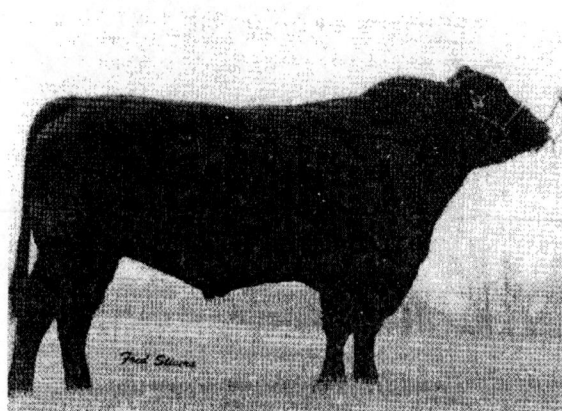

**Figure 22.1B.** Angus 7AN95 SCOTCH CAP 10226429 (Select Sires, Inc., Plain City, OH)

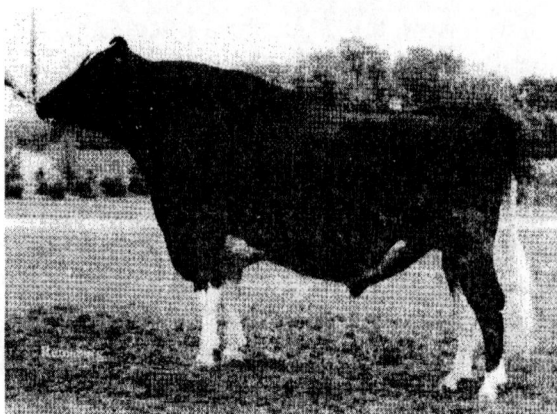

**Figure 22.1C.** Holstein 7H1897 TO-MAR-BLACK-STAR-ET 1929410 (Select Sires, Inc., Plain City, OH)

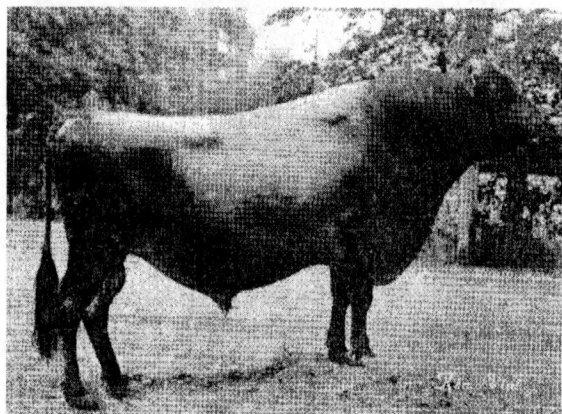

**Figure 22.1D.** Jersey 7J177 HIGHLAND MAGIC DUNCAN 635862 (Select Sires, Inc., Plain City, OH)

they are the best combination of information on the bull's relatives. In dairy, these values are called Parent Averages. Special emphasis should be given to milk and protein. Most bulls with low Parent Averages will sire offspring with below-average production.

In the future, genetic markers may be useful in selection of young sires. A genetic marker is a unique sequence of DNA that is associated with an economically important trait, such as milk production or ribeye area. Simple tests may soon be available that identify which animals carry the favorable genetic markers. The advantage of these markers is that genetic differences in sires can be detected long before information on their performance or their progeny's performance is available.

2. *Genetic evaluations for type or conformation traits*—Genetic evaluations for overall conformation are readily available for dairy cattle. Bulls with high ratings in overall conformation will have increased demand. In addition, genetic evaluations on individual type traits are useful. Special attention should be given to udder traits and to feet and leg traits. Use of these individual type traits will indicate which bulls sire offspring with improved wearability. Genetic evaluations for conformation traits are not readily available for beef cattle. In this case, evaluating the conformation of the bull will provide limited but useful information.

3. *Fertility*—Both the fertility history of the older bull and his reproductive soundness must be considered. In the case of a young bull, he should be a son of a proven bull; his reproductive capacity and family fertility history are very important.

4. *Health*—Only healthy, structurally sound bulls that are free from venereal diseases should be used in the AI program.

5. *Freedom from genetic defects*—Ancestry, and the bull himself if he has offspring, should be free of undesirable genes. A careful check for genetic defects should be made from the standpoint of family history.

6. *Age*—If the bull is proven, how many years of productive life can be counted on? If the bull is young, how long until he is ready for AI service?

7. *Recognized family lines*—Family lines (breeding) are generally recognized by cattle breeders and are important in purebreds. While non-registered herd owners are not as concerned with bloodlines, they usually hear about "the bulls doing the job" and demand them. Also, no matter how desirable a bull might be, the sale of his semen depends upon demand.

8. *Economy*—The purchase price and other costs associated with the bull must be justified.

9. *Breeder*—Is the seller a reputable cattle breeder? Bulls should be acquired only from persons who have the reputation for breeding good cattle and for being honest and fair dealing.

Review Exercise 3. Also, study Figure 22.2 and Tables 22.1 and 22.2. The figure and the tables will be referred to as we discuss use of genetic evaluations in the following sections.

## Using Genetic Evaluations for Sire Selection

Genetic evaluations provide two pieces of useful information. They indicate where a bull ranks within a population, and they indicate the genetic differences between bulls. To produce meaningful information, the evaluation of an individual bull needs to be compared with the evaluations of other bulls of interest or with the population average.

If one trait or index could be identified that summarized all the economically important traits, sire selection would be easy. One could simply select the bulls that ranked the highest for that one trait. However, there are many different opinions as to which traits are important. The skill in sire selection is determining

# NAAB DAIRY SIRE SUMMARY NOVEMBER, 2002

## HOLSTEIN (BY NAAB CODE)

| NAAB CODE | SIRE NAME | ID NUMBER | SAMPLING INFO. NO. HRDS | NO. DAUS | CD | ORG | Net Merit $$ | Net Merit % ile | M | MILK LBS | FAT % | FAT LBS | PROTEIN % | PROTEIN LBS | R | FM $$ | CM $$ | SCS | PL | M | PTAT | R | TPI‡ | CE % DB | CE R |
|---|---|---|---|---|---|---|---|---|---|---|---|---|---|---|---|---|---|---|---|---|---|---|---|---|---|
| 14HO2970 | KINGS-RANSOM D EVENT -TV | USA 17115165 | 68 | 88 | S | 14 | 480 | 88 | | 1228 | -0.17 | 3 | 0.01 | 38 | 89 | 474 | 486 | 2.70 | 4.9 | | 0.33 | 86 | 1449 | 7 | 83 |
| 14HO3023 | ANDERSONVILLE D DELMAN-ET -TV | USA 17163941 | 58 | 68 | S | 14 | 502 | 92 | | 1689 | -0.13 | 29 | -0.02 | 46 | 86 | 536 | 499 | 2.95 | 3.8 | | 1.04 | 85 | 1542 | 9 | 73 |
| 14HO3037 | SHER-EST DUSTER SKIP-ET -TV | USA 17176087 | 87 | 140 | S | 14 | 479 | 88 | M | 1585 | -0.03 | 49 | 0.02 | 53 | 90 | 444 | 492 | 2.93 | 0.9 | | 1.19 | 87 | 1504 | 6 | 77 |
| 14HO3039 | BULLCREST PATRON SABRE -TV | USA 17253930 | 71 | 96 | S | 14 | 498 | 91 | | 1060 | 0.09 | 61 | 0.09 | 54 | 86 | 348 | 538 | 3.12 | 1.9 | | 0.97 | 88 | 1555 | 9 | 80 |
| 14HO3094 | BOWLING-GREEN BENWOOD -TV | USA 120119675 | 65 | 79 | S | 14 | 489 | 90 | | 2624 | -0.18 | 49 | -0.05 | 64 | 86 | 593 | 472 | 2.99 | 0.6 | | 1.11 | 86 | 1521 | 10 | 73 |
| 14HO3099 | TOWERVIEW-ACRES TYCO-ET -TV | USA 17347852 | 41 | 56 | S | 14 | 363 | 57 | | 681 | -0.02 | 21 | 0.07 | 37 | 82 | 251 | 393 | 2.89 | 1.7 | | 1.82 | 80 | 1447 | 10 | 69 |
| 14HO3139 | CHASIN-RAINBOWS LB JACK-TW -TV | USA 17391177 | 52 | 70 | S | 14 | 269 | 29 | | 1016 | 0.02 | 41 | 0.05 | 41 | 84 | 199 | 289 | 3.31 | -0.1 | | 1.23 | 84 | 1301 | 9 | 73 |
| 14HO3148 | ELM-PARK DETROIT-ET -TV | USA 18006909 | 80 | 108 | S | 14 | 455 | 82 | | 1513 | 0.03 | 62 | 0.06 | 60 | 88 | 357 | 483 | 3.24 | 0.6 | | 0.25 | 88 | 1432 | 7 | 73 |
| 14HO3152 | JOHANSSON BW TAI TASKER-ET -TV | USA 120135022 | 57 | 77 | S | 14 | 375 | 60 | | 2105 | -0.24 | 15 | -0.07 | 44 | 84 | 509 | 350 | 2.90 | 0.7 | | 1.35 | 82 | 1395 | 9 | 76 |
| 14HO3154 | CARNATION VIRGO-ET -TV | USA 17391047 | 86 | 116 | S | 14 | 463 | 84 | | 1539 | -0.08 | 37 | -0.02 | 40 | 90 | 507 | 457 | 2.82 | 2.2 | | 1.22 | 90 | 1507 | 10 | 78 |
| 14HO3155 | NEYER JOHNSON MARK-RED-ET -TV | USA 17369359 | 65 | 89 | S | 14 | 299 | 38 | | 1712 | -0.22 | 6 | -0.06 | 37 | 86 | 400 | 280 | 2.97 | 0.8 | | 0.65 | 86 | 1223 | 11 | 83 |
| 14HO3158 | WA-DEL RICE SATURN-ET -TV | USA 120614769 | 60 | 81 | S | 14 | 494 | 91 | | 2079 | -0.14 | 39 | 0.03 | 70 | 86 | 445 | 512 | 3.08 | 0.2 | | 0.67 | 85 | 1474 | 8 | 77 |
| 14HO3160 | CLINITA PATRN FOUNDATION-ET -TV | USA 18062814 | 71 | 98 | S | 14 | 463 | 84 | | 1629 | -0.04 | 48 | -0.01 | 46 | 88 | 485 | 462 | 2.94 | 0.8 | | 2.09 | 87 | 1567 | 7 | 78 |
| 14HO3161 | VANSTRA DEW RUD GALLEON-ET -TV | USA 18053686 | 66 | 88 | S | 14 | 431 | 76 | | 1683 | -0.16 | 22 | 0.00 | 49 | 87 | 443 | 433 | 2.84 | 1.6 | | 1.64 | 85 | 1511 | 8 | 76 |
| 14HO3166 | B-Y-J SCRIBE-ET -TV | USA 18047844 | 77 | 104 | S | 14 | 462 | 84 | | 2403 | -0.12 | 56 | -0.02 | 66 | 88 | 507 | 458 | 3.22 | 0.3 | | 0.43 | 87 | 1439 | 7 | 75 |
| 14HO3182 | PARADISE-R SANCHO -TV | USA 18024147 | 54 | 70 | S | 14 | 427 | 74 | | 2522 | -0.17 | 46 | -0.12 | 44 | 83 | 646 | 381 | 3.29 | 1.2 | | 0.91 | 83 | 1405 | 7 | 72 |
| 14HO3188 | HONEYCREST JOLT LITENING-ET -TV | USA 18037275 | 60 | 91 | S | 14 | 383 | 62 | | 1803 | -0.04 | 54 | -0.02 | 49 | 86 | 420 | 379 | 3.27 | 0.5 | | 1.20 | 87 | 1418 | 8 | 75 |
| 14HO3202 | DREAM&DO-B FORMATION JAREK -TV | USA 120410552 | 41 | 68 | S | 14 | 339 | 50 | | 1333 | -0.12 | 20 | 0.01 | 43 | 81 | 321 | 348 | 3.21 | 0.8 | | 1.41 | 79 | 1385 | 10 | 74 |
| 14HO3204 | PARADISE-D D PATRON PATT -TV | USA 120482928 | 56 | 89 | S | 14 | 496 | 91 | | 1623 | -0.03 | 51 | 0.01 | 51 | 85 | 482 | 504 | 3.04 | 1.5 | | 1.71 | 84 | 1577 | 7 | 73 |
| 14HO3213 | CORYDON AERO GERARD -TV | USA 121206489 | 58 | 75 | S | 14 | 396 | 66 | | 1464 | -0.04 | 42 | 0.00 | 43 | 84 | 404 | 398 | 2.93 | 0.8 | | 1.51 | 82 | 1436 | 8 | 73 |
| 14HO3217 | WIL-HART WADE LON-ET -CV | USA 121149482 | 45 | 62 | S | 14 | 356 | 54 | | 728 | -0.06 | 12 | 0.07 | 37 | 82 | 253 | 383 | 3.11 | 1.6 | | 1.96 | 79 | 1477 | 7 | 70 |
| 14HO3234 | VEEMAN-DAIRY PAW RANGER-ET -TV | USA 18058022 | 67 | 93 | S | 14 | 361 | 56 | | 989 | -0.02 | 31 | 0.05 | 42 | 87 | 279 | 384 | 3.15 | 1.1 | | 1.44 | 83 | 1410 | 7 | 78 |
| 23HO604 | TO-MAR FOREVER-ET -TV | USA 17005513 | 64 | 120 | S | 23 | 374 | 59 | | 1146 | 0.09 | 57 | 0.02 | 35 | 89 | 338 | 387 | 3.10 | 0.6 | | 1.43 | 89 | 1430 | 9 | 95 |
| 28HO582 | MERIT PERFORMER-ET -TV | USA 2235524 | 85 | 133 | S | 39 | 314 | 42 | | 630 | 0.14 | 34 | 0.07 | 7 | 92 | 205 | 343 | 3.21 | 0.2 | | 0.70 | 78 | 1316 | 9 | 96 |
| 28HO583 | LYSTEL LEDUC-ET -TV | CAN 6193092 | 376 | 501 | | 28 | 105 | 5 | M | 38 | 0.14 | -3 | 0.03 | 3 | 90 | 65 | 115 | 3.39 | 0.2 | | 2.25 | 84 | 1218 | 19 | 97 |
| 29HO809 | BLACKCREST KOKOMO-RED -TL | USA 2258099 | 82 | 118 | S | 29 | 286 | 34 | | 1198 | -0.19 | 34 | -0.01 | 32 | 92 | 303 | 289 | 3.03 | 1.8 | | 0.02 | 84 | 1185 | 10 | 76 |
| 29HO812 | FIVE-ALIVE CARUSO-RED-ET -TV | USA 2249017 | 63 | 101 | S | 29 | 181 | 12 | | 1363 | -0.24 | -11 | -0.03 | 33 | 90 | 243 | 170 | 3.19 | 1.5 | | 0.30 | 85 | 1089 | 9 | 77 |
| 29HO819 | COUNTRY-AYRE REDNECK-RED-ET -TL | USA 2289807 | 86 | 123 | S | 29 | 280 | 31 | | 961 | -0.09 | 12 | 002 | 8 | 92 | 253 | 290 | 2.99 | 1.8 | | 0.18 | 84 | 1207 | 10 | 77 |
| 29HO826 | BRIAR SUCCESS STIEVE-RED-ET -TV | USA 2286878 | 41 | 51 | S | 29 | 88 | 4 | | 562 | -0.03 | 13 | -0.03 | 8 | 83 | 149 | 75 | 3.18 | 0.3 | | 1.77 | 77 | 1131 | 14 | 78 |
| 29HO830 | CLOVER-MIST N SCARLET-RED -TV | USA 17019030 | 76 | 117 | S | 29 | 219 | 17 | | 1451 | -0.27 | -13 | -0.07 | 27 | 90 | 333 | 195 | 2.93 | 1.9 | | -0.12 | 79 | 1067 | 8 | 80 |
| 29HO832 | APPLOUIS RJ MYSTERY-RED-ET -TL | USA 17076504 | 65 | 100 | S | 29 | 183 | 13 | | 481 | 0.04 | 26 | 0.03 | 22 | 89 | 132 | 197 | 3.31 | 0.2 | | 0.85 | 79 | 1144 | 10 | 80 |
| 29HO834 | J-W-RUS SHERMAN-RED-ET -TL | USA 17192806 | 155 | 349 | | 29 | 168 | 10 | | 556 | -0.05 | 8 | 0.04 | 26 | 94 | 105 | 185 | 2.89 | -0.7 | | 0.14 | 87 | 1049 | 9 | 87 |
| 29HO6658 | KED JUROR-ET -TV | USA 2124357 | ........ | 69926 | S | 29 | 223 | 18 | | 798 | -0.02 | 24 | -0.05 | 25 | 99 | 230 | 223 | 3.17 | 1.0 | M | 1.91 | 99 | 1306 | 7 | 99 |
| 29HO6735 | EASTVIEW MEADOWLORD-ET -TV | USA 2128554 | 5284 | 17110 | S | 29 | 290 | 35 | | 519 | 0.15 | 55 | 0.00 | 25 | 99 | 227 | 307 | 2.92 | 0.1 | M | 1.56 | 98 | 1333 | 9 | 98 |
| 29HO6822 | BER MARDI GRAS-ET -RC | USA 2140604 | 1524 | 2732 | S | 29 | 66 | 3 | | 302 | 0.06 | 25 | -0.02 | 5 | 97 | 94 | 60 | 3.13 | -1.3 | M | 1.23 | 97 | 1023 | 13 | 94 |
| 29HO6995 | PEN-COL DUSTER-ET -TV | USA 2147486 | 5354 | 26876 | S | 29 | 453 | 82 | | 1264 | -0.18 | 1 | 0.03 | 44 | 99 | 413 | 467 | 2.80 | 4.4 | M | 0.79 | 99 | 1450 | 9 | 99 |

**Figure 22.2.** Excerpt from the NAAB Dairy Sire Summary—Holstein Sires. February, 2002, p. 12 of the NAAB Dairy Sire Summary.

which information should be used in making your selection decisions.

## Selecting Dairy Sires for Herd Use

In Figure 22.2, an excerpt from NAAB's Dairy Sire Summary shows a listing of sires from the November 2002 USDA genetic evaluations. This format lists bulls in NAAB Code order. Notice the many different traits that are summarized. This demonstrates the major challenge in using genetic evaluations. The key is to identify the economically important traits and basically ignore the other information.

A major emphasis in any dairy producer's selection program should be the production traits. The major source of income for all dairy producers is milk sales. Which production traits to use for selection of sires should be determined by the method by which the dairy's milk sales are valued. If milk is paid for totally on the basis of milk volume, then PTA Milk should be the selection trait. The most common situation is for milk to be paid for through some combination of milk, fat, and protein yield. Therefore, economic indexes are calculated by USDA that express profitability based on different markets (see NM$, FM$, CM$ in Exercise 3).

Another important value to consider is reliability. Sires receive evaluations based on different amounts of information. The reliability value indicates the relative accuracy of a sire's evaluation based on the amount of information used in his evaluation. Reliability values range from 50 to 99 percent on proven sires, and the higher numbers indicate increased accuracy. Bulls that rank highly but have reliability values below 80 percent should be used sparingly, in case their evaluations drop when more information is added. See Table 22.1, which indicates the one standard deviation confidence interval for a certain reliability. For a bull with 75% reliability, we would expect 68 out of 100 daughters to be +/- 280 for PTA milk.

There is a difference of opinion over what information to consider in addition to production and reliability. Registered breeders generally prefer to place some emphasis on overall conformation or type. This is summarized in Figure 22.2 as PTA Type (PTAT). PTAT is combined with the production traits in the TPI for Holsteins and PTI for the other breeds, as explained in Exercise 3. Use of these indexes is quite popular among registered breeders.

Use of PTAT and these indexes may not be the optimal selection method for commercial dairy producers. These individuals may better be served by including evaluations of individual linear type traits in addition to production in their selection decisions. Udder traits and feet and leg traits should be emphasized. While these are not provided in the NAAB Sire Summary listing, they are routinely available from AI organizations and breed associations.

Calving ease is a trait that should be considered when breeding virgin heifers. Calving difficulty is not a major problem with mature cows and can be ignored when breeding older animals. To minimize the complications from difficult births, only bulls that have evaluations

**Table 22.1. Magnitude of Possible Changes in Genetic Evaluations of Holsteins at Various Levels of Reliability**

| (Standard Errors of Prediction) | | | | |
|---|---|---|---|---|
| Reliability | PTA Milk | PTA Fat | PTA Protein | PTA Type |
| 75 | 280 | 11 | 10 | 0.35 |
| 80 | 250 | 10 | 8 | 0.31 |
| 85 | 217 | 9 | 7 | 0.27 |
| 90 | 177 | 7 | 6 | 0.22 |
| 95 | 125 | 5 | 4 | 0.16 |
| 99 | 56 | 2 | 2 | 0.07 |

of 9 percent Difficult Birth in Heifers (DBH) or lower should be used on virgin heifers.

Dairy cattle breeders should keep in mind that due to the use of superior sires, the genetic potential for milk production is increasing with each generation. Therefore, selection standards need to be adjusted continually to allow for new, more highly evaluated bulls. By doing this, dairy producers will be taking advantage of gains in production each succeeding year.

Several warnings need to be mentioned so that common selection mistakes are avoided. Including too many traits in the selection decision will lead to only limited progress in any one trait. Dairy producers will best be served by choosing two to four of the most economically important traits and ignoring the information on the other traits. Changing selection criteria each generation will also limit genetic improvement. Significant genetic gains can be made only through consistent selection over several generations. Change your selection criteria only if it is clear that what you were previously using is no longer appropriate.

## Selecting Beef Sires for Herd Use

Beef producers should select sires based on the economical production of beef of high quality and minimum waste. Beef breed associations have developed measures and terminology for ranking beef sires on their own performance and the performance of their progeny. The measures are called Expected Progeny Differences (EPD's). EPD's usually considered in selection are:

1. *Birth weight*—Useful on progeny in terms of avoiding calving problems with first-calf heifers. Low to average birth weights are preferred.

2. *Weaning weight*—Usually 205 days adjusted. High weaning weights are preferred.

3. *Yearling weight*—Useful in evaluating growth and ability to gain. It is of value in selecting both heifers and bulls. The 365-day yearling weight is more applicable to bull selection. Heifers may be selected on a 550-day adjusted weight at the end of the first grazing season. High yearling weights are preferred.

4. *Maternal traits*—Most breed associations summarize milk production and maternal calving ease, but these values may not be available for all breeds. Evaluations of maternal traits are important for maintaining adequate reproductive performance in a cow herd, because such performance is closely linked with profitability. Intermediate values for milk production and high values for maternal calving ease are preferred.

5. *Carcass traits*—Genetic evaluations for these traits are available only on a limited basis at this point. It is likely that in the future, availability of this information will improve. These traits are important, for they are a direct measure of the end-product. Traits evaluated may include carcass weight, marbling, and ribeye area.

Each beef breed association runs a separate genetic evaluation for its breed. The average evaluations on sires from various breeds are included in Table 22.2. Since cross-breeding is a common practice among beef producers, it is likely that genetic evaluations from several different breeds will be used. It is important to keep these averages in mind to help determine which bulls are superior for a specific trait. For example, an evaluation of 20 for weaning weight may be above average for one breed but below average for another. Evaluation on bulls of differ-

**Table 22.2.** Average EPD's of Current Sires in Various Beef Breeds from Spring 2002 Genetic Evaluations

| Breed | Birth Weight EPD | Weaning Weight EPD | Yearling Weight EPD | Milk EPD |
|---|---|---|---|---|
| Angus | 1.80 | 14.7 | 26.3 | 6.6 |
| Gelbvieh | 1.9 | 35.0 | 62.0 | 18.0 |
| Hereford | 4.0 | 35.0 | 60.0 | 13.0 |
| Limousin | 1.5 | 11.9 | 22.5 | 3.9 |
| Simmental | 3.4 | 35.9 | 58.9 | 7.8 |

ent breeds cannot be directly compared. This is also true for the dairy breeds. The averages listed in Table 22.2 will change as new sires are added to the evaluations.

The AI organizations are emphasizing performance- and progeny- tested beef sires. Most have extensive testing and proving programs to provide genetically superior sires to beef producers. The use of such sires, selected on the basis of their ability to transmit the genetic potential for more rapid growth and superior carcass traits while maintaining reproductive performance, is destined to play an important role in beef production for the future.

## The Young Sire Sampling Program

Most of the dairy bulls entering AI centers today have been developed through what is commonly known as "the young sire sampling program." Essential features of this program are:

1. Young sires, backed by high-production ancestors with good conformation (type), are selected and used for inseminating 300 to 600 cows or more so as to obtain 50 to 100 production-tested (Dairy Herd Improvement Test [DHI]) daughters in many herds. Many of these young bulls are "bred to order" by agreements between an AI organization and a dairy cattle breeder to inseminate the best cows to the highest production AI-proven bulls available.

2. A young bull is usually moved to the AI center when he is a few months old and grown to semen-producing age. After the specified number of cows are inseminated, he is held in waiting until his daughters come into production. Some semen may be collected and stored during this time. For the breeds with limited demand, an option that may be considered is to collect and store 15,000 to 30,000 units of semen from a young bull while awaiting his first progeny proof. The bull could then be slaughtered. It may be cheaper in some cases to pay the cost of semen storage than to feed and house a bull awaiting proof.

3. The USDA includes all sires with at least 10 milking daughters in its quarterly genetic evaluations. However, AI organizations usually wait for records to be reported on at least 30 daughters

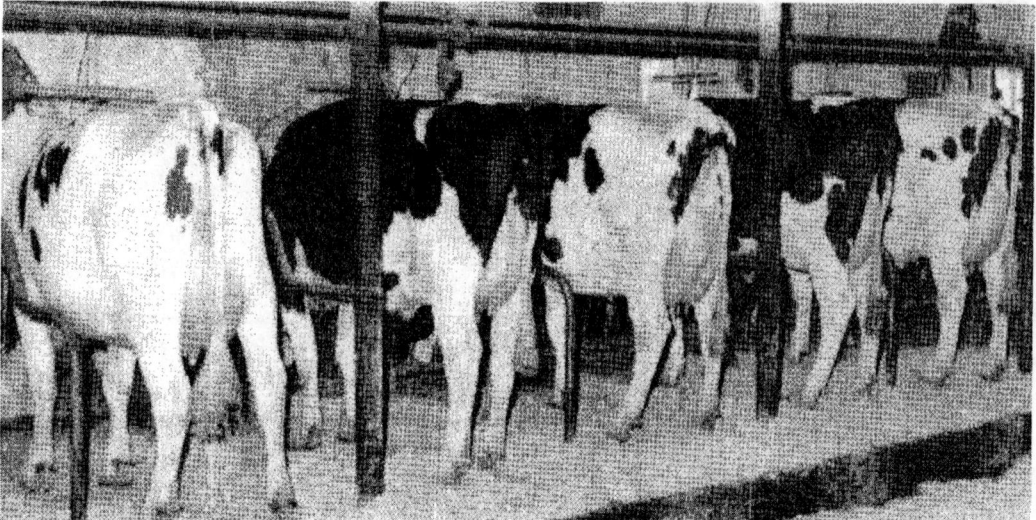

**Figure 22.3.** A group of daughters by a bull selected for AI use. Note the uniformity of tightly-attached, well-shaped udders. (Courtesy, Genex Cooperative, Shawano, WI)

before determining whether a sire should be placed in regular AI service or slaughtered, Figure 22.3.

4. Approximately 10 young bulls are sampled for every 1 expected to be put into use. Some bull studs exceed this ratio. The progeny test is the only way a bull's transmitting ability can be determined with reasonable accuracy. Providing young sires requires a large investment and about six years before it begins to pay off.

5. A sampled young sire is sufficiently proven to begin heavy use, if so merited, at 5½ to 6 years of age. Thus, his useful life will be two to three years longer than the naturally proven sire, which is usually at least eight years old before production proof is available.

6. Many young sires result from selected matings. Outstanding cows in production and conformation, sired by an AI-proven bull with a high PTA, owned by a reputable breeder(s), are mated to top-ranked AI-proven bulls to produce sires for the future. Breeders cooperate in this program, as their best cows may be inseminated to an outstanding AI-proven sire, and they have a built-in market for the resulting bull calves.

7. Syndicates, composed of several to many breeders, often buy outstanding young bulls and sample them. In most cases, a young bull is placed in an AI center, by suitable business arrangements, for sampling and assembling proof. The AI organization may carry an option to purchase the bull if his progeny proof is high. The purchase price is generally based on the volume of semen sold.

In some cases, a group of breeders will syndicate a bull and use him, by means of artificial insemination, in their herds. The bull, in these instances, may be housed on a breeder's farm, and custom-collected semen used. Having daughters of the bull in several herds will result in a repeatability factor more dependable than having the daughters all in one herd.

# QUESTIONS

1. What are the main objectives to consider in selecting dairy bulls for AI purposes?

2. What are the most important factors to consider in selecting young bulls for sampling?

3. What are the chief advantages of the young sire sampling program? What are the advantages from the standpoint of cooperation between the breeder and the AI organization?

4. What are the most important measures of a sire's genetic potential to use in selecting a bull available through artificial insemination for your herd?

5. What is the value of PTA in choosing a sire for your herd? Just what does PTA tell you?

6. What information does reliability provide? Why is it important?

7. How much attention would you pay to the conformation (type), size, disposition, ease of milking, and other physical characteristics of the daughters of an AI bull for use in your herd? Which type traits would you emphasize most? Why?

8. What are the advantages of an AI-proven sire with 100 daughters located in many herds compared to a naturally proven bull with 10 daughters in one herd?

9. What items would you stress most in selecting a beef bull for AI use?

10. Can a young sire sampling program aid in providing better gain-transmitting beef bulls? If so, how?

11. How important is the fertility level of bulls used in artificial insemination? What final measures are used to determine fertility in beef and dairy bulls used in artificial insemination?

12. What precautions would you follow to insure the purchase of only healthy, disease-free bulls? To determine freedom from genetic defects?

# REFERENCES

Campbell, J. R. and R. T. Marshall. 1975. Science of Providing Milk for Man. McGraw-Hill, New York.

Guidelines for Uniform Beef Improvement Programs. Extension Service, USDA, Washington, DC.

Lasley, J. F. 1986. Genetics of Livestock Improvement (4th Ed.). Prentice-Hall, Englewood Cliffs, NJ.

Proceedings—Annual Conferences on Artificial Insemination of Beef Cattle, 1967 to 1986. National Association of Animal Breeders, Inc., P.O. Box 1033, Columbia, MO 65205.

# WEB SITES

Dairy Genetic Evaluations
    *http://aipl.arsusda.gov/*
    *http://www.holsteinusa.com/*
    *http://www.naab-css.org/*
    *See Appendix D*
Beef Genetic Evaluations
    *http://www.beefimprovement.org*
    *See Beef Breed Registry Association's web sites in Exercise 17*
    *See Appendix D*

# EXERCISE 23

# Bull Management and Care

## OBJECT

To become familiar with some of the basic practices involved in the proper management of bulls used for artificial insemination.

## DISCUSSION

Artificial insemination is an important aid to dairy and beef producers because it makes superior genetics more readily available. The animals selected for entrance into controlled AI programs represent an elite segment of the total cattle population. A great deal of effort and expense is involved in their selection and sampling, in order to increase the productivity of the cattle and the income of herd operators using these AI bulls. For the AI business to be successful and render the greatest possible service to its customers, all bulls used must be in good physical condition, free of disease, and maintained in good health for their productive lives. These valuable animals that are selected to parent the succeeding generations are fed carefully formulated rations, undergo continuing health appraisal, and are tested and monitored routinely to prevent the introduction of disease. They also receive husbandry considerations that provide clean, well-lighted/ventilated housing, monitoring of body condition, and adequate exercise. The management and care given the bulls can have a significant impact on their fertility and breeding life.

## PROCEDURE

This exercise will deal with on-farm bull management, feeding and nutrition, bull housing, exercise, frequency of semen collection, and health and general management. These considerations will be studied as they apply to the AI business and as they influence the well-being and productivity of AI center bulls.

### Care and Management

Proper care and management of the bull destined for AI service should actually begin on the farm of origin long before the animal's entry into an AI center. All efforts should be made to reduce exposure of the calf to disease-producing organisms. Even though a bull calf may have the potential to become a genetic leader in his breed, normally he will not qualify to enter an AI program unless he has a clean bill of health and does not have antibody titres for certain diseases.

An important disease agent of concern during the gestation period is Bovine Viral Diarrhea Virus (BVDV). A fetus infected transplacentally from its dam during the first trimester of pregnancy does not elicit an immune response and becomes persistently infected. If the calf survives, it will shed BVDV throughout its life into all body secretions, including semen. It is important to test bulls for BVDV before they enter an AI center and to eliminate those that are viremic for this pathogen.

When the calf is born, the calving area should be clean, have been previously disinfected, and be well bedded. It is also highly recommended that the newborn calf's umbilicus be disinfected with an iodine solution immediately. These practices will reduce the chances of infection through the calf's navel.

Additionally, it is important that the calf receive colostrum within the first several hours of life. Colostrum contains protective antibodies (which confer passive immunity) against infectious disease agents. However, the calf is able to absorb colostral antibodies only during about the first 12 hours of life. It should be noted here that bovine leukosis virus (BLV) in colostrum from BLV-infected cows can infect calves that are fed such colostrum. Therefore, it is prudent to feed calves colostrum only from BLV-negative cows. A supply of colostrum from negative cows can be frozen and maintained for use in those cases where the calf's dam is BLV-positive. Guidelines for the prevention of BLV infection are presented in Table 23.1.

Another calfhood management concern is the prevention of infection with paratuberculosis (Johne's disease). Cattle are most susceptible during the first few months of life, and

infection occurs by ingesting fecal material or feedstuffs that are contaminated with *Mycobacterium avium* subsp. *paratuberculosis.* Older cattle are less susceptible to this infection. Keeping the maternity pen clean, preventing contact with a contaminated environment or dam, and feeding the calf carefully collected colostrum are important preventive measures (Table 23.2).

After receiving adequate colostrum, the bull calf should be moved from the maternity area to an individual calf hutch or pen that is clean, well ventilated, and separate from the cow herd. Rearing a calf in an individual pen allows for better monitoring of the bull's health status and growth rate and avoids possible contact transmission of diseases from other calves.

Other on-farm management practices can include administering an injection of vitamins A, D, E, and K during the first week of the calf's life, dehorning the bull calf at an early age, taking scrotal circumference measurements to monitor the growth and size of the bull calf's testicles, and administering internal/external parasite control products as necessary. Although vaccination may be appropriate for protection against some diseases, bull

**Table 23.1.** Guidelines for Prevention of Bovine Leukosis Virus (BLV) Infection in Calves[a]

---

1. Feed calves colostrum and milk collected from cows that have tested negative to the leukosis (BLV) test. Thereafter, feed the calves a high-quality milk replacer.
2. House calves in individual pens.
3. For blood collection, TB testing, treatments, and vaccinations, use needles that are sterile and that have not previously been used.
4. Thoroughly wash and disinfect all veterinary instruments and calf identification tools after each use. Acceptable disinfectants are chlorhexidine (Nolvasan Solution, Fort Dodge Laboratories) and sodium hypochlorite (Clorox).
5. Use an electric dehorning iron to dehorn calves when they are young. If older calves are dehorned, wash and disinfect the gouge dehorner or other instrument after each animal. Use an electric dehorning iron to control hemorrhage. Spray the base of the horn with insect repellant.
6. For embryo transfer, use recipient heifers that have tested negative to the leukosis (BLV) test.

---

[a]D. R. Monke and R. J. Milburn. 1988. On-farm management of bulls intended for AI service. Proc. 12th Tech. Conf. on Artificial Insemination and Reproduction. NAAB. p. 68.

**Table 23.2.** Guidelines for Prevention of *Mycobacterium avium* subsp. *paratuberculosis* Infection in Calves[a]

1. Clean and disinfect the maternity pen prior to calving time.
2. Move the calf to a clean facility immediately after birth.
3. Do not permit natural nursing.
4. Thoroughly wash the udder and teats of the cow before collecting colostrum to feed the calf.
5. Raise the calf apart from adult animals in the herd.
6. Wear clean clothing and footwear in the calf-rearing area. Perform calf-related chores before handling adult cows.
7. Use only clean utensils for feeding the calf.
8. Feed a quality milk replacer.
9. Be sure that feed is not contaminated with animal waste.
10. Protect calf-rearing areas from adult cow quarters.

[a]D. R. Monke and R. J. Milburn. 1988. On-farm management of bulls intended for AI service. Proc. 12th Tech. Conf. on Artificial Insemination and Reproduction. NAAB. p. 68.

calves that are destined for AI programs should *not* be vaccinated against brucellosis, leptospirosis, paratuberculosis, or infectious bovine rhinotracheitis (Bovine Herpes Virus-1). Vaccination antibody titres can interfere with the interpretation of several diagnostic tests, and this may prohibit a bull from qualifying for entrance into an AI center.

Before a bull calf can enter an AI center, a physical examination must be conducted by an accredited veterinarian, and specific health tests need to be completed on the farm of origin. It is also important that the bull calf be accurately identified and possess an appropriate registry certificate, if applicable.

## Feeding and Nutrition

Many aspects of a bull, such as growth, disease resistance, onset of puberty, libido, testis size, longevity, and ability to produce quality semen can be affected by nutrition. Nutrition management of the bull is an ongoing process from the time he is a calf throughout his productive life at the AI center. The bull's nutrient requirements are generally based on age, body weight, body condition, reproductive development, and environmental conditions. AI centers typically have the available feed components analyzed for nutrient content, and they often consult with nutritional experts in formulating bull rations. In addition, the bulls are monitored continually for body condition and body weight to insure that nutritional levels are optimal for periods of growth, maintenance, or regular semen production.

Often overlooked is the importance of the feeding and care that a bull calf receives on the farm. Proper attention must be given so that the calf grows adequately and is not susceptible to disease. Following the feeding of colostrum, the newborn calf should receive whole milk or high quality milk replacer. It is recommended that milk or milk replacer be fed twice a day. The protein level should be at least 20 percent, with fat at least 10 percent. In addition, milk replacer should contain vitamins A, D, and E, B complex vitamins, vitamin $B_{12}$, and appropriate minerals. Extra energy will be required during the cold seasons by calves raised in unheated areas.

A calf starter ration containing at least 16 percent protein can be offered to the calf as early as three days of age. High-quality, fine-stem hay can be fed beginning at one or two weeks of age. Any time feed is offered, fresh water should also be readily available.

A 6- to 18-month-old bull calf must be fed liberally in order to reach the maximum size for his age and breed and to produce sperm as early as possible. Young bulls that are underfed during the major growth period (birth to two years of age) attain puberty and sperm production later than those that are furnished proper nutrition.

The young bull should receive all of the good-quality roughage, such as legumes or mixed hay, that he will readily clean up and sufficient concentrate (grain feed) to supply the energy, protein, minerals, and vitamins to keep him growing rapidly but not fatten. Pasture and silage may be used in the feeding program for young bulls, but adequate grain feed should be given to keep the animals growing steadily.

A satisfactory grain ration for the young bull should be balanced with respect to its protein and energy content, and should be palatable and economical.

The roughage fed to bulls should preferably be mixed legume and non-legume hay. Silage, such as grass silage, or haylage in limited amounts is desirable. Feeding bulls an overabundance of alfalfa hay can result in a mineral imbalance because of the high calcium content of alfalfa. Excess calcium in the diet may result in osteopetrosis, vertebral ankylosis, and osteoarthritis, causing lameness, an unwillingness to mount, and poor muscular coordination. Usually a calcium to phosphorus ratio of 1.5:1 is recommended where indicated for most bull concentrate rations. In areas where the soil is deficient in trace minerals, these elements may be supplied by the use of trace-mineralized salt.

Water and salt should be available to the bulls at all times. Where pasture is not available, the young bulls should have access to exercise pens and sunshine as much as possible.

After a bull is 20 to 30 months of age, feeding should be less liberal. At this time, the bull is not growing as rapidly and must be kept in good breeding condition to assure normal fertility and normal quantity of semen. The bull should never be allowed to become over-conditioned or fat! Corn, silage, and feeds high in fat content should not be used in the bull ration in large amounts. Such grains as oats, barley, bran, and wheat are recommended. A mixture of early-cut grass hay (for vitamin D) and a mildly cured, early-cut legume hay (for vitamin A) is a very good roughage ration. Bulls should be fed so that they remain in good working condition. Too much roughage will cause the bulls to become paunchy. About 1 to 2 pounds of hay per 100 pounds of body weight is generally satisfactory. Special feeds such as wheat germ oil, etc., have proved of little value in improving the fertility of dairy bulls.

With proper nutritional management, bulls of a large dairy breed should obtain a mature weight of 2,200 pounds by 48 months of age (Table 23.3).

### Table 23.3. Bull Nutrition: Goals[a]

| Age (months) | Large Breed | |
| | Body Weight (lb.) | ADG[b] (lb.) |
| --- | --- | --- |
| Birth | 96 | — |
| 3 | 275 | 1.92 |
| 6 | 450 | 1.92 |
| 12 | 850 | 2.19 |
| 24 | 1550 | 1.92 |
| 36 | 2000 | 1.23 |
| 48 | 2200 | 0.55 |

[a]N. A. Jorgenson. 1988. Bull nutrition. Proc. 12th Tech. conf. on Artificial Insemination and Reproduction. NAAB. p. 88.

[b]ADG = Average daily gain.

## Housing

A variety of indoor and outdoor housing systems are used to provide for the needs of AI bulls. The type of housing system used will generally vary with geographic location, age, and semen collection status of bulls. The housing system should be considered acceptable if the basic needs of animals are met, including shelter from inclement weather, physical comfort, disease control, provision for adequate nutrition, and safety. AI center facilities are typically constructed with durability, safety, efficiency, economy, and convenience as important considerations. The internal surfaces of the housing and pens should allow for effective cleaning and disinfection, and there should be provisions made for the segregation of sick or injured animals. It is also important that the essential mechanical equipment of the housing facility be maintained in good working order.

The basic housing components of an AI center generally consist of (1) a separate isolation barn in which to house incoming bulls and collect semen while the animals undergo various health tests and examinations prior to being admitted to the resident-herd population, (2) sire-in-waiting barn(s) for housing bulls during the progeny-testing period, and (3) the semen production center for housing the resident-herd population of bulls that are on a regular semen collection schedule. Additional bull housing facilities may also be established to meet organizational objectives or qualify for particular export markets. Figure 23.1 illustrates an example of a production center layout.

## Exercise

Bulls should have sufficient exercise to maintain good muscle tone. Exercise can be obtained by access to an exercise lot or by use of mechanical exercisers. However, there seems to be little correlation between the amount of exercise and the quantity and quality of semen produced by a bull. Exercise is a factor affecting the bull's appetite and muscle tone, and it can help promote proper hoof wear. The amount of exercise given bulls will vary among AI organizations.

## Frequency of Semen Collection

The frequency of semen collection for AI center bulls is largely based on the individual bull's market demand and physical condition. Generally, beginning at 10 to 12 months of age, dairy bulls are collected to obtain the required number of units (i.e., 800 to 1,500 straws) for distribution to progeny test herds. During this period it may be necessary to collect several ejaculates at weekly intervals before a bull has produced the required quality and quantity of semen for release to progeny test herds. In addition, all health testing requirements for the "isolation" period must be completed. Depending upon their age, size, and individuality, young bulls can be collected once or twice a week. However, after the initial semen collections for progeny testing, young dairy bulls are not routinely collected. When a bull has attained a reliable genetic evaluation based on his daughters' production information (normally after 3.5 years), he then will be placed on a regular semen collection schedule to meet the commercial demand. A regular semen collection schedule for mature bulls generally consists of a total of four to six ejaculates collected per week (on two to three collection days).

There are no set recommendations for frequency of collection, because different bulls vary widely in their capacity. However, AI laboratories carefully monitor weekly sperm output levels of bulls in regular semen production as well as establish collection goals for individual

# PRODUCTION CENTER
## Floor Plan

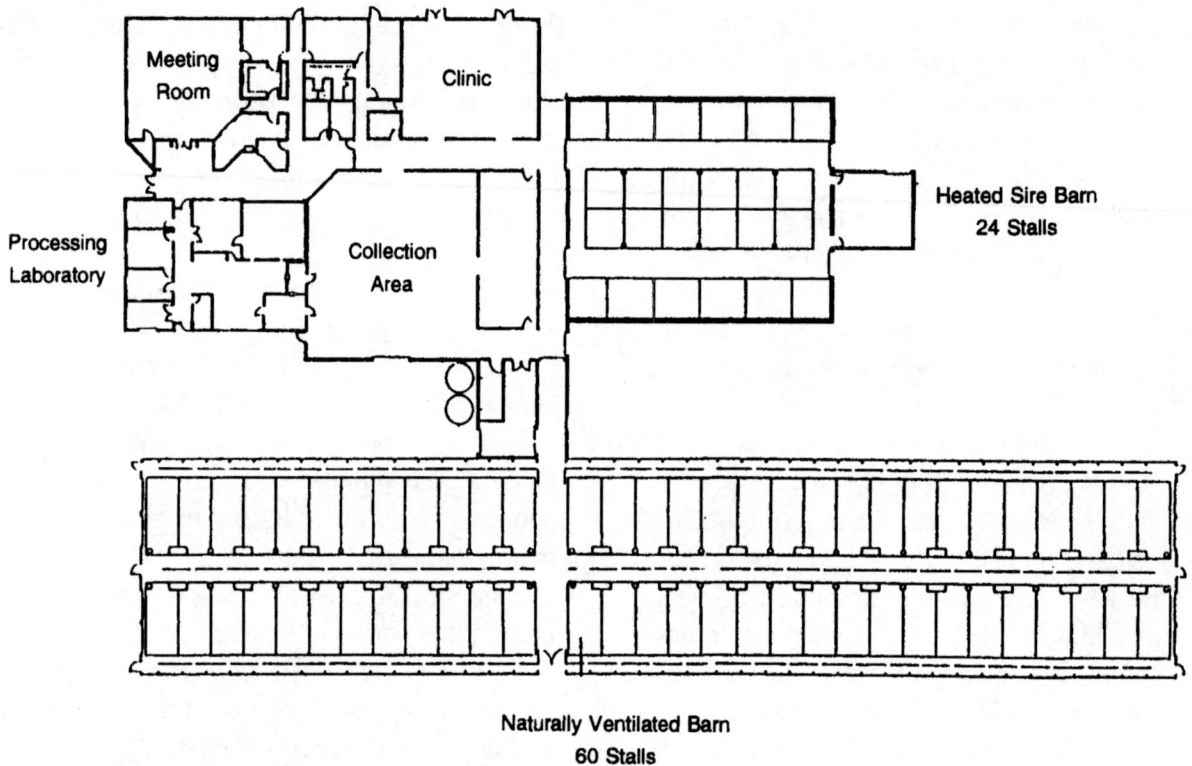

**Figure 23.1.** Floor plan for an efficient modern semen production facility designed to house both young bulls and proven sires. (Courtesy, Genex Cooperative, Ithaca, NY)

bulls. Experience indicates that most bulls in AI use could be safely collected more frequently if the demand for semen so dictated. The semen quality as determined by laboratory evaluations (see Exercises 7 through 15), the behavioral characteristics of the animal, and the judgment of the semen collection personnel should be the primary factors in deciding the frequency of collection for a particular bull.

## Health Management

AI centers have established comprehensive health monitoring programs that are de-signed to insure that the population of bulls is maintained in a disease-free state and that infectious organisms of concern are not transmitted in the semen. The "CSS Minimum Requirements for Disease Control of Semen Produced for AI" provides a minimum industry standard for AI center health management. These requirements include testing and examination of bulls prior to their entry into isolation, during an isolation period, and semiannually throughout their residency at the AI center (see Exercise 24). Additional health testing protocols are frequently followed as well to qualify for various export markets.

## General Management of Bulls

The selection, sampling, and proving of bulls requires a significant investment in labor, feed, and facilities by the AI business. Once a bull is proven to be genetically superior, every effort should be made to keep him productive. The elimination of bulls from AI service can be due to many factors. Some of these are poor production of offspring, disease processes, degenerative physical conditions, and hoof and limb disorders. The culling rate for genetic reasons increases over time as younger proven bulls of higher genetic merit replace the older proven bulls.

The following are pertinent general recommendations in bull care and handling:

1. Handle all bulls carefully, and use two people when leading bulls. Human safety and animal safety are prominent concerns.

2. Keep a strong ring in each bull's nose.

3. Tie bulls by their collars or halters, not their nose rings.

4. Keep all pens or stalls clean, sanitary, and well bedded.

5. Keep bulls clipped. Groom them daily if possible.

6. Keep bulls' feet properly trimmed as necessary. Hoof care is important.

7. Maintain a healthy environment. Test all bulls routinely for disease.

8. Treat bulls humanely. Avoid all situations that might cause the animals stress, fright, or discomfort.

For additional information on AI center management practices, refer to Appendix H.

## QUESTIONS

1. List several of the on-farm bull management considerations that are important in order to qualify for entrance into an AI program.

2. How should young bulls be fed and handled? Why is it important to grow a young bull fairly rapidly?

3. Why should bulls in service be fed so as to be in thrifty condition but not overconditioned?

4. What is the correlation between age and fertility of a bull? Between frequency of service and fertility? Do bulls vary greatly in this respect? Explain.

5. How often should semen be collected from mature bulls in AI use?

6. Why is exercise of importance for bulls? Does exercise influence the fertility of bulls? Explain.

7. Explain why hoof care is important for AI bulls.

8. Speculate on why bulls in AI use should be kept clipped and groomed regularly.

9. What safety precautions should be followed in handling bulls?

10. What are some of the principal reasons why bulls are eliminated from AI centers?

11. Do you believe that movement of bulls from one AI center to another could affect libido and fertility? Explain. Under what circumstances do you think that a bull might be moved at an AI center?

12. What are the essential requirements for housing a large number of bulls at an AI center? Describe the various bull housing environments that are frequently used.

## REFERENCE

Monke, D. R., and R. J. Milburn. 1988. On-farm management of bulls intended for AI service. Proc. 12th Tech. Conf. on Artificial Insemination and Reproduction. NAAB. p. 68.

Monke, D.R. 2002. Bull management: artificial insemination centers. In Encyclopedia of Dairy Sciences., H. Roginski, J. W. Fuquay, P. F. Fox. (Eds.). Academic Press. pp. 198–204.

# EXERCISE 24

# Health Requirements for Sires in AI Use

## OBJECT

To become familiar with the importance of using only healthy and disease-free sires for production of semen used for artificial insemination; the importance of proper hygiene in the collection and processing of semen; and the role of AI in controlling the transmission of venereal diseases in livestock.

## DISCUSSION

Artificial insemination plays a multipurpose role in livestock production. It not only affords an effective means of genetic improvement for the production of milk and meat, but it also greatly reduces the possibility of disease transmission, eliminates the need for maintaining a dangerous bull(s) on the farm or ranch, and can improve reproductive efficiency. By using AI, a herd owner can avoid introducing sires from other herds, thus eliminating a possible source of infection.

Artificial insemination is effective in controlling the spread of disease only if all semen comes from fertile, disease-free sires. It is well known that certain diseases can be transmitted through semen from an infected bull. Of greatest importance are those diseases that may be primarily or opportunistically transmitted through semen. Unless effective health standards for bulls producing semen for AI are followed, the use of AI could itself be a factor in widely disseminating disease. This is because the freezing of semen does not necessarily

destroy pathogenic microorganisms. Consequently, disease surveillance of donor sires is of utmost importance to guard against the spread of disease. The collecting, processing, and freezing of semen from bulls located in private herds and in contact with cows that are often of unknown health status is a considerable risk from a disease standpoint. If such semen is shipped to other herds or through trade channels, the potential for spreading disease can be magnified.

Artificial insemination has succeeded in establishing an enviable record in supplying fertile semen of high genetic potential for herd improvement without apparent spread of disease. Such results come about only through diligent attention to technical details and a comprehensive and effective sire health program. There should be no relaxation of effort in this connection, and our past success should not lull us into a state of carelessness.

The tabulation in Figure 24.1 summarizes the potential for the possible spread of disease through semen from infected bulls.

As early as 1954, the AI organizations in the United States, in cooperation with a committee of the American Veterinary Medical Association, drafted and put into effect, on a voluntary basis, a Sire Health Code. The recommendations in this code were updated from time to time and in 1979 were incorporated into the Certified Semen Service's sire health program. They serve as a guide for the AI industry, cattle breeders, and animal health regulatory officials.

| Pathogen or Disease | Usual Means of Transmission | Aberrant Transmissibility at Coitus? | Aberrant Transmissibility by AI? | Survives Semen Processing with Antibiotic & Freezing? | Available Methods to Prevent Spread of Pathogens Through AI | Are Sufficient Facts Established to Justify Commitment to Specific Programs? |
|---|---|---|---|---|---|---|
| **(A)** Mycobacterium tuberculosis subsp. bovis | Ingestion Inhalation | Remote possibility | Highly improbable | Yes | Disease-free bulls Repeated testing with tuberculin | Yes |
| Mycobacterium avium subsp. paratuberculosis | Ingestion | Genital lesions typical in bulls | Low under current AI center management | Yes | Disease-free semen Repeated fecal culture of bulls | Yes, in herd |
| Brucella abortus | Ingestion | Rare, if ever | Yes, if genital lesion | Yes | Disease-free bulls Repeated testing, serum agglutination test, CF, PCFIA, semen plasma agglutination test | Yes |
| Leptospira sp. | Ingestion Contamination of abraded surfaces | Yes | Yes | Yes/No | Disease-free bulls Repeated testing with interpretation Culture | Yes |
| Campylobacter fetus subsp. venerealis | Coitus | Typical transmission at coitus | Yes | Yes/No | Prophylactic treatment of semen during processing with antibiotics Disease-free bulls through systematic diagnosis & treatment | Yes |
| Tritrichomoniasis foetus | Coitus | Typical transmission at coitus | Yes | Yes | Disease-free bulls through systematic diagnosis & treatment | Yes |
| **(B)** Corynebacterium pyogenes<br><br>Pseudomonas<br><br>Staph. Strep. | Direct contamination of susceptible tissues | Probable | Probable | Yes/No | Lesion-free bulls leucocyte-free semen Selectively withholding semen | No |
| **(C)** Mycoplasmas (PPLO) | "Contact" Venereal? | Possible | Possible | Yes/No | Control by treatment of semen with antibiotics | No |
| Ureaplasmas | "Contact" Venereal? | Possible | Possible | Yes/No | | No |
| Haemophilus somnus | "Contact" Venereal? | Possible | Possible | Yes/No | | No |
| Chlamydia Psittacosis lymphogranuloma venereum–like agent (PLGV) (epizootic bovine abortion) | Vector? Venereal? | Possible | Possible | Yes/No | ? | No |

**Figure 24.1.** Infectious agents of importance in bulls. (A) Traditional diseases of importance in AI. (B) Pathogens of uncertain importance in AI. (C) Intermediate pathogens of uncertain importance in AI. (D) Viruses of importance. (E) Diseases of importance only to general health. (Modified from D. E. Bartlett. 1972. A responsible health program for AI. Proc. 4th Tech. Conf. on Artificial Insemination and Reproduction. NAAB. p. 49)

| Pathogen or Disease | Usual Means of Transmission | Aberrant Transmissibility at Coitus? | Aberrant Transmissibility by AI? | Survives Semen Processing with Antibiotic & Freezing? | Available Methods to Prevent Spread of Pathogens Through AI | Are Sufficient Facts Established to Justify Commitment to Specific Programs? |
|---|---|---|---|---|---|---|
| (D) IBR-IPV (Herpes group) | "Contact" | Yes | Yes | Yes— demonstrated or assumed for all viruses when in semen at collection | Lesion-free bulls Serological/virus isolation testing | No |
| BVD-MD (Myxovirus group) | "Contact" | Possible | Yes, if persistently infected bull | | Disease-free bulls Virus isolation testing to identify persistent infection | Yes |
| Para-influenza III (Myxovirus group) | "Contact" | Highly improbable | Highly improbable | | Symptom-free bulls | No |
| Fibropapillomas (Papovirus group) | "Contact," especially if skin abrasions | Probable | Possible | | Lesion-free bulls | Yes |
| Catarrhal vagino-cervicitis (ECBO Picornavirus group) | "Contact" | Possible | Probable | | ? | No |
| Foot-&-mouth disease (Picornavirus group) | "Contact" | Yes | Yes | | Foot-&-mouth-free cattle population | Yes |
| Bluetongue (Orbivirus group) | Insect borne | Possible | Possible | | Serological/virus isolation testing | No |
| Bovine leukosis virus (BLV) | "Contact" with infected lymphocytes | Remotely possible | Highly improbable | | Competent semen collection technique to prevent blood contamination Serological testing | No |
| (E) Anaplasmosis | Blood borne by insects & instruments | Highly improbable | Highly improbable | Possible, if ever in semen | — | — |
| Rabies | Bites of skunks or dogs | Highly improbable | Highly improbable | Possible, if ever in semen | — | — |
| Internal worm & external insect parasites | Ingestion; "Contact"; Proximity | | | — | — | — |
| Others | — | — | — | — | — | — |

Certified Semen Services (CSS) is mainly concerned with reducing the risk of disease and also preventing sire and semen misidentification. CSS provides an objective auditing (inspection) program in these areas for participating AI businesses that enter into a contractual agreement for services. As indicated in a previous exercise, all regular members of the NAAB participate in the CSS program as well as some other semen-processing businesses that are concerned with sire health and semen identification procedures.

The following CSS Minimum Requirements outline specific testing procedures for bulls and mount animals before they enter the AI center's isolation facilities, for animals during isolation, and for bulls housed in a central location after completing isolation (resident herd). Figure 24.2 depicts preparation of blood samples for diagnostic testing in a CSS-approved

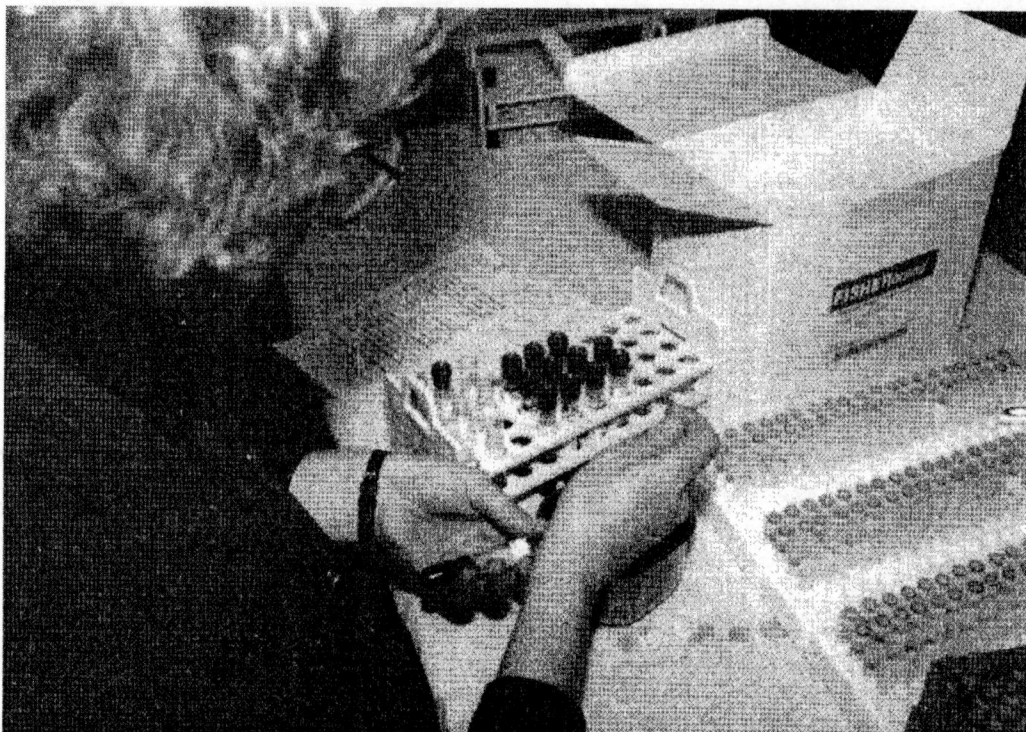

**Figure 24.2.** Blood serum samples from bulls and mount animals housed at a CSS-approved AI center are prepared for shipment to a veterinary diagnostic laboratory for "isolation" testing and routine "resident herd" testing. (Courtesy, the former Atlantic Breeders Cooperative, Lancaster, PA)

AI center. General sanitary conditions and antibiotic procedures and conditions for semen are also included. The main concept underlying the CSS Minimum Requirements is to reduce the likelihood of disease transmission in AI by maintaining healthy bulls in a risk-reduced environment during the period of seminal collection and residency.

## CSS Minimum Requirements for Disease Control of Semen Produced for AI

The "CSS Minimum Requirements for Disease Control of Semen Produced for AI" provides a minimum standard for the health monitoring and disease surveillance of bulls prior to entering isolation, during an isolation period, and throughout residency at an AI center. This is a comprehensive standard for those diseases proven to be a significant threat to be seminally transmitted by artificial insemination. Furthermore, it outlines proper sanitary procedures and includes requirements for the addition of appropriate antibiotics to semen and extender to control specific microorganisms. The goal of these requirements is to protect the health of the seminal donors and the herds in which the semen is used.

## General Sanitary Conditions

1. Semen collection equipment which comes in contact with the bull or his secretions or excretions shall be thoroughly disinfected after each use.

2. New, disposable plastic gloves shall be used by the collector on each bull to assure that the collector's hands cannot serve as a means of transmitting infectious, contagious material from bull to bull.

264

3. The laboratory used for semen processing shall be fully enclosed and partitioned from bull housing and semen collection areas, and structured to provide for hygienic handling and storage of semen.

4. The health tests to be conducted in accordance with the following requirements shall be conducted in a manner generally consistent with the procedures described in "The Recommended Uniform Diagnostic Procedures for Qualifying Bulls for the Production of Semen" as published by the American Association of Veterinary Laboratory Diagnosticians (AAVLD) or other diagnostic procedures recognized as being at least equal to the AAVLD published procedures.

5. Attention shall be given to liquid nitrogen refrigerators returning from foreign countries not declared free of foot-and-mouth disease by USDA, to determine if they have been disinfected at the port of entry. If they have been properly disinfected, there will be a tag attached indicating this fact. If disinfection has not been done, the USDA/APHIS veterinarian in the state involved shall be notified, and appropriate action shall be taken immediately to have the refrigerators properly disinfected.

## Mount Animals

Mount animals (teasers) used during semen collection shall be submitted to the same regimen of periodic health tests as bulls in semen production and be maintained continuously in a health testing status equivalent to the CSS bulls. Mount animals shall not be interchanged between the CSS resident herd and the CSS isolation testing environments. Areas of contact by the erect penis or of genital secretions upon the hair coat or skin of a mount shall be effectively and thoroughly disinfected between successively mounting bulls.

## Pre-entry to Isolation

Bulls and mount animals that are intended to enter a CSS-approved AI center shall be healthy and free of infectious or contagious diseases and shall not originate from a herd under quarantine. Subsequent to the pre-entry testing described below, the bulls and mount animals should not be used for natural service and should be isolated from other cattle. Isolation means no direct contact or fence line contact with other cattle.

The following pre-entry examination and diagnostic tests shall be conducted and results received for each bull and mount animal prior to starting the isolation interval. These tests are preferably conducted prior to arrival at the isolation facilities of the AI center. However, these tests may be conducted in a separate facility at the AI center, as described below, but the animal isolation interval shall not start until results of the pre-entry tests are known.

For purposes of these requirements, pre-entry testing performed at the AI center shall mean that bulls and mount animals must be housed in a pre-isolation facility that is effectively separated from facilities occupied by resident bulls and mount animals, and also separate from bulls and mount animals housed in isolation facilities. Any equipment used to handle bulls and mount animals for semen collection, feeding, watering, and cleaning in isolation or resident herds shall **not** be used at the pre-isolation facility.

1. *Physical examination*—A physical examination shall be conducted by an accredited veterinarian within 30 days prior to entry to determine that the bulls or mount animal do not display

265

any clinical symptoms of any infectious, contagious disease.

2. *Tuberculosis*—An intradermal tuberculin test shall be conducted within 60 days prior to entry; the result should be negative.

3. *Bovine brucellosis*—A buffered brucella antigen test (Card or BAPA) or a complement fixation (CF) test shall be conducted within 30 days prior to entry; the result shall be negative. The brucellosis test should comply with applicable regulations if the animal must be transported interstate.

4. *Bovine leptospirosis*—A blood test for serotypes L. pomona, L. hardjo, L. canicola, L. icterohaemorrhagiae, and L. grippotyphosa shall be conducted within 30 days prior to entry. Any animal with a significant titer may be subjected to a second blood test within two to four weeks after the first. An end or limiting titer (1:100 or greater) may be run on both samples. Cattle with a stabilized low titer (negative at 1:400) on both tests may be considered satisfactory to enter the isolation facility.

5. *Bovine viral diarrhea virus (BVDV)*— A blood test for BVDV shall be conducted within 30 days prior to entry; the result shall be negative. The test for BVDV shall be a viral isolation test of whole blood or serum (see Isolation,1.,f.,ii.) performed in bovine cell culture followed by staining of the cell culture by immunofluorescence (FA) or immunoperoxidase (IP) methods, or an antigen capture ELISA.

## Isolation

Each bull and mount animal shall be held in isolation throughout the period of time necessary to conduct the tests listed below. Each bull and mount animal shall successfully complete the isolation protocol before being permitted to enter the facilities occupied by resident bulls and mount animals and before any semen from the bull is released for use.

For purposes of these requirements, isolation shall mean that the bulls and mount animals are housed in facilities under the control (supervision) of the AI company. These facilities are effectively separated from facilities occupied by resident bulls and mount animals, and any equipment used to handle the bulls and mount animals for semen collection, feeding and watering, and cleaning the facilities occupied by the bull or mount animal shall not be used for both isolation and resident herds. Further, semen collection areas for bulls in isolation shall be effectively separated from areas used for resident bulls.

1. The following tests shall be conducted on all bulls and mount animals while resident in the isolation facility.

   a. *Tuberculosis*—One intradermal tuberculin test; the result shall be negative. This test shall be conducted at least sixty (60) days after the date of a pre-entry test for tuberculosis.

   b. *Bovine brucellosis*—One buffered brucella antigen test (Card or BAPA) and one complement fixation (CF) test with negative results. These serological tests shall be conducted not sooner than thirty (30) days after the date of the pre-entry test for brucellosis.

   If a result other than negative is received for a bull, it is recommended that another official USDA brucellosis test be conducted. A negative result on retest or on additional official brucella tests may permit the bull a negative brucella classifica-

266

tion, but final classification remains the prerogative of the state veterinary officials.

c. **Bovine leptospirosis**—Serological test for serotypes L. pomona, L. hardjo, L. canicola, L. icterohaemorrhagiae, and L. grippotyphosa. This test shall be conducted not sooner than thirty (30) days after the date of the pre-entry tests for leptospirosis. A negative result is preferred. However, if the result is not negative (that is positive at 1:100 or higher), the bovine must have at least one retest conducted at least 14 days following the previous test. Cattle that are negative at 1:400 on at least two consecutive tests are considered to have a stabilized low titer.

d. **Bovine campylobacteriosis**—Preputial material shall be cultured and examined for Campylobacter fetus venerealis; the result shall be negative. As an alternative procedure, the preputial material may be examined using the flourescent antibody (FA) technique as a screening test. Any positive FA test shall be followed by a culture of preputial material, the result shall be negative.

Bulls and mount animals may be placed on the following variable testing schedule:

| Age of sire when entering isolation | Minimum number of tests (at weekly intervals) |
| --- | --- |
| Less than 180 days* | 1 |
| 180–364 days | 3 |
| 365 days and over | 6 |

*Providing AI center veterinarian can certify that bull has not been housed with female cattle since reaching the age of thirty (30) days.

e. **Bovine venereal trichomoniasis**—Microscopic examinations of cultured preputial material collected from the fornix shall be negative. The frequency of testing shall be the same as that listed under Isolation 1.d. Bovine Campylobacteriosis.

f. **Bovine viral diarrhea virus (BVDV)**—All bulls and mount animals entering CSS-approved AI centers must be tested for viremia to persistent BVDV infection with negative results before entry into the AI center's resident herd. Furthermore, all bulls are to be evaluated by a testing program to detect persistent testicular infection.

The following test methods and schedules are to be used to test for persistent BVD viremic infection:

i. **Diagnostic test**—The animal must be subjected to a virus isolation test performed in bovine cell culture with a negative result as demonstrated by staining of the cell culture by immunofluorescence (FA) or immunoperoxidase (IP) methods.

ii. **Diagnostic specimens**—either whole blood or serum. Whole blood must be used for animals less than 6 months of age.

iii. **Confirmation of persistent BVDV infection**—If BVDV is demonstrated by FA or IP in cell culture, the animal is to be isolated from other cattle and retested in not less than 21 days by inoculation of bovine cell cultures with an appropriate specimen (whole blood or serum). Demonstration of BVDV a second time is considered confirmation of persistent infection, and the animal is not eligible to enter the resident herd of the CSS-approved AI center.

iv. ***Confirmation that an animal is not persistently infected***—Animals from which BVDV has been isolated or demonstrated must remain in isolation apart from other cattle until proven free of BVDV by two consecutive negative virus isolation tests conducted at least 10 days apart and performed on the appropriate specimen (whole blood or serum).

Bulls from which BVDV has been isolated but are later proven to be free of persistent infection (as stated above in *iv.*) must have samples of any semen that were collected and processed within the 30 days preceding and following the date of positive virus isolation, subjected to BVDV isolation tests with negative results from each collection code before distribution.

2. The following test shall be conducted for all bulls before their semen is released. If the bulls are not of semen producing age during the CSS isolation period, this test may be conducted after the isolation period is completed:

## Bovine Viral Diarrhea Virus (BVDV)

One of the following test methods and schedules is used to test for persistent testicular BVDV infection.

i. Test all bulls at any time during the isolation interval for BVDV by the serum neutralization (SN) test. All bulls that test positive must have one virus isolation test of processed semen performed in bovine cell culture with a negative result as

demonstrated by staining of the cell culture by immunofluorence (FA) or immunoperoxidase (IP) methods. Processed semen is semen that is completely extended and frozen.

–or–

ii. All bulls must have one virus isolation test of processed semen performed in bovine cell culture with a negative result as demonstrated by staining of the cell culture by immunofluorence (FA) or immunoperoxidase (IP) methods. Processed semen is semen that is completely extended and frozen.

(Any bulls with a positive virus isolation test of semen should have additional processed semen tested to confirm persistent testicular infection.)

**Note: Any bull that has a persistent testicular infection for BVDV is not eligible for semen collection and is not permitted to remain in the resident herd.**

3. All semen shall be treated with the antibiotics gentamicin, tylosin, and Linco-Spectin (GTLS) as described by Shin, et al (1) Lorton, et al (2) and Lorton, et al (3). Details of the procedures to be used are listed in Appendix 1.

## Resident Herd

Once a bull or mount animal has completed the isolation testing outlined above, the animal may enter the resident herd where it shall continue to be tested in accordance with the below listed test procedures.

1. The following tests should be conducted for all bulls and mount animals at six-(6)-month intervals:

268

a. **Tuberculosis**—The official intra-dermal tuberculin test, with negative result.

b. **Bovine brucellosis**—One buffered brucella antigen test (Card or BAPA) and one complement fixation test with negative results. If result of either test is not negative, refer to Isolation 1. b. Bovine Brucellosis for additional information.

c. **Bovine leptospirosis**—Serological test for serotypes L. pomona, L. hardjo, L. canicola, L. icterohaemorrhagiae, and L. grippotyphosa. If result is not negative, the bull must have a stablized low titer. Refer to Isolation 1.c. Bovine Leptospirosis.

d. **Bovine venereal trichomoniasis**—A single microscopic examination of cultured preputial material with negative result.

e. **Bovine campylobacteriosis**—A single culture test of preputial material with negative result. As an alternative procedure, the preputial material may be examined using the fluorescent antibody (FA) technique. Any positive FA test result shall be followed by culture of preputial material, and the desired result shall be negative.

Antibiotics shall be added to all processed semen as described above (refer to Isolation 3.).

2. All bulls or mount animals in the resident herd shall be maintained in continuous isolation from all cloven-hoofed animals that have not completed all of the test procedures outlined herein with negative results. At any time that an individual bull or mount animal from the resident tested herd is permitted contact with an untested animal, he shall be removed immediately from the resident tested herd and shall not be permitted re-entry until such time as he has completed another cycle of isolation and the tests prescribed therefor, except as provided for in paragraph 3 below.

3. It is not required that a bull temporarily held out of semen production be tested for bovine trichomoniasis and bovine campylobacteriosis provided he is at a location effectively separated from the resident herd. However, he shall be maintained in a herd which otherwise meets all conditions of a resident herd. The routine testing regimen as defined for the resident herd must be resumed prior to the release of semen that was processed after the bull's return to production.

## Antibiotics and Semen Processing

1. Antibiotics will be added to the neat semen and extender to provide effective microbiological control of:

   Mycoplasmas
   Ureaplasmas
   Haemophilus somnus
   Campylobacter fetus subsp.
   venerealis

2. Effective microbiological control is the condition in which the number of organisms potentially present are reduced to below the threshold of infectivity.

3. An acceptable protocol is the treatment of semen and extender with the antibiotics gentamicin, tylosin,

lincomycin and spectinomycin (GTLS) as described by Shin, et al (1) Lorton, et al (2) and Lorton, et al (3). Details of the procedures to be followed are described in, Section I of Appendix 1.

4. Acceptable alternative protocols must provide effective microbiological control (of organisms in 1 above) based on scientific evidence, submitted to Certified Semen Services, Inc. An example of an approved alternative protocol is the 1-step procedure as described by Shin and Kim (4). Details are described in Section II of Appendix 1.

# REFERENCES

(1) Shin, S. J., D. H. Lein, V. H. Patten, and H. L. Ruhnke. 1988. A new antibiotic combination for frozen bovine semen. 1. Control of mycoplasmas, ureaplasmas, *Campylobacter fetus* subsp. *venerealis* and *Haemophilus somnus*. Theriogenology. 29:577.

(2) Lorton, S. P., J. J. Sullivan, B. Bean, M. Kaproth, H. Kellgren, and C. Marshall. 1988. A new antibiotic combination for frozen bovine semen. 2. Evaluation of seminal quality. Theriogenology. 29:593.

(3) Lorton, S. P., J. J. Sullivan, B. Bean, M. Kaproth, H. Kellgren, and C. Marshall. 1988. A new antibiotic combination for frozen bovine semen. 3. Evaluation of fertility. Theriogenology. 29:609.

(4) Shin, S. J. and S. G. Kim. 2000. Comparative efficacy study of bovine semen extension: 1-step vs. 2-step procedure. Proceedings 18th Technical Conf. on Artificial Insemination and Reproduction, NAAB, Columbia, MO. pp. 60–62.

**Appendix 1**

## GTLS ANTIBIOTIC PROCEDURES/CONDITIONS

### I. Standard CSS Protocol (2-Step Method)

#### A. Antibiotics/Stock Solutions

1. Antibiotics:

   a. Gentamicin sulfate: powder, micronized, non-sterile, U.S.P. (veterinary grade), 100 grams per bottle.

   b. Tylosin: labeled as Tylan Soluble, product of Elanco Products Company, 100 grams per bottle.

   c. Linco-Spectin: product of the Upjohn Company, 20 ml per vial, each ml contains 50 mg lincomycin and 100 mg spectinomycin.

**NOTE: Antibiotics obtained from some sources have not been tested and may contain deleterious agents that may harm or kill sperm cells. For recommended sources, contact Certified Semen Services.**

2. Stock solutions of individual antibiotics (gentamicin and tylosin) may be prepared and stored separately at 41°F (5°C) for eight days or stored frozen in LN vapor for up to six months. Linco-Spectin as supplied by distributor should be maintained at 41°F (5°C) after it is opened.

3. Stock solutions of individual antibiotics will be combined on day of use, and not held over.

4. Extenders must be used on the day the combined antibiotics are added.

#### B. Neat Semen Treatment

1. 100 µg of tylosin, 500 µg gentamicin, and 300/600 µg of Linco-Spectin dissolved in .02 ml of double-distilled sterile water will be added and carefully mixed with each ml of neat semen.

**NOTE: All of the antibiotic concentrations expressed herein are for active units of antibiotic. Potency values may vary between**

batches of antibiotic. Therefore, amounts of raw material have to be adjusted for each batch in order to obtain the required concentrations of active antibiotic.

2. The addition of these antibiotics should be scheduled so as to allow a three- to five-minute time period for the antibiotics to be in contact with the neat semen before the addition of any extender.

## C. Non-Glycerol Fraction of Extender

1. All non-glycerol fractions of any of the five extenders listed below will be prepared to contain the following concentrations of antibiotics before being added to semen:

| | |
|---|---|
| tylosin | 100 µg per ml |
| gentamicin | 500 µg per ml |
| Linco-Spectin | 300/600 µg per ml |

2. A volume of this extender (up to 50 percent of the planned final extended volume) is added to the neat semen prior to cooling. All semen must be held in contact with the non-glycerol extender for a minimum of two hours prior to the addition of any glycerol containing extender.

## D. Glycerol Containing Fraction of Extender

1. This fraction of the extender may contain 5-10 percent of the antibiotic concentration listed under C. (1) Non-Glycerol Fraction of Extender.

2. The glycerol fraction of the extender should be added to the non-glycerol fraction of extender plus semen at a 1- to 1-ratio.

## E. Final Concentration of Antibiotics

Following the above procedures will yield a final concentration of 50 µg tylosin, 250 µg gentamicin, and 150/300 µg of Linco-Spectin in each ml of frozen semen.

## F. Required Processing Procedures

It has been shown that processing procedures, extender composition, and antibiotic combinations may affect efficacy of microbial control or fertility. Therefore, deviation from the following may require the organization to conduct additional efficacy testing:

1. Use of extender other than one approved by CSS.

2. Antibiotic/neat semen contact of less than three minutes.

3. Cooling of semen and non-glycerol fraction less than two hours to 5°C.

4. Glycerol is not an extender component until after cooling to 5°C.

## G. Deviation from Required Processing Procedures

If there is deviation from any of the procedures listed under Section F:

1. A written request for an exception will be made to the Service Director of CSS.

2. The CSS Service Director will determine whether the deviation will require testing for efficacy. Appropriate efficacy testing may be done at a laboratory approved by CSS that has demonstrated competency for carrying out these analyses.

3. The test results will be returned from the laboratory to the CSS Service Director and the requesting organization.

4. If the results demonstrate efficacy equal to or greater than that obtained by Shin (1) then permission to use the procedure will be granted.

5. All fees and expenses for these tests will be paid by the organization making the request.

## H. Tested and Approved Extenders

The following five extenders have been tested for efficacy of control of microbial organisms. Use of the antibiotic combination in extenders 1 and 3 did not adversely affect post-thaw motility or fertility (extenders 2, 4, and 5 were not evaluated). Other extenders may be approved by the CSS Service Director by following the procedures outlined in Section G. Antibiotics dissolved in double distilled sterile water should be included in the preparation of extenders to yield the final volumes shown under Section I, E of Appendix 1.

The final composition of each extender is as follows:

1. Egg Yolk Citrate

   20% egg yolk
   2.12 gm % sodium citrate dihydrate
   0.183 gm % citric acid monohydrate
   7.0% glycerol

2. 20% Egg Yolk-Tris

   20% egg yolk
   2.42 gm % tris (hydroxymethyl
       aminomethane)
   1.38 gm % citric acid monohydrate
   1.0 gm % fructose
   7.0% glycerol

3. Heated Whole Milk

   7.0% glycerol

4. Plus-X

   Plus-X, as supplied by distributor.
   7.0% glycerol

5. 28% Egg Yolk-Tris

   28% egg yolk
   1.92 gm % tris (hydroxymethyl
       aminomethane)
   1.10 gm % citric acid monohydrate
   1.00 gm % glucose
   7.0% glycerol

# REFERENCES

(1) Shin, S. J., D. H. Lein, V. H. Patten, and H. L. Ruhnke. 1988. A new antibiotic combination for frozen bovine semen. 1. Control of mycoplasmas, ureaplasmas, *Campylobacter fetus* subsp. *venerealis* and *Haemophilus somnus*. Theriogenology. 29:577.

## II. Alternative CSS Protocol (1-Step Method)

### A. General Description

As described by Shin and Kim (4), this processing protocol is approved only for 20% Egg Yolk Tris extender (see Section I, H, 2 of Appendix 1). It requires the same preparation of antibi-

otics/stock solutions (see Section I, A of Appendix 1); and neat semen treatment (see Section I, B of Appendix 1) as the standard 2-step protocol. However the main differences from the standard CSS 2-step protocol are as follows:

1. The extender is not fractionated into a non-glycerol and glycerol component. The complete extender contains 7.0% glycerol.

2. The concentration of GTLS antibiotics in each ml of extender is the same as that prescribed for neat semen treatment (i.e., 100 μg tylosin, 500 μg gentamicin, 300/600 μg Linco-Spectin). Thus the final concentration of antibiotics is essentially doubled compared to the standard 2-step protocol.

### B. Neat Semen Treatment

Identical to that for the standard 2-step protocol. See Section I, B, 1 and 2 of Appendix 1.

### C. Final Concentration of Antibiotics

The 1-step protocol will yield a final concentration of 100 μg tylosin, 500 μg gentamicin, and 300/600 μg of Linco-Spectin in each ml of frozen semen.

### D. Required Processing Procedures

It has been shown that processing procedures, extender composition, and antibiotic combinations may affect efficacy of microbial control or fertility. Therefore, deviation from the following may require the organization to conduct additional efficacy testing:

1. Use of extender other than one approved by CSS and described by Shin and Kim (4).

2. Antibiotic/neat semen contact of less than three minutes.

### E. Deviation from Required Processing Procedures

If there is deviation from any of the procedures listed under Section D above:

1. A written request from an exception will be made to the Service Director of CSS.

2. The CSS Service Director will determine whether the deviation will require testing

for efficacy. Appropriate efficacy testing may be done at a laboratory approved by CSS that has demonstrated competency for carrying out these analyses.

3. The test results will be returned from the laboratory to the CSS Service Director and the requesting organization.

4. If the results demonstrate efficacy equal to or greater than obtained by Shin (1) or Shin and Kim (4) then permission to use the procedure will be granted.

5. All fees and expenses for these tests will be paid by the organization making the request.

# REFERENCES

(1) Shin, S. J., D. H. Lein, V. H. Patten, and H. L. Ruhnke. 1988. A new antibiotic combination for frozen bovine semen. 1. Control of my- coplasmas. ureplasmas. *Campylobacter fetus* subsp. *venerealis* and *Haemophilus somnus.* Theriogenology. 29:577.

(4) Shin, S. J. and S. G. Kim. 2000. Comparative efficacy study of bovine semen extension: 1-step vs 2-step procedure. Proceedings 18th Technical Conf. on Artificial Insemination and Reproduction, NAAB, Columbia, MO. pp. 60–62.

## Apppendix 2
## Basic AI Center Testing Protocol

The basic health testing program is outlined in the "CSS Minimum Requirements for Disease Control of Semen Produced for AI." These requirements have been developed over the years by the AI industry to help ensure semen used in AI is not a vehicle for transmitting those disease agents of concern.

Following is a summary of the CSS testing program:

**TESTING ENVIRONMENTS**

| | Pre-entry to Isolation (Within 30 days prior to entering isolation facilities) | Isolation (Testing before entry into a resident herd and semen release) | Resident herd (Semen collection center) |
|---|---|---|---|
| *Physical Examination* | Conducted by accredited veterinarian. | | |
| *Tuberculosis* | Negative intradermal tuberculin test. (Within 60 days prior to entry) | Negative intradermal tuberculin test at least 60 days after pre-entry test. | Negative intradermal tuberculin test at 6-month intervals. |
| *Brucellosis* | Official test of state where bull is located. Blood serum test (CF, BAPA or Card). | Complement fixation (CF) and one BAPA or Card test at least 30 days after pre-entry testing. | Complement fixation (CF) and one BAPA or Card test at 6-month intervals. |
| *Bovine Viral Diarrhea Virus* | One negative virus isolation test performed on either whole blood (animals less than 6 months of age) or serum, **or** an antigen capture ELISA | One negative virus isolation test performed on either whole blood (animals less than 6 months of age) or serum. Negative virus isolation test of processed semen before release for use, or negative virus isolation test of processed semen for any donors testing BVDV positive by SN test. | |

*(continued)*

273

| | | |
|---|---|---|
| *Leptospirosis* | Blood test for 5 serotypes important in USA.* | Blood test for 5 serotypes important in USA*. No sooner than 30 days after pre-entry test. | Blood test for 5 serotypes important in USA* at 6-month intervals. |
| *Campylobacteriosis* | | Series of negative culture tests of preputial material or screening by fluorescent antibody (FA) with any positive FA tested by culture for final determination. | Negative single culture test of preputial material or FA for screening test at 6-month intervals. |
| | | Bulls under 180 days of age —negative on 1 test▼. | |
| | | Bulls 180–364 days of age —negative on 3 weekly tests. | |
| | | Bulls 365 days or older tested negative on 6 weekly tests. | |
| *Trichomoniasis* | | Series of negative microscopic examinations of cultured preputial material. | Negative single microscopic test of cultured preputial material at 6-month intervals. |
| | | Bulls under 180 days of age— negative on 1 test.▼ | |
| | | Bulls 180–364 days of age— negative on 3 weekly tests. | |
| | | Bulls 365 days or older tested negative on 6 weekly tests. | |

*L. pomona, L. hardjo, L. canicola, L. icterohaemorrhagiae, L. grippotyphosa.

▼Providing AI center veterinarian can certify that bull has not been housed with female cattle since reaching the age of 30 days.

## Antibiotic Treatment of All Semen and Extender

1. Neat Semen Treatment   100 µg of tylosin, 500 µg gentamicin, and 300/600 µg of Linco-Spectin dissolved in 0.02 ml of double distilled sterile water, added and mixed with each ml of neat semen.

2. CSS Approved Semen Extender (Standard 2-Step Method)   The same antibiotics are added to the extender such that the final concentration is 50 µg tylosin, 250 µg gentamicin, and 150/300 µg of Linco-Spectin in each ml of frozen semen.

3. CSS Approved Semen Extender (Alternative 1-Step Method)   The same antibiotics are added to the extender such that the final concentration is 100 µg tylosin, 500 µg gentamicin, and 300/600 µg of Linco-Spectin in each ml of frozen semen.

---

(Certified Semen Services (January 2002)

The CSS sire health program is designed to make a distinction between semen from bulls meeting the CSS Minimum Requirements and semen from those that do not. This is accomplished through use of the CSS block-style logo:

**CSS®**

Semen from bulls that are maintained under conditions complying with or exceeding the CSS Minimum Requirements may be designated as CSS "Health Certified Semen." The CSS logo may be imprinted *only* on semen packages (straws) containing "Health Certified Semen." The logo may also be displayed in advertising if *all* semen advertised and sold by the AI business is in compliance with the CSS Minimum Requirements (see Appendix I).

## Paratuberculosis (Johne's Disease)

Testing for paratuberculosis was previously a CSS program requirement. However, by action of the CSS Board of Directors in 1987, paratuberculosis was deleted from the CSS Minimum Requirements because under prevailing AI center management practices, there is a lack of evidence of its transmitability through semen. Nevertheless, it is still recommended that AI center animals receive a fecal culture test for paratuberculosis every 12 months as a general herd health surveillance practice. Paratuberculosis is typically spread by ingestion of fecal material from an infected animal.

In addition to the health tests required in the CSS program, the following diseases are often of importance for international trade.

## Bluetongue

Bluetongue is a disease of sheep that may be carried by cattle and transmitted by specific blood-sucking insects. Serological and virus culture tests for bluetongue are available.

## Infectious Bovine Rhinotracheitis (IBR), Infectious Pustular Balanoposthitis (IPB), Infectious Pustular Vulvovaginitis (IPV)

Infections are caused by strains of Bovine Herpesvirus–1 (BHV–1), resulting in respiratory disease, abortion, and infertility. Vaccination is one control measure. Serological and virus culture tests are available.

## Leukosis

Leukosis is a virus infection of lymphocytes transmitted either (1) pre-natally through ingestion of positive colostrum or (2) by contact or procedures that could transfer blood from one animal to another. Malignant neoplasms (lymphosarcoma) develop in a relatively small percentage of those animals infected with bovine leukosis virus. A serological test is available.

## Foot-and-Mouth Disease

Foot-and-mouth disease (FMD) is a highly contagious viral disease and can be transmitted through semen. Although the United States is free of this disease, the virus has been found to withstand semen processing and freezing. Serological and virus culture tests are available. Because of the contagious nature and economic importance of foot-and-mouth disease, USDA/APHIS has very strict protocols to prevent the entry of FMD virus into the United States. Laboratory diagnosis of the virus should be conducted at a national disease-secure laboratory, such as the Foreign Animal Disease Diagnostic Laboratory in Greenport, New York.

The 2001 outbreaks of FMD in the United Kingdom, France, and the Netherlands have underscored the need for heightened biosecurity. For specific information on the current status of FMD refer to the USDA/APHIS and OIE websites at http://www.aphis.usda.gov and http://www.oie.int, respectively.

## BSE ("Mad Cow Disease")

Bovine Spongiform Encephalopathy (BSE) is a chronic degenerative disease affecting the central nervous system of cattle. More commonly known as "mad cow disease," BSE belongs to a family of diseases called Transmissible Spongiform Encephalopathies (TSEs). TSEs are known to affect cattle, sheep, goats, mink, cats, deer, elk, and humans. These diseases have a long incubation period (several months to years), involve progressive neurological disorders, and are always fatal. The causative agent of BSE has not been completely characterized, but it is apparently smaller than the smallest known virus. BSE is believed to be transmitted through the ingestion of contaminated meat and bone meal. BSE was first identified during an epidemic outbreak in Great Britain in the late 1980's. Since then, it has been diagnosed in several other countries, but it has never been found in the United States. Although evidence indicates that BSE is not transmitted in semen, USDA/APHIS has in place import protocols requiring semen donors to be free of BSE and to be from herds having no incidence of BSE for the previous five years.

## QUESTIONS

1. From a disease control standpoint, what procedures are necessary when adding new bulls for AI use?

2. Why are isolation of bulls and the testing period necessary? What tests should be conducted while bulls are in isolation?

3. How often should bulls furnishing semen for AI use be tested or examined for brucellosis? Tuberculosis? Trichomoniasis? Leptospirosis? Campylobacteriosis? BVD virus?

4. How is *Campylobacter fetus* controlled in an AI program?

5. Why should bulls located in private herds, if custom collected and semen is used outside the home herd, be health tested and not permitted contact with the cow herd?

6. Can frozen semen from countries infected with foot-and-mouth disease be imported into the United States? Explain.

## REFERENCES

Bartlett, D. E., et al. 1976. Specific pathogen free (SPF) frozen bovine semen: A goal? Proc. 6th Tech. Conf. on Artificial Insemination and Reproduction. NAAB. p. 11.

Barto, D. 2001. On patrol for BSE. BEEF. September 2001. p.52.

CSS Minimum Requirements for Disease Control of Semen Produced for AI. 2002. Certified Semen Services, Columbia, MO.

Diseases Transmissible by Semen and Embryo Transfer Techniques. 1985. Technical Series No. 4. Office of International des Epizooties, Paris.

Doak, G. A. 1986. CSS implementation of new antibiotic combination. Proc. 11th Tech. Conf. on Artificial Insemination and Reproduction. NAAB. p. 42.

Elliott, F. I., D. M. Murphy, and D. E. Bartlett. 1961. The use of Polymyxin B sulfate with dihydrostreptomycin and penicillin for the control of *Vibrio fetus* in a frozen semen process. Proc. IV International Congr. of Animal Reproduction (The Hague). p. 539.

Howard, T. H. 1985. Vibriosis and trichomoniasis: Old foes back as 'New Diseases.' The Dairyman 85:28.

Howard, T. H. 1986. CSS sire health: Present and future. Proc. 11th Tech. Conf. on Artificial Insemination and Reproduction. NAAB. p. 19.

Lein, D. 1986. The current role of ureaplasma, mycoplasma, and *Haemophilus somnus* in bovine reproductive disorders. Proc. 11th Tech. Conf. on Artificial Insemination and Reproduction. NAAB. p. 27.

Lorton, S. P., et al. 1988. A new antibiotic combination for frozen semen. II. Evaluation of seminal quality. Theriogenology 29:593.

Lorton, S. P., et al. 1988. A new antibiotic combination for frozen semen. III. Evaluation of fertility. Theriogenology 29:609.

Lyle, W. E., et al. 1973. Recommended uniform diagnostic procedures for qualifying bulls for the production of semen. In: Committee of the AAVLD. Proc. 16th Ann. Mtg. Am. Assoc. Vet. Lab. Diag. and 77th Ann. Mtg. U.S. Anim. Health Assoc. p. 455.

Manual of Recommended Diagnostic Techniques and Requirements for Biological Products for Lists A and B Diseases. 1990. Vol. II. Office of International des Epizooties, Paris.

Manual of Recommended Diagnostic Techniques and Requirements for Biological Products for Lists A and B Diseases. 1991. Vol. III. Office of International des Epizooties, Paris.

Morrow, D. A. 1970. Bovine diseases and the AI industry. Proc. 3rd Tech. Conf. on Artificial Insemination and Reproduction. NAAB. p. 79.

Orthey, A. E., and H. L. Gilman. 1954. The antibacterial action of penicillin and streptomycin against *Vibrio fetus,* including concentrations found in naturally infected semen. J. Dairy Sci. 37:416.

Shin, S. J., et al. 1988. A new antibiotic combination for frozen bovine semen. I. Control of mycoplasmas, ureaplasmas, *Campylobacter fetus* subsp. *venerealis* and *Haemophilus somnus.* Theriogenology 29:577.

## WEB SITES

Certified Semen Services, Inc.
   *http://www.naab-css.org*

USDA-APHIS/VS—International Regulations
   *http://www.aphis.usda.gov/vs/ncie/iregs/animals/*

# EXERCISE 25

# The AI Business—Organizations

## OBJECT

To study the organization and conduct of AI and to become familiar with the operation of an AI business.

## DISCUSSION

Artificial insemination has undergone revolutionary changes in the past 60 years. Technological developments, particularly the freezing of semen and the long-distance shipping of semen, have been contributing factors. Economic pressure, due to the decline of the dairy cattle population from some 30 million head of cows and heifers of breeding age in 1945 to about 13.1 million in 2001, has forced a reorganization of AI businesses and a restructuring of their service programs in many areas. While the sales of total units per 100 cows have remained steady since the late 1980's, the number of herds has declined some 12 percent, with individual herds becoming much larger. One consequence of these developments is a reduction in the number of full-time AI technicians. Because their businesses simply "dried up," many AI organizations have discontinued technician service except in the heavily-populated dairy cattle areas. Also, during the past 40 years, many dairy operations have converted to beef cattle. The increasing cost of operation and a scarcity of dairy workers are both contributing factors.

With fewer but larger dairy herds, the practice of selling semen to herd owners for "do-it-yourself" insemination has increased. Training schools, with courses of short duration to instruct herd owners or their employees to handle the insemination in their herds, have become a part of AI. Direct selling of semen has increased the area served by many AI organizations. The use of frozen semen and its longtime storage in liquid nitrogen containers on the farm or ranch accounts for increased competition among organizations. Not only privately-owned or proprietary organizations, but also farmer-owned cooperatives, are doing business in all states. A steady growth in the number of beef cattle artificially inseminated is also a factor in organizations expanding their operational areas.

## How AI Organizations Function

The artificial insemination of farm animals, largely cattle in the United States, is carried out under the marketing programs of several major centers (organizations). Each organization maintains a battery of both dairy bulls and beef bulls in regular service. In addition, each organization will have from a few to hundreds of young bulls being sampled, in waiting for proof, or under contract with dairy or beef cattle breeders.

The present AI organizations consist of farmer-owned cooperatives and privately-owned or proprietary organizations. America is unique in the number of privately-owned and operated AI organizations. At the start of the organized AI program in 1938, and for several years following, most organizations were farmer-owned cooperatives. Over the years, privately-owned businesses have become more numerous and have claimed a larger share of the cows artificially inseminated. At the present time, two of the large AI organizations in the United States, in terms of units of semen sold, are privately-owned by interests outside the United States. ABS Global is owned by Genus, a United Kingdom corporation and Alta Genetics is owned by a Dutch corporation, Alta Pon.

The farmer-owned cooperative AI businesses, in many cases, have merged and established centrally located headquarters, with the merging members carrying on sales and service programs. Two of the largest are Select Sires, Inc., Plain City, Ohio, resulting from the merging of 12 smaller cooperatives in 11 states; and Genex Cooperative, Shawano, Wisconsin, resulting from the federation of 5 AI cooperatives. The advantages of such mergers are greater volume of business per employee and per bull; more efficient use of facilities, management, and work force; and greater gross income. The success of any AI business is highly dependent upon the volume of business efficiently conducted.

The trend since 1950, when there were 97 AI businesses, has been toward larger AI organizations. The volume of business an organization does is an important factor in attaining maximum efficiency and lowering unit costs. The use of frozen semen has made it possible for an AI organization to include the entire United States and foreign countries in its sales area. Prior to 1954, when liquid semen was used exclusively, the operational area of an AI center was limited because semen had to be utilized one or two days after collection. The shipping of liquid semen was limited to relatively short distances accessible by car, bus, train, and occasionally plane. Small organizations, particularly the cooper-

atives, survived under these conditions because competitors could not enter their service areas unless they built local bull housing facilities. This proved to be highly uneconomical. Today, with frozen semen utilized almost exclusively, the production and distribution of semen and the artificial insemination of cows in the field is carried out as follows:

**Central Production Facility—** Bulls are maintained in the bull housing facilities (Figure 25.1). Semen is collected, processed, stored, or delivered to the trade area. Delivery of semen to technicians and distributors is largely by truck. Delivery by truck makes it possible to furnish the field operators semen, liquid nitrogen, and supplies. Large AI organizations maintain a fleet of trucks that make regularly scheduled runs to each service area. The technicians and the distributors meet the trucks at scheduled stops and obtain their supplies. Some organizations maintain distribution centers in the heavily populated cattle areas (Figure 25.2).

The cooperative organizations distribute semen to their regularly employed AI technicians, who service the cows in the area. Most cooperatives also sell semen to distributors or representatives in other areas.

As a rule, the privately-owned AI organizations do not directly employ many AI technicians. The general plan is to have a distributor or a representative in each area who handles relations with the customer and the service representative. The distribution and sales program for semen and AI service assumes a pattern similar to that of any large business—i.e., population, distribution, sales promotion, supervision, and public relations.

The majority of semen is sold by organizations, both cooperative and privately owned, directly to herd owners for "do-it-yourself" AI in their herds. This is particularly

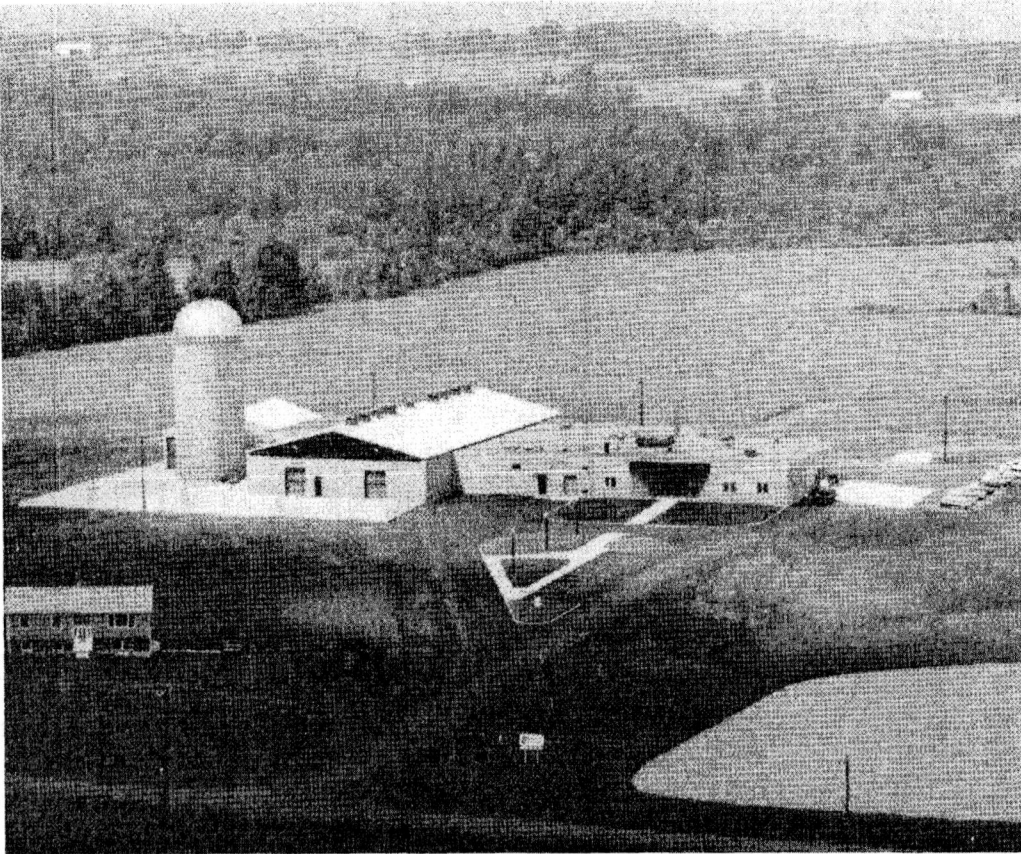

**Figure 25.1.** Aerial view of large AI center production facility for resident herd bulls. Shown are bull-housing barn, feed storage, semen-processing laboratory, and supervisor's residence. (Courtesy, Genex Cooperative, Ithaca, NY)

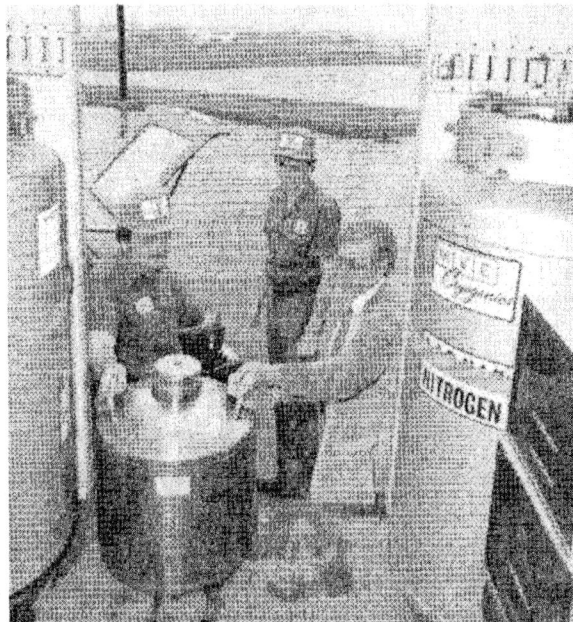

**Figure 25.2.** A COBA/Select Sires AI technician gets a supply of semen and liquid nitrogen from the supply truck. (Courtesy, C. Harold Johnson, COBA/Select Sires, Columbus, OH)

true in the artificial insemination of beef cattle, where the breeding is seasonal and nearly all inseminations are made by ranch or farm personnel. The sale and use of semen in "do-it-yourself" AI herds is generally done under the supervision of the AI organization's area distributor or local representative. It has become more common for AI representatives to provide "turnkey" programs for beef operations. The AI representative provides all services from estrus synchronization through breeding.

## QUESTIONS

1. Why have AI organizations become fewer in number but larger in the volume of cows serviced?

2. What are the advantages of merging or consolidating AI organizations?

3. How are semen, liquid nitrogen, and supplies delivered to local distributors for an AI business?

4. Why has the total number of bulls now owned by AI organizations increased dramatically compared to 40 years ago?

5. How do AI businesses conduct progeny-proving programs? Why is it necessary to sample many young bulls for genetic evaluations?

6. How would you promote and "sell" AI to dairy cattle breeders? To beef cattle breeders?

7. Do you think the distribution of liquid semen will ever become popular again? What would be the advantage of using liquid semen? Explain.

## REFERENCES

Herman, H. A. 1981. Improving Cattle by the Millions. Univ. of Missouri Press, Columbia.

Losh, D. J., and B. L. Erven. 1985. Study of Artificial Insemination Practices on U.S. Dairy Farms—Implications for Increased Semen Sale. Dept. of Agr. Economics and Rural Sociology, *Ohio State Univ., Columbus.*

## WEB SITES

Artificial Insemination Organizations
   *http://www.naab-css.org*

# EXERCISE 26

# Records, Accounting, and Regulations Pertaining to Registered Cattle—Important Concerns in Operating an AI Business

## OBJECT

To become familiar with the financial records, semen and laboratory records, regulations for registered cattle, and other records used in the conduct of an AI business.

## DISCUSSION

There are numerous records involved in operating an AI and semen sales and service business. These include records relating to bull purchases and bull sales; equipment and supplies; personnel, payroll, and fringe benefits; semen sales; shipping costs; travel expenses; in the case of cooperatives, patronage statements; and often refunds. There are records of the registration and transfer of bulls, records of blood typing, regulations for the insemination of registered cattle, and sire health records. There are also records on building costs, maintenance, and repairs of the physical plant; feed and veterinary costs; and often farm operations. The efficient and successful AI business must have a complete accounting system for use by management in guiding the financial destiny of the business. Most AI businesses today utilize electronic processing and follow the general office procedures of any modern business. Artificial insemination is in the realm of big business. A recent annual balance sheet of a major coop-

erative AI business is presented in this exercise to give an idea of the assets and liabilities of a large AI organization.

Records, bookkeeping procedures, and financial reports vary with each organization. Cooperatives have a membership sign-up program and the distribution of patronage dividends, while privately-owned businesses have stockholder reports and dividend distributions.

The most important fact to point out is that management must know both the cost of providing an insemination dose of semen delivered to the buyer and the cost of service in the field. The ability to balance income against expenses and to show a gain over a period of years is the mark of a successful business. If there is a criticism of AI in the United States, it is that its services have been priced too low. The philosophy of "low-cost service" has been the undoing of some farmer-owned cooperatives over the years. Be reminded that any successful AI business progresses on the caliber of sires utilized and the service rendered and that where there are no profits, there is no progress. It is the margin above costs that permits expansion programs, better sires, research, promotion, and, above all, constantly improved service. The business that survives in a highly competitive market does so on the basis of the quality of the products and the services rendered.

## BALANCE SHEET

_____ **Breeders Cooperative**
**for the period ending** _____, 20_____

### ASSETS

**CURRENT ASSETS:**

| | |
|---|---|
| Cash on Hand & in Bank | $1,475,204 |
| Accounts Receivable | 3,069,270 |
| Inventories | 1,992,018 |
| Prepaid Expenses | 70,616 |
| Accrued Interest Receivable | 46,422 |
| Total Current Assets | $6,653,530 |

**FIXED ASSETS:**

| | |
|---|---|
| Land & Land Improvements | $577,556 |
| Buildings | 5,369,489 |
| Sires | 2,167,209 |
| Equipment | 4,941,428 |
| | $13,055,682 |
| Less Depreciation | 6,340,572 |
| Net Depreciated Value | $6,715,110 |
| Construction in Progress | 338,865 |
| Total Fixed Assets | $7,053,975 |

**OTHER ASSETS:**

| | |
|---|---|
| Investments at Cost | $500,960 |
| Notes Receivable | 668,183 |
| Cash Value of Life Insurance & Annuities | 383,988 |
| Deferred Income Tax Benefit | 50,000 |
| Total Other Assets | $1,603,131 |

| | |
|---|---|
| TOTAL ASSETS | $15,310,636 |

### LIABILITIES & MEMBERSHIP EQUITY

**CURRENT LIABILITIES:**

| | |
|---|---|
| Current Maturities of Long-Term Liabilities | $300,920 |
| Accounts Payable | 763,708 |
| Accrued Taxes, Insurance, Retirement & Travel | 1,060,932 |
| Members' Future Services | 156,235 |
| Income Payable to Members | 281,319 |
| Total Current Liabilities | $2,563,114 |

**LONG-TERM LIABILITIES: LIABILITIES & MEMBERSHIP EQUITY**

| | |
|---|---|
| Deferred Compensation | $370,168 |
| Retirement Contribution | 717,907 |
| Other | 298,860 |
| Total Long-Term Liabilities | $1,386,935 |

| | |
|---|---|
| MEMBERSHIP EQUITY | $11,360,587 |
| TOTAL LIABILITIES & MEMBERSHIP EQUITY | $15,310,636 |

The difference of a few dollars in the price of semen or service from an average sire as compared to that from a distinctly superior bull means little when there might be as much as a $100-a-year difference in the returns from milk per cow, plus the added breeding value of the progeny.

In the laboratory, records are kept of each semen collection, its quality, extension, storage time, and so forth. Records of sire performance, sire health, and semen production are also regularly kept.

Summaries are maintained of semen sales, supplies, and number of cows inseminated per

| | | | | BREED CODES | | | | | | | | | | | | | |
|---|---|---|---|---|---|---|---|---|---|---|---|---|---|---|---|---|---|

**ATLANTIC BREEDERS COOPERATIVE**
# MEMBERSHIP ACTIVITY

BREED CODES
1. AYRSHIRE 5. BROWN SWISS 9. GOATS 22. SIMMENTAL
2. GUERNSEY 6. ANGUS 10. BRAHMAN 23. BEEFALO
3. HOLSTEIN 7. HEREFORD 14. CHIANINA
4. JERSEY 8. CHAROLAIS 14. SHORT HORN

| SERVICE DATE | RECEIPT NO. | TAG OR REG. NO. | 1-G 2-R | STUD | BREED | BULL | PRES. TECH. | SER. NO. | REPEAT DATE | STUD | BREED | BULL | PREV. TECH. | CHARGE | CASH | MEMBER NO. |
|---|---|---|---|---|---|---|---|---|---|---|---|---|---|---|---|---|
| | | | | | | | | | | | | | | | | |

**Figure 26.1.** Membership activity report (herd breeding record sheet). (Courtesy, Atlantic Breeders Cooperative, Lancaster, PA)

territory and per inseminator. Sire efficiency compilations are made regularly, and the percentage of non-returns is computed. Reports are sent regularly to the members of cooperatives, and most associations have a monthly newsletter. Financial records consist of money received, cash disbursements, etc. Most organizations follow a standard bookkeeping system and employ a controller.

Typical record forms used and a brief note concerning each follow. These will acquaint a manager-to-be with only a part of the record-keeping set-up. Actual experience will have to provide the remainder.

## PROCEDURE

Read the preceding discussion and the explanation of the various records used in the conduct of an AI business. Study the requirements for the registration of purebred cattle

resulting from artificial insemination and the responsibility of the herd owner and the inseminator (technician).

The herd breeding record sheet, Figure 26.1, may be used for listing each cow in a herd, services, sire used, collections for services, and so forth. This form is computer generated from the inseminator's receipts.

The inseminator's daily record and call sheet (Figure 26.2) is kept in duplicate by the inseminator. One side lists calls, mileage, collections, and so forth. The other side lists expenses, semen destroyed, etc. This sheet, properly filled out and accompanied by breeding receipts and money collected, is mailed to the local or central headquarters at regular intervals.

A laboratory record of semen, Figure 26.3, is of value in evaluating the fertility of a sire. Some permanent records should be kept on each sire. Following is some information about what should be recorded, as provided by the Purebred Dairy Cattle Association.

## Inseminator's Daily Record and Call Sheet

Inseminator _____     Date _____ 19 ____

| Order No. | Mileage | Name | Call Taken By | Time Call Taken | Number and Breed | Noticed In Heat | | First Service | Repeat | Time Bred | Payment | | Charge |
| | | | | | | PM | AM | | | | Cash | On Acct. | |
|---|---|---|---|---|---|---|---|---|---|---|---|---|---|
| | | | | | | | | | | | | | |
| | | | | | | | | | | | | | |
| | | | | | | | | | | | | | |
| | | | | | | | | | | | | | |
| | | | | | | | | | | | | | |
| | | | | | | | | | | | | | |
| | | | | | | | | | | | | | |
| | | | | | | | | | | | | | |
| | | | | | | | | | | | | | |
| | | | | | | | | | | | | | |
| | | | | | | | | | | | | | |
| | | | | | | | | | | | | | |
| | | | | | | | | | | | | | |
| | | | | | | | | | | | | | |
| | | | | | | | | | | | | | |
| | | | | | | | | | | | | | |
| | | | | | | | | | | | | | |
| | | | | | | | | | | | | | |
| | | | | | | | | | | | | | |
| | | | | | | | | | | | | | |

**Figure 26.2.** Inseminator's daily record and call sheet.

## Requirements Governing Artificial Insemination of Purebred (Registered) Dairy Cattle

The respective breed registry association AI rules are not totally uniform, but the rules are quite similar. The following information is based solely on information provided in published form by the respective breed registry association and is believed to be complete and accurate. However, all regulations are subject to change and interpretation by the respective breed registry association.

This information is provided as a guideline to interested persons. It is the responsibility of anyone planning to register cattle of a specific breed to obtain complete details of all regulations pertaining to registration from the respective breed registry association.

**PUREBRED DAIRY CATTLE ASSOCIATION**

Tom McKittrick, Administrator
Suite 101
2820 Walton Commons West
Madison, WI 53718
Tel: 608/224-0400

286

# SEMEN PRODUCTION RECORD

Date _____  Coll. Code_____

| Collector | Bull Code | Bull Name | Sample Number | Semen Volume | Semen Conc. | Pre/Fr. Motility | Dilution Rate | Units Calculated | Units Frozen | Post/Fr. Motility | PIA | PABN | Remarks |
|---|---|---|---|---|---|---|---|---|---|---|---|---|---|
| | | | | | | | | | | | | | |
| | | | | | | | | | | | | | |
| | | | | | | | | | | | | | |
| | | | | | | | | | | | | | |
| | | | | | | | | | | | | | |
| | | | | | | | | | | | | | |
| | | | | | | | | | | | | | |
| | | | | | | | | | | | | | |
| | | | | | | | | | | | | | |
| | | | | | | | | | | | | | |
| | | | | | | | | | | | | | |
| | | | | | | | | | | | | | |
| | | | | | | | | | | | | | |
| | | | | | | | | | | | | | |
| | | | | | | | | | | | | | |
| | | | | | | | | | | | | | |
| | | | | | | | | | | | | | |
| | | | | | | | | | | | | | |
| | | | | | | | | | | | | | |
| | | | | | | | | | | | | | |
| | | | | | | | | | | | | | |
| | | | | | | | | | | | | | |
| | | | | | | | | | | | | | |

**Figure 26.3.** Laboratory semen production record. (Courtesy, Select Sires/PA, Tunkhannock, PA)

# U.S. DAIRY BREED REGISTRY ORGANIZATIONS

**THE AMERICAN GUERNSEY ASSOCIATION**

7614 Slate Ridge Blvd, P.O. Box 666
Reynoldsburg, OH 43068-0666
Tel: 614/864-2409
Fax: 614/864-5614
*www.usguernsey.com*

**THE AMERICAN JERSEY CATTLE ASSOCIATION**

6486 E. Main St.
Reynoldsburg, OH 43068-2362
Tel: 614/861-3636
Fax: 614/861-8040
*www.usjersey.com*

**AMERICAN MILKING SHORTHORN SOCIETY**

P.O. Box 449, 800 Pleasant Street
Beloit, WI 53511-5456
Tel: 608/365-3332
Fax: 608/365-6644
*www.agdomain.com/web/
usmilkingshorthorn/*

**AYRSHIRE BREEDERS' ASSOCIATION**

267 Broad St.
Westerville, OH 43081
Tel: 614/882-1057
Fax: 614/895-3757
*www.usayrshire.com*

**THE BROWN SWISS ASSOCIATION**

800 Pleasant Street
Beloit, WI 53511_5456
Tel: 608/365-4474
Fax: 608/365-5577
*www.brownswissusa.com*

**HOLSTEIN ASSOCIATION USA, INC.**

1 Holstein Place
Brattleboro, VT 05302-0808
Tel: 800/952-5200
Fax: 802/254-8251
*www.holsteinusa.com*

## REQUIREMENTS FOR REGISTRY AND IDENTIFICATION OF HOLSTEIN CATTLE RESULTING FROM ARTIFICIAL INSEMINATION OF DAM

1. APPLICANT RESPONSIBLE: The applicant identifying an artificially-conceived animal assumes full responsibility for the accuracy of all information required by The Holstein Association on appropriate application forms for the issuance of a Certificate of Registration, Recording or Identification.

   The Holstein Association may at any time request the owner of dam at time of service or owner of dam at time of calving, whichever is applicable, to provide a proof of ownership of semen or the availability of semen of the indicated sire on the application for identification.

   a. Such proof may be in the form of a breeding receipt which identifies the semen used when inseminating the identified dam of the animal for whom an application for registry or identification has been filed.

   b. In instances where the semen used was involved in a transaction (sale, purchase or gift) for future use (not applicable under "a." above), the first owner or seller should provide the second owner or buyer with a Bill of Sale or equivalent document identifying the semen, the date of the transaction, quantity involved and source of such semen. A copy of the Bill of Sale or equivalent document may be requested at any time by The Holstein Association as evidence of availability of semen for use. The Bill of Sale or equivalent document need not necessarily be from the original producer or supplier, but should be traceable to the original source through a series of such documents involving each ownership of the semen available and used.

2. IDENTIFICATION OF SEMEN: The vial, straw or other package carrying the semen from which the dam conceived shall have been accurately labeled with the following information:

   a. The name and registration number of the bull registered in the Herd Book of Holstein Association USA, Inc. This may be supplemented by the unique identification code of the sire placed on file with The Holstein Association by the semen producing and/or freezing business or owner of sire.

   b. The date of semen collection or a semen collection code which is unique and identifiable with the business or organization collecting and/or freezing the semen. Such code shall be available to The Holstein Association for reference on request.

   c. The identification code of the business or organization collecting and/or freezing semen as assigned by NAAB may be shown at the option of the owner of the sire. When a code is used, adequate information must be on file with The Holstein Association to completely and accurately identify it with the business or organization collecting and/or freezing the semen; otherwise, the name of such business or organization shall be included on the inseminating unit.

3. BLOOD TYPE:

   a. At such time as semen is frozen, the bull from which collected will be blood typed with his living unblood-typed sire and/or dam. Approval of the laboratory from which a certified blood type will be accepted must be obtained from The Holstein Association. Specifications for the blood type and form of report are available from The Holstein Association. Under extenuating circumstances, The Holstein Association reserves the right to grant exceptions to this requirement.

   b. BLOOD TYPING SERVICE AVAILABLE: The Holstein Association provides a blood typing service to meet these requirements through an arrangement with a blood typing laboratory qualified to meet all provisions set forth in 3a. (above). A $45.00 service fee will be charged by The Holstein Association for each animal involved in such blood typing service.

4. CANADIAN SEMEN: Semen originating in Canada and produced by a sire(s) registered in the Herd Book of The Holstein Association of Canada, shall have met all requirements of the Joint Dairy Breeds Committee of Canada for use in artificial insemination in Canada before importation. In addition, provisions 1 and 3 above shall apply.

## REQUIREMENTS GOVERNING AYRSHIRE, BROWN SWISS, GUERNSEY, JERSEY, AND MILKING SHORTHORN[1]

1. BLOOD TYPING:

   a. Any registered dairy bull from which semen is frozen must be blood typed along with his liv-

---

[1] As summarized by Certified Semen Services, Inc., P.O. Box 1033, Columbia, MO 65205.

ing unblood typed parents at the expense of the owner or lessee.

b. Blood typing to be acceptable must be conducted at a laboratory approved by and operating under Agreement with the National Society of Livestock Record Association of which PDCA member organizations are members.

c. Blood typing fees are payable to the respective breed organization for administering, recording, and maintaining such data.

d. If in the opinion of the breed registry organization, there is a question of parentage as represented by the application for registry, the offspring in question must be blood typed with the dam and the results of blood typing by the designated laboratory in all matters of identification and parentage will be accepted as official.

2. LISTING BULLS: A registered dairy bull from which semen has been collected and used for the artificial insemination of dairy cows must be listed with the respective breed registry organization by the owner or lessee before the resulting offspring are eligible for registration.

Compliance of essential Listing shall consist of:

a. The AI business immediately sending a Semen Freezing Report to the respective breed organization of any registered dairy bull from which semen is collected for the first time.

b. The name and registration number given on the Semen Freezing Report must agree with the name and registration number recorded in the breed registry records to avoid the assumption of mislabeling.

c. The owner or lessee at time of first collection is responsible for having the bull blood typed with his living unblood-typed parents to verify parentage. This procedure is initiated by contacting the respective breed organization for proper forms and instructions.

d. The listing procedure is completed when a one-time listing fee of $30 (AJCC's listing fee is $40) is paid to the respective breed registry organization prior to accepting Applications for Registration of offspring resulting from artificial insemination.

3. SEMEN IDENTIFICATION: Positive identification of semen is essential for accuracy of records to register the resulting offspring. The breeder submitting the application is responsible for proof of identification of semen used to produce the offspring for which application is being made.

a. Acceptable identification requirements for each breeding unit (i.e., ampules, straws, etc.) of semen used is considered as follows:

1. The name and number of the bull as registered in the records of the respective breed registry organization

2. Collection code

3. AI Center (stud) code

4. Breed code

5. Bull's number assigned by the AI Business

b. When a Sale Invoice or Bill of Sale is accepted by a purchaser of frozen semen as substantiating evidence of ownership of the semen, the Sales Invoice or Bill of Sale should include the following, in addition to the semen identification under (a) above.

1. Name and address of seller

2. Name and address of purchaser

3. Date of purchase

4. Number and type of individual breeding units

4. REGISTRATION PROCEDURE: Each Application for Registration must be submitted with one of the following conditions to be considered for registry when the sire and dam are not owned by the same person at the time of breeding:

a. An acceptable breeding receipt issued by an Employed or Affiliated Technician of a recognized AI business may accompany the application. This breeding receipt must include the following data:

1. Breed, name and registration number of cow, or

2. Breed, name and positive identification for a cow eligible to register such as tattoo or other identifying number; or sketch of color markings. (Brown Swiss, Jersey and Milking Shorthorn require tattoo in lieu of sketch.)

3. Owner's name and address

4. Name of bull and registration number

5. Bull code including AI Center (stud) code and breed code

6. Collection code

7. Service number

8. Date of breeding
9. Previous service information
10. Inseminator's signature

b. In lieu of a breeding receipt, the owner may certify to accepting full responsibility for any damages resulting from inaccurate breeding information as specified by the respective breed registry organization.

5. Each breed registry organization reserves the privilege of establishing separate conditions for the artificial insemination of animals within its respective breed.

## Blood Typing—A Must!

All dairy breed registry organizations require that the blood type of a bull and his living ancestors not previously blood typed be on file in the registry office. To meet blood-typing requirements, the owner of the animal should contact the proper breed registry association office and obtain the necessary forms, collection vials, and instructions for handling and mailing the blood sample.

In the future, it is likely that DNA typing of individuals will play a prominent role in parentage qualification and identity verification. Registry associations may adopt DNA typing as methods and procedures become more standardized on a worldwide basis. Such was the case with blood typing.

## Semen Sales

There is no standard form used to record the sale of semen from one party to another, but anyone who buys semen from another party should have a bill of sale or an invoice of the purchase. For information to be listed, see Item 3(b), "Semen Identification," in the breed registry AI requirements. The breed registry organization may demand a copy of the bill of sale or invoice on any given lot of semen.

## Semen Freezing Report

A form for reporting semen collected and frozen, Figure 26.4, is used by AI and custom freezing businesses. This form should be mailed

**SEMEN FREEZING REPORT**
Submit to respective breed office

Bull ............................................................................................ No. ........................

Breed .............................. Owner ........................................................................

Date frozen ........................... Address .............................................................

I hereby certify that the above named bull was identified with his certificate of registry when the above semen was collected and that the owner was informed of the blood typing requirement.

Signed (Organization) .......................................................................

By (Authorized person) .......................................................................

.............................................................................................................

PDCA Form 14 — Available from PDCA or Breed Registry Office.

**Figure 26.4.** Semen freezing report. (Courtesy, Purebred Dairy Cattle Association)

21st CENTURY GENETICS®
100 MBC Drive · P.O. Box 469 · Shawano, WI 54166

Breeding Receipt ______

Owner ______

Address ______

Date of Breeding ______ Breed of Cow ______ Ser. No. ______

Unit No. ______ Farm No. ______

**SIRE USED**

Name of Bull ______

Registration No. ______

Bull I.D. 21 ______ Coll. Code ______

**FEMALE SERVICED**

Name of Cow ______

Reg. No. ______ Tatoo or Tag ______

**PREVIOUS SERVICE**

Date ______ Prev. Bull 21 ______

Bull Reg. No. ______

I hereby certify that I am duly authorized by the above named business to issue this receipt in its name which is given as evidence for service rendered and also a certification of date of service and identity of semen used for service of animal identified hereon.

______ (INSEMINATOR SIGNATURE) ______ (INSEM. NO.)

Form A 98

**Figure 26.5.** A standard breeding receipt form. (Courtesy, Genex Cooperative, Shawano, WI)

immediately to the breed registry office when a dairy bull is collected for the first time.

## Breeding Receipts

A breeding receipt may be used if the animal is inseminated by a technician who is employed by or affiliated with a recognized AI business.

In lieu of a breeding receipt, the owner of the animal inseminated may certify to accepting full responsibility for any damages or losses resulting from inaccurate breeding information. Figure 26.5 is a breeding receipt form used by technicians for AI organizations. Figure 26.6 is a form that may be used if more than one animal is being bred in a herd on the same day.

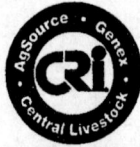

**Genex Cooperative Inc.**
A subsidiary of Cooperative Resources International
PO Box 469 • Shawano, WI 54166-0469

397021

| SU Number | | Acct. Number | |
|---|---|---|---|
| Owner Name | | Date of Breeding | |

**1**

| Animal ID. | | Heifer | ☐ Yes | ☐ No |
|---|---|---|---|---|
| Animal Reg. No. | | Last Calving Date | | |
| Sire Code | Sire Name | | QCN | |
| Service Fee | | Semen Fee | | |

**2**

| Animal ID. | | Heifer | ☐ Yes | ☐ No |
|---|---|---|---|---|
| Animal Reg. No. | | Last Calving Date | | |
| Sire Code | Sire Name | | QCN | |
| Service Fee | | Semen Fee | | |

**3**

| Animal ID. | | Heifer | ☐ Yes | ☐ No |
|---|---|---|---|---|
| Animal Reg. No. | | Last Calving Date | | |
| Sire Code | Sire Name | | QCN | |
| Service Fee | | Semen Fee | | |

**4**

| Animal ID. | | Heifer | ☐ Yes | ☐ No |
|---|---|---|---|---|
| Animal Reg. No. | | Last Calving Date | | |
| Sire Code | Sire Name | | QCN | |
| Service Fee | | Semen Fee | | |

**5**

| Animal ID. | | Heifer | ☐ Yes | ☐ No |
|---|---|---|---|---|
| Animal Reg. No. | | Last Calving Date | | |
| Sire Code | Sire Name | | QCN | |
| Service Fee | | Semen Fee | | |

| BREEDING PROGRAM SPECIALIST Signature | Number | Paid on Account |
|---|---|---|
| | | |

**OFFICE COPY**

**Figure 26.6.** A multiple-animal breeding receipt. (Courtesy, Genex Cooperative, Shawano, WI)

292

These forms can be used for both grade and registered cows. Triplicate copies are made. The original is given to the herd owner and may accompany the application for registry in case of a purebred. The other copies are retained by the AI business for internal use.

## Instructions to Inseminators (Technicians)

Technicians filling out breeding receipts should be familiar with the requirements listed under Item 3, "Semen Identification," and Item 4, "Registration Procedure," and do their part in seeing that the owner of a cow inseminated has complete and accurate information. While the animal owner assumes full responsibility for the information submitted on the registry application, the inseminator who is careless and omits information on the breeding receipt will probably not be welcome in the future.

## Helpful Information for Inseminators

1. When completing the breeding receipt, use the full registered name and number of the cow, taken directly from the registration certificate. Give the same information for the bull, taken from the semen package label.

2. Always use indelible pencil or ink.

3. Give the original breeding receipt to the owner at the time of insemination. The breeding receipt may be retained for later use by the owner as a service certificate when applying for registration of a resulting calf or transfer of the animal inseminated.

4. Receipts are numbered; account for each one. If you spoil one, mark it "void" and send it with your regular report.

## Herd Operators Assure the Accuracy of Parentage Records

With bulls in artificial service siring thousands of calves a year in many herds, every herd owner should use precautions to prevent errors and faulty records that may prevent the resulting progeny from qualifying for registration. As a rule, both purebred and non-purebred animals resulting from artificial insemination are from well-above-average sires and command higher prices at the marketplace. Careless record keeping, failure to identify the offspring accurately, and errors due to inadvertently choosing the wrong sire when removing the semen unit from the storage container at the time of insemination cause grief for herd owners and breed registry associations. Some safeguards to prevent these disappointments are:

1. Be sure that every bull used for artificial insemination, as well as his sire and dam, are blood typed in the laboratory approved by the respective breed association.

2. Make sure that every ampule, straw, or other semen dose is clearly and permanently labeled. Never use unlabeled semen.

3. Know your semen supplier. Don't buy or use semen offered by individuals or organizations that have not attained a record for confidence and reliability.

4. Systematically record every insemination, and file the breeding receipt. If repeat breedings are necessary, be sure to obtain the proper receipt for subsequent inseminations. Make certain that

the breeding receipt pertaining to the insemination that produced the calf for which you are making registry is available for the breed association.

5. Check the requirements governing artificial insemination for your respective breed association. Don't guess about requirements. Contact your breed association to obtain current information. Requirements of beef registry associations vary a great deal. Get the specific requirements for your breed before you submit an animal for registration.

6. Identify every animal at the time of insemination by color, diagram, tattoo, brand, or other permanent identification.

## Registering Beef Cattle Resulting from Artificial Insemination

The requirements for registering purebred beef cattle resulting from artificial insemination of the dam vary from breed to breed. Some breeds have an unrestricted AI policy. Some limit the number of calves registered to a sire in any one year. Breeding permits, also called "AI certificates," are sold by some beef breed associations in specific numbers for each sire.

The breeder of purebred beef cattle who plans to register calves resulting from artificial insemination should write to the respective breed organization for AI requirements. A list of beef breed associations can be found at the end of Exercise 17.

## QUESTIONS

1. Why are accurate cost-account records necessary in the conduct of an AI business?

2. Why is it necessary for any successful AI business to have a margin of profit?

3. What is the general relationship between the volume of business and the net profit of an AI business?

4. What is the responsibility of the herd owner in making information on the identity of cattle available to the inseminator?

5. When is a breeding receipt required for registered dairy cattle? When is such a receipt not necessary?

6. Why do most breeds (beef and dairy) require that a bull be blood typed if his semen is frozen and used for artificial insemination?

7. How would you proceed in having a bull blood typed?

8. Where would you obtain the precise requirements for registering calves resulting from artificial insemination in beef cattle?

## REFERENCES

Artificial Insemination Regulations of Beef Breed Associations. 2000. Certified Semen Services, Columbia, MO.

A Summary of Artificial Insemination Requirements of Members of the Purebred Dairy Cattle Association. 2000. Certified Semen Services, Columbia, MO.

# EXERCISE 27

# Career Opportunities in the AI Industry

## OBJECT

To become familiar with the opportunities for a career in livestock improvement, the various positions in the field of AI, and the qualifications for each.

## DISCUSSION

Artificial insemination as a means of improvement of livestock is well established in the agricultural community. Today, its adoption by dairy farmers ranks second only to the use of hybrid seed corn as the highest utilization program (99 percent) ever recorded in modern agriculture.

The improvement of farm animals through the genetic selection of superior sires is an important phase of livestock production. Artificial insemination is an effective means of maximizing the superior sire's genetic potential through widespread distribution. A 1998 study indicated that the total economic activity in the U.S. economy from bovine artificial insemination was more than 600 million dollars annually. Overall, improved breeding adds billions of dollars annually to the income from livestock in the United States. Since 1945, the average milk production per cow has increased from 4,500 to over 18,139 pounds annually. Beef producers are increasing weaning weights of calves from 50 to 75 pounds in a single year by breeding to superior, progeny-tested beef bulls. Through the use of artificial insemination, an outstanding sire can be used for several thousand matings, in many herds, each year. Some highly outstanding dairy and beef sires have produced over 100,000 offspring. And a select group of dairy sires have each produced in excess of 1 million units of frozen semen.

Artificial insemination in swine breeding has increased tremendously in the past few years, particularly with liquid boar semen. Horse breeders, turkey growers, sheep and goat breeders, and dog breeders also utilize artificial insemination. It is regularly used in turkey hatching egg production and in the fertilization of queen bees, as well as in the production of small animals for laboratory use.

As an established part of worldwide agriculture, AI will continue to be a source of employment for thousands of workers. Most of the key jobs in the AI field are filled by college graduates who have practical livestock and business experience.

In the ever-changing world of genetic improvement, artificial insemination personnel provide critical support and are key management consultants to livestock producers. They play significant roles in each producer's genetic success.

Men and women employed by an AI organization, regardless of their position, contribute to the organization's total efforts.

### Key Jobs and Their Requirements

### Office Management

**General Manager (CEO)**—The general manager of an AI organization oversees all aspects of the organization. This individual possesses strong leadership and communication skills to effectively perform this comprehensive task. The manager's skills are highly developed and come from years of leadership experience in the industry.

**Finance Manager**—The organization's business administrator is the finance manager. This person creates and follows the company's budget and handles all financial matters. Training in business is essential to the success of the finance manager.

**Data Processor**—With the increased use of computers to maintain genetic records, production data, inventories, and financial information, the person with computer skills is very valuable. From writing computer programs to data entry, the responsibilities of a data processor are diverse.

**Support Staff**—For an office to operate smoothly and efficiently, a strong support staff is essential. This staff includes office assistants, receptionists, and clerical staff. The staff provides an invaluable foundation for all office co-workers.

## Marketing Department

**Technician**—This professional provides insemination service for producers who choose AI technician service over breeding their own cows. A technician must maintain a flexible schedule to accommodate customers' needs, yet structure each day to be as efficient as possible.

The successful technician properly handles and thaws frozen semen and practices insemination techniques to produce optimum results for customers. Many AI organizations offer refresher courses in these areas to keep the technician up to date on correct procedures.

Technicians are key people in the organization's marketing efforts because they are in direct contact with the customers. They are of-

ten asked for advice on which bulls to use and therefore need to be knowledgeable of the organization's sires. The technician is a typical entry-level position in the AI industry.

**Direct Herd Sales Representative**—Selling skills play a vital role in direct herd sales. The representative sells semen to livestock producers who breed their own cows. In addition, the sales representative delivers liquid nitrogen and supplies.

The direct herd sales representative also provides producers with valuable information on the organization's sires. The sales representative is an important resource of information for the producer and helps him or her determine the sires that will best meet the goal of optimum genetic improvement. The sales representative is another typical entry-level position in the AI industry.

**Sales Manager**—The sales manager supervises the technicians and direct herd sales representatives for a specific geographic area. This person is the communication link between the organization's headquarters and the field personnel. The sales manager delivers vital information to the technicians and salesmen on the organization's sire lineup and marketing philosophy. In addition, customer information is conveyed to headquarters through the sales manager.

The sales manager is also responsible for the growth and development of these employees and therefore needs to be a strong motivator.

**Training School Instructor**—The training school instructor plays a key role in teaching producers and technicians how to properly handle and thaw frozen semen and effectively inseminate cows. For a successful AI program, the instructor also emphasizes general reproductive physiology, techniques of heat detection, principles of genetics, technician hygiene, and disease prevention.

The instructor supports the organization's marketing efforts. Through the training school, the instructor sells the advantages of a total AI program to livestock producers.

**Marketing Manager**—The marketing manager of an AI organization is responsible for its semen merchandising program. The marketing manager establishes the strategy and direction of the marketing program, along with short- and long-term goals for the marketing team.

Experience in sales and marketing is essential to the success of the marketing manager. This person usually has past work experience as a sales representative or area manager.

**International Marketing Director**—The person working with international marketing aids the organization in merchandising semen worldwide. This position may involve extensive travel. Speaking several foreign languages can be a strong asset to success in this marketing position.

## Communications Department

**Advertising Coordinator**—One of the key persons responsible for sire promotion is the advertising coordinator. The advertising coordinator's main duties include creating and placing all advertisements. To further publicize the organization's sires, sire catalogs and brochures are generated. In addition, the advertising coordinator publishes a national newsletter to keep the organization's customers informed.

Creativity is a definite asset to the advertising coordinator. Furthermore, a working knowledge of computers and desktop publishing are credentials of a successful coordinator.

**Public Relations Coordinator**—As the title indicates, this position involves both customer and employee relations. The coordinator organizes the visitor tour program so customers and prospective customers have the opportunity to observe the AI center operations. In addition, this person develops the employee newsletter and edits and distributes news releases on company events. The public relations coordinator is also responsible for trade show exhibits and for organizing local and regional membership meetings.

**Progeny Photograph Coordinator**—Daughter photos are key tools for marketing sires. The photograph coordinator organizes picture-taking efforts between headquarters and employees to produce quality pictures of the bulls' best daughters. This person is also responsible for sire photographs and the development of sire videos.

## Production Department

**Production Manager**—This individual is responsible for overall sire management and semen production. The production manager also works closely with the center veterinarian in administering the sire health program. This person is involved in administrative planning for long-range company goals.

**Sire Manager**—This individual and assistants feed and care for the organization's sires and are responsible for the semen collection activities. These efforts are crucial to a sire's health, longevity, and semen-producing ability. In addition to sire care, the sire manager also maintains the physical appearance of the sire barns on a daily basis.

**Farm Manager**—The person involved in farm management plants, cultivates, and harvests the crops for the organization. Other duties include maintaining and caring for the grounds, buildings, and farm equipment.

**Laboratory Supervisor/Technician**—After sire management collects the semen, the lab technician processes the collection. This includes evaluation, extension, cooling, packaging, and freezing. After processing, the frozen semen is quality checked and placed into inventory and/or shipped to the sales force. The lab technician insures that each straw of semen meets the organization's standards for hygiene, identification, and quality. The laboratory supervisor is responsible for overseeing all phases of semen processing.

**Researcher**—The person involved in research is constantly investigating improved methods to produce, process, package, and evaluate bull semen. This individual often provides key support to the production department, processing laboratory, quality control program, and technician or field force. The researcher is also interested in the latest developments in other fields related to AI.

**Veterinarian**—AI centers now maintain an average of about 100 bulls in active use, although some have from 200 to over 1,000 sires, if young bulls being sampled or awaiting proof and beef sires are included. One or more veterinarians are employed full time by the large organizations. Responsibilities of a veterinarian are extensive and are an important part of an AI organization. The veterinarian's tasks involve conducting sire health tests, treating ailments, inspecting bulls to be purchased and evaluating the herd of origin, keeping a watchful eye on the physical condition and fertility of each sire, caring for the feet and limbs, and performing other duties concerned with the maintenance of valuable sires. An increasingly important role of the AI center veterinarian is that of dealing with regulatory requirements for the exportation of semen.

## Genetics Department

**Herd Evaluator**—The evaluator offers advice to producers on sires that can improve their herds. The job includes evaluating each cow's strengths and weaknesses and suggesting sires that will correct the worst faults. The evaluator possesses a trained eye for cattle evaluation.

**Sire Analyst**—In sire procurement, the individual acquires young sires for the organization's sampling or progeny test program. As future sires, these young bulls must meet certain genetic, health, and semen quality standards. A sire analyst is highly trained and experienced in cattle genetics and evaluation. The sire analyst's selection of these young bulls determines the future strength of the company's sire lineup.

**Sire Sampling**—Once the young bulls have entered the program, they must be accurately sampled. This involves the random distribution of semen to many progeny test herds. The person responsible for sire sampling administers the progeny test program and evaluates the resulting young sire daughters. This person also must be knowledgeable in cattle genetics and be a trained evaluator.

## For a Successful Career in AI

**Education**—Educational requirements can vary from position to position, depending on job qualifications, but all require a high-school diploma. In addition, "on-the-job training" is also a means of learning job skills.

Technical training, usually a two-year program, is valuable to learn specific job requirements. The lab technician and the data processor would be examples.

Bachelor of Science degrees in Dairy or Animal Sciences, Agricultural Economics, Production, and Communications are valuable for positions in the Marketing, Communications, Genetics, and Production Departments.

A Masters degree in Business Administration may be required for leadership positions in Marketing or Management. A Master of Science or a Ph.D. degree may be required for key positions in the Genetics or Production Departments and for certain research positions.

**Internships**—Many AI organizations offer internships to provide an individual with the opportunity to experience the industry before committing to a specific career. Most are offered during the summer, and some are offered during the school year. They can involve any phase of the organization. Internships provide a very valuable background for potential employment within the AI industry.

## Keys to Success

The keys to success in any position are self-motivation and strong people skills. Utilizing these talents in one position can lead to growth in other areas of the organization.

## Salaries and Benefits

The pay scale for workers in the AI field is generally adequate for services performed and is competitive with the pay scale for workers in other positions requiring similar technical training and special abilities. The salaries of managers, assistant managers, and other key personnel are equal to, or in some cases higher than, those paid in other areas of the livestock field. Retirement, major medical benefits, and insurance (both accident and life) are among the fringe benefits accorded most employees in the AI industry.

# QUESTIONS

1. What are the positions offering career opportunities in the AI industry? List them.

2. What are the essential qualifications for a herd evaluator? Production manager? Sales manager? General manager? Public relations coordinator?

3. How would you suggest one proceed to qualify as a capable technician, or inseminator? Why is this a good position in which to begin a career in the AI field?

4. Are technicians adequately paid? Are there other compensations besides salary? Explain.

5. How does a technician, supervisor, manager, etc., obtain training in "selling the program"?

6. Should technicians combine farming with their activities? If so, how and in what areas? (Give your own ideas in answering.)

7. What is the advantage of having a veterinarian on the AI organization's staff?

8. How do salaries, retirement, hospitalization, and other fringe benefits for workers in the AI field compare with those for other positions in the fields associated with agriculture?

# WEB SITES

Exciting Career Opportunities in AI. National Association of Animal Breeders, Columbia, MO.
*http://www.naab-css.org/*

Contacts
See Appendix D

# PART FIVE

# Artificial Insemination

# of Dairy Goats

# and Other Farm Animals

# EXERCISE 28

# Artificial Insemination of Dairy Goats and Sheep

## OBJECT

To become acquainted with the techniques and advantages of using artificial insemination as a means of improving dairy goats and sheep.

## INTRODUCTION

Dairy goat breeders can well afford to give consideration to the use of artificial insemination as a means of improving milk production, type or conformation, and dollar value in their herds. Early results of artificial insemination in goats are shown in Figure 28.1. The use of artificial insemination in sheep has been quite limited in North America. However, the basic techniques for sheep are similar in many ways to those for goats, as will be explained later.

Interest in artificial insemination has increased with goats because of its outstanding success with cattle and also because, in some localities, fewer milk goats are kept and bucks of good quality are not available. The techniques used in the artificial insemination of goats are similar to those used with cattle. The factors that have made artificial insemination programs a valuable tool in the genetic improvement of cattle also apply to the dairy goat industry.

One of the most important contributions made possible by the artificial insemination of dairy goats is the effective sampling and proving of young bucks for the transmission of economical traits. AI is the most practical way

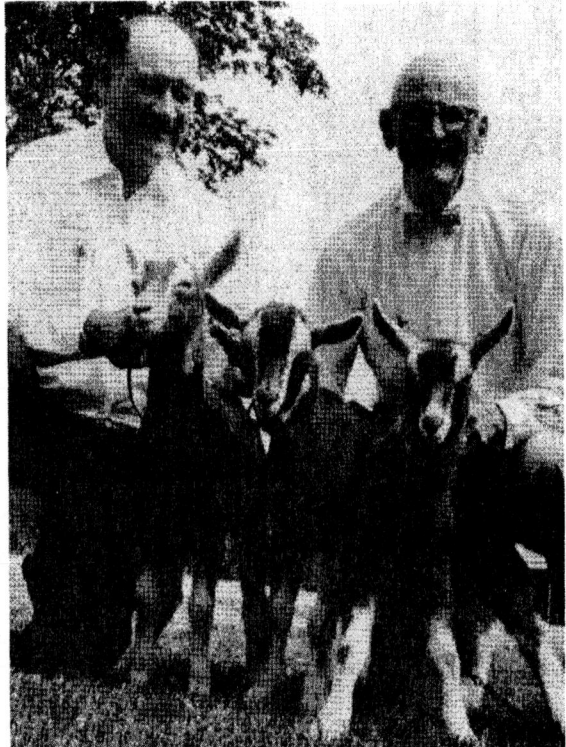

**Figure 28.1.** Triplet Toggenburg kids were among the first resulting from artificial insemination using frozen semen in Missouri. They are pictured with their owner, the late Dr. A. J. Durant (right) and Dr. H. A. Herman, of Columbia, MO. Sire of the kids, Laurelwood Acres Seafarer II, was housed in Ripon, CA, where semen was collected and frozen.

that genetic improvement can be made effectively in the dairy goat population.

The doe must kid yearly if she is to produce a desirable amount of milk. Goat owners, on the average, find it necessary to use the most readily available bucks. Often a buck that offers little hope for improved milk production in the progeny is the only one available. The use of purebred bucks to improve grade or native dairy goats was studied by workers in New Mexico. The results are shown in Figure 28.2.

## ARTIFICIAL INSEMINATION OF DAIRY GOATS

### Advantages

1. Dairy goat herds, for the most part, are fairly small. In many cases, only one to several does are kept. Often, milk goats are pets for the children and a source of diversion for the parents. In small herds, few people can afford to keep a really good buck, or in many cases any buck. Bucks are the chief culprits as far as "goat smell" is concerned. Through the use of artificial insemination, owners can utilize the kind of bucks that will make improvement in their herds at a reasonable cost. The breeding fees involved will be less than the cost of feeding and housing a buck. The small goat herd owner is spared the expense, trouble, and often the nuisance of keeping a buck on the premises.

2. Well-proven bucks, which have been found superior by the progeny test, are not plentiful. Only three to four years of active service may be expected on the average after they are proven. A few dozen offspring—or at best about a hundred in large herds—are possible through natural service. Through the effective use of AI, several hundred to several thousand offspring are possible from one buck.

3. The owner of a small herd can secure the genetic potential for improvement in milk production in a system-atic manner if superior bucks are used through artificial insemination.

4. Bucks of outstanding merit may be used for the breeding of many does. Semen can usually be extended from 5 to 20 times its original volume, allowing the insemination of many does from one ejaculate compared to only one doe in natural service. Owners of superior bucks can use them fully in their own herds rather than depending on less desirable bucks. Such bucks may also supply semen for use in many other herds and bring additional revenue to the owners.

5. The mating of outstanding bucks and does, even though they are located hundreds of miles apart, is possible. Such matings create new lines, reduce inbreeding, invoke some hybrid vigor, and can lead to production of highly outstanding individuals.

6. Among goats, the incidence of breeding troubles resulting from infections of the genital tract is not very great. However, it is well known that males vary widely in fertility. The systematic examination and evaluation of semen, which is a part of the AI process, soon locates the males that are subfertile. Diseases of a genital nature that may be carried by the buck in natural service are virtually eliminated when artificial insemination, using semen from disease-free bucks, is utilized.

7. Eliminates the trouble and expense of transporting does to be mated. Frozen buck semen may be stored for years, may be shipped thousands of miles, and can be readily available when needed.

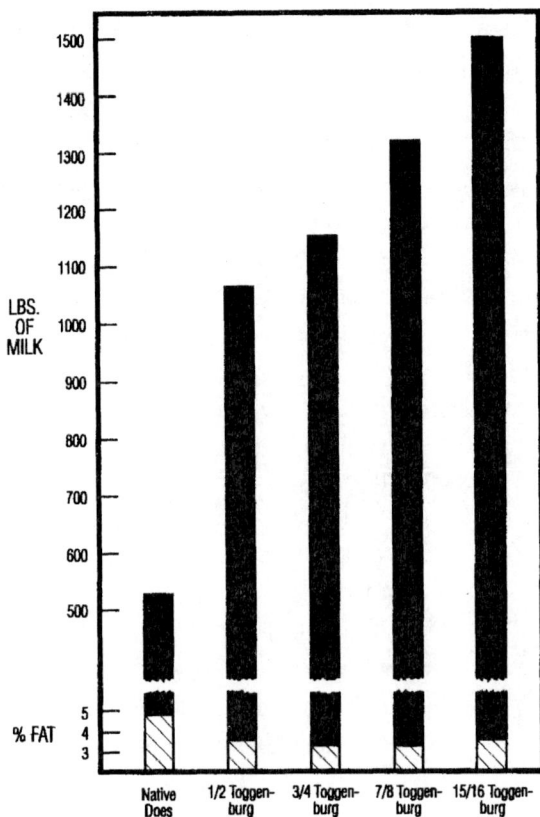

**Figure 28.2.** Improvement in milk production resulting from use of good purebred bucks on grade or native does. (New Mexico Agr. Exp. Sta.)

## Artificial Insemination Techniques

The artificial insemination of goats may be divided into two distinct phases: (1) collection, processing, storage, and transportation of semen, and (2) artificial insemination of the doe in estrus.

Only the goat breeder who maintains bucks for artificial insemination in his or her own herd and furnishes semen for use in other herds will be vitally concerned in semen collection and processing (Phase 1). The herd owner who purchases semen from outside sources will be concerned chiefly with insemination techniques (Phase 2) and will need to exercise proper precautions in care and handling of semen after it reaches

him or her. The success of AI depends upon the efficiency with which Phases 1 and 2 are carried out. Highly viable semen, properly handled to preserve its fertility, and does inseminated using correct techniques at the proper stage of heat are necessary for good conception rates.

## Collection, Processing, and Storage of Semen

The role of the male in reproduction is chiefly one of producing fertile spermatozoa and, under natural breeding, fertilizing the ova (eggs) shed by the female after estrus. Where artificial insemination is used, semen, which contains the spermatozoa, is collected, processed, and introduced into the female by mechanical means. Since some understanding of the anatomy and the physiology of the male reproductive system is helpful to those persons who undertake the collection and processing of semen, this subject will be briefly reviewed.

## Structure and Function— Male Reproductive Organs

The organs for reproduction are quite similar in all farm animals. A diagrammatic view of the reproductive organs of the ram, which are similar to those of the buck, is shown in Figure 28.3.

The primary organs of reproduction are the *testicles,* two in number, which are carried outside the body wall in the scrotum. The testicles have at least two functions: (1) the production of *spermatozoa* (male germ cells) and (2) the production of *endocrine* substances, *male hormones (testosterone,* particularly) that markedly affect the development and behavior of the male. The development of the

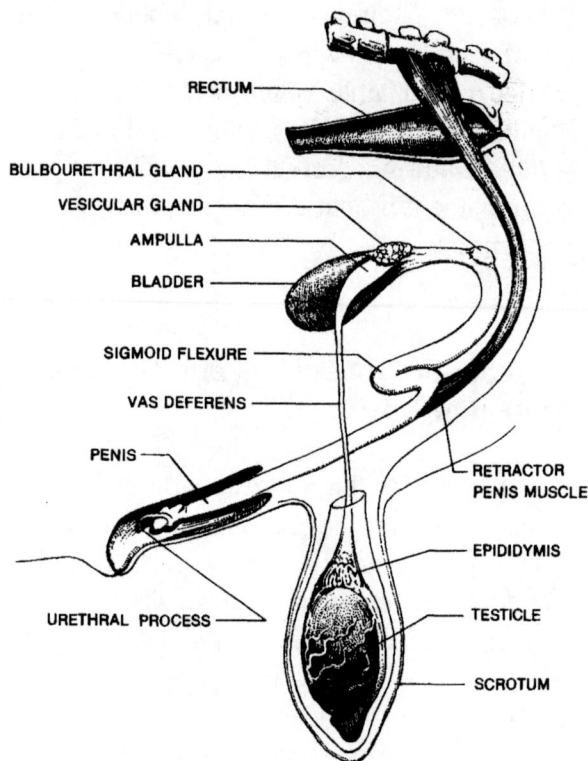

**Figure 28.3.** Diagrammatic view of reproductive organs of the ram. (Those of the buck are similar.) Reproductive structures in small ruminants (ram, buck) are much the same as in the bull (see Exercise 5). Notable differences are that small ruminants have relatively larger testicles, the prostate is entirely disseminate, bulbo-urethral glands are relatively larger, and the free end of the penis has a distinct urethral process. (M. E. Ensminger. 1986. Sheep & Goat Science [5th Ed.]. Interstate Publishers, Inc., Danville, IL. p. 350)

beard, masculine neck and body structure, as well as sex drive, is due to the male hormones.

Attached to each testicle is a convoluted duct, the *epididymis,* which extends down the outside of the testicle to its base. The epididymides have a secretory function involving hormones and enzymes necessary for maturing of the sperm. The spermatozoa, after being formed in the testicles, pass to the epididymides, where they undergo the maturing process and are subsequently stored.

Leading upward from the epididymides are the *vasa deferentia,* muscular ducts that pass through the inguinal canal into the abdominal cavity and open into the pelvic urethra. The urethra extends through the penis and pro-

vides an opening for the ejaculation of the semen. The vasa differentia enlarge to form the *ampullae,* where sperm and glandular secretions collect prior to ejaculation. Lying on either side of the ampullae are the *vesicular glands* (seminal vesicles), usually considered accessory organs. They secrete a thick, alkaline, globulin-containing fluid that becomes a part of the ejaculate and serves as a carrier for the spermatozoa.

Additional accessory glands are:

1. The *prostate,* located near the neck of the bladder and surrounding the urethra. Its function is the secretion of alkaline fluids. This gland is believed to be involved in neutralizing adverse substances in the urethra and the vagina. In the ram and the buck, the prostate gland is small and disseminated, and the body of the prostate is missing.

2. The *bulbo-urethral* or *Cowper's glands,* two in number, located on either side of the urethra. The secretions of these glands are relatively thin and watery. A part of the function is to lubricate the urethral canal and aid in transporting spermatozoa during ejaculation.

The *penis* has the function of draining the bladder and is also an organ of copulation, thus serving to introduce spermatozoa into the artificial vagina during semen collection or into the vagina of the female in natural service.

*Semen* is the normal discharge of the reproductive organs ejaculated by the male. It is a whitish-colored, somewhat thick fluid and contains spermatozoa and accessory gland secretions. The amount of semen ejaculated by a buck varies from 0.5 to 2.0 ml. The average is about 1.0 ml. The quantity varies with the age and size of the buck and is influenced by the sexual stimulation prior to ejaculation. The number of spermatozoa per milliliter varies widely but ranges from 1 to 5 billion. Goat spermatozoa typically exhibit a high rate of motility. Methods for evaluation of motility and sperm numbers will be discussed in connection with semen processing.

## Health Requirements— Bucks in AI Use

Bucks providing semen for artificial insemination purposes should be health tested regularly and be free of disease.

The principal diseases for which bucks in AI service should be tested are those that can be transmitted through semen. The following tests should be conducted routinely as long as a buck is having semen collected for AI use:

Tuberculosis—Negative intradermal tuberculin test every six months.

Brucellosis—Negative blood serum and semen plasma agglutination tests every six months.

Leptospirosis—Blood serum agglutination test for various leptospirosis serotypes every six months.

Trichomoniasis—Negative by culture microscopic examination every six months.

Campylobacteriosis (Vibriosis)—Negative by culture examination every six months.

Other health tests for various diseases may be required for the export of frozen semen. Check with regulatory authorities for specific country import health requirements for semen.

If an AI facility for bucks is maintained, new bucks that are added should be tested off the premises and be isolated until all health requirements are met before admittance and before distribution of semen.

**Figure 28.4.** Type of artificial vagina used to collect goat semen. Note the stopcocks for admission or release of air to control pressure.

Bucks maintained in private herds and furnishing semen for AI use in other herds should be kept in isolation. It is better also that they not be used for natural service.

## Collection of Semen

Semen may be obtained by one of three methods: (1) the artificial vagina (Figure 28.4), (2) electrical stimulation, or (3) collection from a doe that has been served.

Of these methods, collection by means of the artificial vagina is distinctly superior from the standpoint of obtaining normal, uncontaminated, viable semen. It is the method recommended for routine use.

Electrical stimulation works successfully in sheep and goats and is similar to procedures described for the bull (see Exercise 6). Small rectal probes for rams and bucks are commercially available for this purpose. Semen obtained by electrical stimulation is usually lower in sperm numbers and thinner in consistency than that obtained with the artificial vagina. The equipment used for electrical stimulation is cumbersome, requires skill in using, and should only be used by individuals with proper training and experience.

The collection of semen from the vagina of a recently-bred doe is possible by use of a soft-nozzle syringe. However, such semen is mixed with mucus, sloughed cells, and debris. *This is not a recommended procedure.*

## Equipment for Collection by Artificial Vagina and Equipment for Insemination

The artificial vagina used in collecting goat semen is very similar to that used with cattle except smaller. It consists of a medium-hard rubber casing about 8 inches (~20 cm) in length and about 1½ inches (~4 cm) in diameter, with a soft rubber inner liner. The inner liner of latex rubber, about 10 inches (~25 cm) in length, is placed in the casing, and each end folded over the edges and held in place by rubber bands. A stopcock may be fitted on the vagina to control air pressure. A rubber collection funnel fitted with a semen collection tube is placed on one end of the casing. The assembled artificial vagina is shown in Figure 28.4.

Before collections or inseminations are undertaken, all equipment and materials should be carefully cleaned and sterilized, laid out on a clean, dry table, and covered with a clean towel or with clean paper. The artificial vagina should be thoroughly washed in water, the casing and liner sterilized with alcohol or autoclaved, and everything allowed to dry before use. The equipment needed includes the following:

1. The artificial vagina (as described above).

2. A plastic insemination tube and poly bulb or syringe, available from AI equipment suppliers. The syringe is attached to the tube with a short piece of rubber tubing. An AI gun is used for semen packaged in straws.

3. Small sterile test tubes, 2 to 5 ml in capacity and preferably of Pyrex glass, for holding fresh semen.

4. A doe-size speculum. A Pyrex glass tube 6 inches long with inner diameter of 3/4 inch, the closed end of which has been cut off, makes a very serviceable speculum. The sharp ends of the glass speculum should be smoothed by fire-polishing before use. A metal or plastic speculum of the duckbill type may be used if desired. This speculum provides greater visibility.

5. A battery-powered headlight or penlight.

6. A funnel with rubber tubing, or a kettle with a spout for filling the artificial vagina.

7. A thermometer for checking temperature of the artificial vagina, water, and so forth.

8. Spare collection vials and liners.

## Collecting Semen by Artificial Vagina

A doe is generally used as a mount for the buck in collecting semen with the artificial vagina (Figure 28.5). If a doe in heat is available, she should be used, particularly for a young buck. After a buck has become accustomed to being collected by the artificial vagina, a doe not in heat may be used. Obviously, the buck should not be permitted to serve the doe.

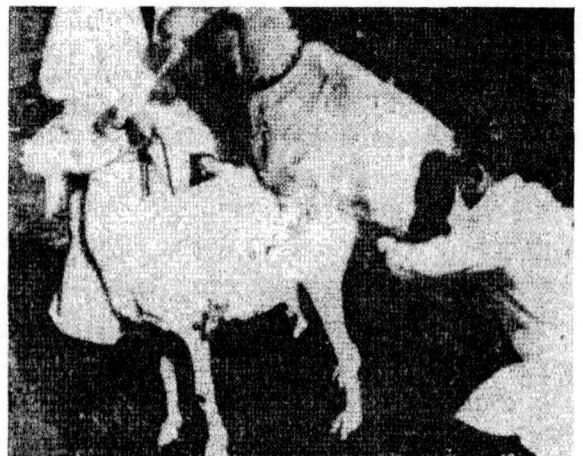

**Figure 28.5.** Collection of semen with the artificial vagina.

If possible, all collections should be made in the same quarters, as a buck quickly learns to anticipate service and will usually mount the doe, or a dummy, more quickly and readily than if in strange quarters. A breeding rack mounted on a stand 18 to 20 inches high facilitates the collection of semen but is not essential. The advantage of using a rack is that it may be set at a convenient level for collecting semen with the artificial vagina. If a rack is not used, the doe should be placed in a stanchion, be tied to a post or fence, or be held by an assistant.

The artificial vagina should be partially filled with water that has been heated to 122°F (50°C). This may be accomplished by using a rubber tube and funnel or a teakettle. The pressure inside the apparatus is properly adjusted with the right amount of water and air (introduced by mouth or attached rubber bulb). After filling, care should be taken to see that the outer surfaces of the apparatus are dry. The surface of the inner liner should then be lightly lubricated with a thin coat of non-toxic lubricant, such as K-Y jelly. A thermometer should be inserted into the artificial vagina to measure temperature. Allowance should be made for some fall in temperature between the time of preparation and collection. The temperature of the artificial vagina at the time of collection should be between 106° and 111°F (41° and 44°C). If the temperature drops below 104°F (40°C) or is above 113°F (45°C), it may inhibit ejaculation. Pressure in the artificial vagina, if too great, may be adjusted by opening a valve or, if too low, by introducing more air through the valve. The pressure needed will vary from one buck to another, but with a little experience, an operator will soon determine the proper pressure.

When the artificial vagina is ready, the operator usually holds it in the right hand, with the open end down at an angle of about 45 degrees, and stands close to the right flank of the doe. As the buck mounts, the penis is directed into the artificial vagina with the left hand,

which is grasping the sheath, care being taken not to touch the penis itself. When the penis contacts the warm, lubricated surface of the artificial vagina, the buck thrusts upward, and the semen is ejaculated into the upper end of the artificial vagina and then collected in the vial. As the buck withdraws, the apparatus is held upright to permit all of the semen to drain into the vial. The vial is then removed and stoppered. Subsequent treatment of the semen will depend on whether the semen is to be stored or used immediately.

The collector should wear new disposable plastic gloves for collecting each buck or wash hands thoroughly with soap and water between different bucks to avoid transmission of potentially infectious disease agents.

## Evaluation of Fresh Semen

The fresh semen should be checked immediately for motility (Figure 28.6). This is done by placing a drop of the semen on a glass slide that has been kept at body temperature and examining the sample under a microscope at low power. A cover slip may be used over the drop of semen if desired. Semen may be also be evaluated after addition of semen extender, which allows for better observation of individual spermatozoa. Experience soon enables the operator to roughly estimate the number of viable sperm producing the swirling current characteristics of good quality semen. Motility ranges from excellent to zero. A simple evaluation system used by workers in the Netherlands is as follows:

| Mass Motility | Percentage of Progressive Motility |
|---|---|
| 4+ Rapid cloud formation | 90–100% |
| 3+ Good cloud formation | 80–90% |
| 2+ Strong flow currents | 70–80% |
| 1+ Poor flow | 60–70% |
| — No motility | 40–60% |

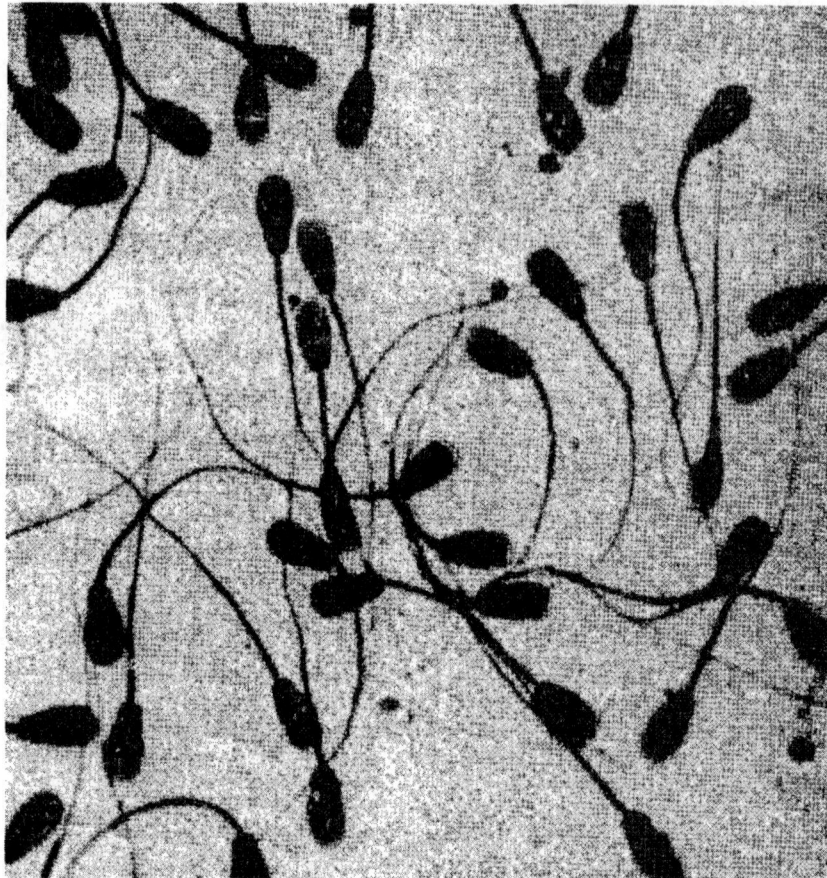

**Figure 28.6.** A sample of semen showing stained spermatozoa ×900.

Only samples with a 4+ or 3+ mass motility and above 60 percent progressive motility can be depended on for good fertilization. While motility is a good indication of viable sperm, it is not a guarantee of fertility. Several fields of view should be observed under the microscope to obtain an accurate motility estimate.

### Extension, Storage, and Shipment of Goat Semen

Goat semen may be used in the fresh state (neat semen) soon after collection; however, this is not efficient use. Semen may be extended several times the original volume so that many does can be inseminated from each ejaculate. Bucks may be collected from two to three times per week. The semen can be extended from 5 to 20 times, depending on the number of sperm present in its original volume. As many as 40 does can be bred with a single ejaculate, and during the heavy breeding season, as many as 300 per week to a single buck.

Extended semen may be used in the liquid state within one to two days after collection, or it may be frozen and stored for months. Each of these methods is outlined.

**Preparation of Liquid Semen**—Soon after collection, the semen should be gradually cooled. One volume of semen is mixed with two or three parts of the extender to be used. Both the semen and the extender should be at room temperature at the time of mixing to prevent "cold shock." A sterile glass flask, such as an Erlenmeyer flask or other suitable vessel, is used to hold the extended semen.

310

Cooling should be at a controlled rate until a temperature of 35° to 41°F (2° to 5°C) is reached. This can be conveniently accomplished by placing the flask of extended semen in a beaker of 90° to 95°F (32° to 35°C) water and setting it in the refrigerator for about two hours. The temperature can be checked at intervals by inserting a thermometer into the water surrounding the flask.

## Extenders

Semen extenders provide some nutrients for the metabolic processes of the sperm, protect against cold shock, buffer the effects of toxic substances produced by sperm metabolism, and aid in maintaining the proper osmotic pressure and mineral balance. Extenders also expand the semen volume so that many females can be inseminated. Commonly used extenders for liquid buck semen are:

1. *Milk extender*—Either fresh homogenized milk or pasteurized skimmed milk can be used. The milk is prepared by heating it to 198° to 203°F (92° to 95°C) in a covered double-boiler. Hold at 198° to 203°F (92° to 95°C) for 10 minutes. Cool to room temperature, remove scum by filtering, and add the antibiotics. Mix the milk diluent with semen at the rate described below.

2. *Yolk-citrate buffer*—This buffer is made up by preparing a solution of sodium citrate in distilled/ultrapure water. If $Na_3C_6H_5O_7 \cdot 5\frac{1}{2}H_2O$ is used, weigh out 36 g per 1,000 ml of water. If $Na_3C_6H_5O_7 \cdot 2H_2O$ is used, weigh out 30 g per 1,000 ml of water. Prepare aseptically, and mix amounts needed at one time with the addition of 20 percent by volume of fresh egg yolk.

3. *Yolk-phosphate buffer*—This is made up by dissolving 2 g $Na_2HPO_4 \cdot 12H_2O$ and 0.2 g $KH_2PO_4$ per 100 ml distilled/ultrapure water. Fresh egg yolk is added in an amount equal to 20 percent by volume of the final extender.

## Antibiotics

As a back-up to health-testing and disease-surveillance programs, for the control of potential pathogenic organisms, antibiotics should be added to the semen extender and possibly to the neat semen before extension (see Exercises 13 and 24). The addition of 1,000 μg of dihydrostreptomycin and 1,000 units of penicillin per ml of the completed extender has been recommended. Other combinations of antibiotics may be substituted following efficacy and toxicity studies.

The fully prepared extender should be used within two days after preparation and kept stored at 41°F (5°C).

## Rate of Extension

The semen may usually be extended about 5 to 20 times by volume. However, this can vary depending upon the buck. Under controlled laboratory conditions, the number of sperm is determined by means of a hemacytometer (calibrated slide of known sample volume used for blood cell counts) or by use of a photoelectric colorimeter (see Exercise 9). The total sperm (volume H concentration) multiplied by the percentage of observed motility gives the number of motile sperm per ejaculate. For example:

Volume of ejaculate = 1.5 ml
Concentration of sperm =
 3,000,000,000 per ml
Percentage of motile sperm = 80

Then, 1.5 ml of semen
 3,000,000,000 sperm per ml =
 4,500,000,000 total sperm 80%
 = 3,600,000,000 motile sperm.

Desirable numbers of motile sperm per insemination to achieve good fertility in the doe are about 150 million for liquid semen and 200 million for frozen semen[1] when deposition is in the cervix. These numbers of required sperm are much greater than for the cow, where semen is deposited in the uterus. It is likely that these numbers could also be reduced substantially for uterine insemination in the doe.[2,3] However, uterine insemination is more difficult.

If the desired inseminate volume is 0.25 ml, for this example a concentration of 600 million motile sperm per ml of extended buck semen is needed for liquid use, or 800 million motile sperm per ml is needed for use as frozen semen. The extension rates for this example are calculated as follows for liquid and frozen semen use:

### Liquid semen

3,600,000,000 motile sperm in ejaculate ÷ 600,000,000 motile sperm per ml desired = 6 ml

Thus, 1.5 ml of neat semen can be extended to 6 ml. With an insemination volume of 0.25 ml, this collection could be used to inseminate 24 does. Each inseminate would contain 150 million live sperm for cervical deposition.

### Frozen semen

3,600,000,000 motile sperm in ejaculate ÷ 800,000,000 motile sperm per ml desired = 4.5 ml

Thus, 1.5 ml of neat semen can be extended to 4.5 ml for frozen semen. With an insemination volume of 0.25 ml, this collection could produce 18 straws. Each straw would contain 200 million live sperm, the recommended inseminate number for frozen semen when deposition is in the cervix.

For different inseminate volumes or desired concentrations, the extension rate is adjusted accordingly.

**Handling Liquid Semen**—Liquid semen may be stored for a day or two in a household refrigerator at 41°F (5°C). Semen can be placed in a small vial (2 ml) filled to the top so as to exclude air. If the semen does not fill the tube, a layer of mineral oil can be placed on top of the semen. Liquid semen may also be packaged in sealed straws.

Shipping may best be done by placing the small vial, properly stoppered, labeled, and wrapped in cotton, in a large test tube. The test tube is then placed in a vacuum bottle containing cracked ice. The amount of ice varies with the time of storage or shipment. The vacuum bottle must be securely packed to avoid breakage during shipment. Alternatively, liquid semen in straws or vials may be shipped in polystyrene-foam-insulated containers with commercially available refrigerant gel packs.

Liquid semen should be used within 24 to 48 hours after collection. Bucks vary greatly in the time sperm fertility survives.

**Preparation of Frozen Buck Semen**—The successful freezing of goat semen and a desirable conception rate with thawed frozen semen were reported in the early 1960's by Drs. C. A. V. Barker[4] and A. F. Fraser[5] at the Ontario Veterinary College, Guelph, Ontario, Canada.

[1] G. Evans and W. M. C. Maxwell. 1987. Salamon's Artificial Insemination of Sheep and Goats. Butterworths, Sidney, Australia. p. 115.

[2] J. A. Fougner. 1976. Uterine insemination with frozen semen in goats. Proc. 8th International Congr. Animal Reproduction and Artificial Insemination (Krakow, Poland) 4:987.

[3] J. Aamdal. 1982. Artificial insemination in goats with frozen semen in Norway. Proc. 3rd International Conf. on Goat Production and Disease. p. 149.

[4] C. A. V. Barker. 1963. Frozen semen for A.I. in dairy goats and swine. Proc. Ann. Conv. Assoc. Anim. Breeders. p. 132.

[5] A. F. Fraser. 1962. A technique for freezing goat semen and results of a small breeding trial. Can. Vet. J. 3:133.

1. Evaluate semen for motility as described for liquid semen.

2. Wash buck sperm cells. In general, seminal plasma is detrimental to the *in vitro* survival of buck and ram semen. An enzyme contained in buck semen, in particular, acts on the phospholipids of the extender to form compounds toxic to spermatozoa. It is advisable to discard seminal plasma in buck semen as soon as possible following collection. This is accomplished by mixing the semen with the washing solution and then centrifuging it. The washing solution is usually the same as the final extending fluid *but without egg yolk.* The semen should be extended at a ratio of one volume of semen to nine volumes of the washing solution. The tube containing the mixture is centrifuged for 15 minutes at 500 to 600 µg. The supernatant is withdrawn by using a pipet and then discarded. A new volume of extender is added, and the mixture centrifuged a second time. Again, the supernatant is withdrawn and discarded. The necessary amount of the extender at 68°F (20°C) is added, and the semen is ready for processing in the fresh form or for freezing. After cooling, the final extension is made with an extender containing glycerol.

## Extenders

Semen extenders provide some nutrients for the metabolic processes of the sperm, protect against cold shock, buffer the effects of toxic substances produced by sperm metabolism, and aid in maintaining the proper osmotic pressure and mineral balance. An extender also makes possible the extension of the volume of semen so that many females can be inseminated. Commonly used extenders for buck semen are:

**Milk extender**—Either fresh homogenized milk or pasteurized skimmed milk can be used by the following treatment: Heat the milk to 198° to 203°F (92° to 95°C) in a covered double-boiler. Hold at 198° to 203°F (92° to 95°C) for 10 minutes. Cool to room temperature, remove scum by filtering, and add the antibiotics. Mix the milk extender with semen at the prescribed rate. Skimmed milk extender can also be prepared by autoclaving at 15 pounds pressure for five minutes. Many operators prefer sterile skimmed milk as an extender.

Semen is mixed with the appropriate volume of non-glycerolated skimmed milk at room temperature. This can be 1:1 or 1:2 dilution. The partially extended semen is then cooled to about 41°F (5°C) as described for liquid semen.

In order to protect sperm from damage during the freezing process, glycerol, at the rate of 14 percent by volume, is added to one-half of the final volume of the skimmed milk extender. The glycerol-containing extender is then added to the semen mixture, in four serial increments, at 10-minute intervals, to bring about the desired total extension. The quantity of glycerol-containing extender added by steps should be 10, 20, 30, and 40 percent, respectively. It is desirable to have a glycerol volume of 7 percent in the final extended glycerolated semen.

**Tris extender**—The tris extender is successfully used by several laboratories in the United States and in some other countries.

The basic tris–citric acid buffer solution should be prepared aseptically and may be stored at 41°F (5°C) for one to two weeks. The formulas for Buffer I and Buffer II follow:

| Ingredients | Buffer I | Buffer II |
|---|---|---|
| Tris | 30.28 g | 30.28 g |
| Citric acid monohydrate | 17.0 g | 17.0 g |
| Fructose or glucose | 12.5 g | 12.5 g |
| Double-distilled/ultrapure water | 1,000 ml | 840 ml |
| Glycerol | — | 160 ml* |

---

*175 ml or 14% may also be used. Volume of water is adjusted accordingly.

To prepare for use, add 250 ml of egg yolk to each liter (1,000 ml). The egg yolk should be from fresh eggs (not over 24 to 48 hours old), and the white (albumin) and the yolk membrane must be completely removed. The buffer composition is then 20 percent egg yolk. Antibiotics—1,000 µg (1 mg) of dihydrostreptomycin per ml and 1,000 units of penicillin per ml—are added. The extenders should be stored at 41°F (5°C) and be used within two days of preparation.

Semen, after collection and evaluation, is added to Extender I (Buffer I + egg yolk), which has been warmed to the same temperature as the semen. After the mixture has been cooled to 41°F (5°C), additional Extender I is added to make ½ the final volume. Or, if desired, sufficient extender to make ½ the final volume may be added initially. Then, to glycerolate, before freezing, an equal volume of Extender II (Buffer II + egg yolk) is either added by fractions over a one-hour period or added all at one time. If the sperm are washed before extension, the extender used should be the same one in which the semen will be cooled.

After the glycerol addition and equilibration, the semen is packaged, usually in 0.25-ml or 0.5-ml straws, and frozen.

***Skimmed milk extender***—There is evidence that egg yolk may be harmful to goat sperm. Chemineau[6] reports that French workers do not use extenders containing egg yolk but instead employ a physiological solution (Krebs-Ringer-Phosphate-Glucose) diluent for washing the sperm. The extender for buck semen recommended by the French workers is as follows:

Dissolve 194 mg of anhydrous glucose in 100 ml of double-distilled/ultrapure water. Add 10 g of skimmed milk powder to the sugar solution. Boil in a water bath for 15 minutes. Cool to room temperature. Add 50 mg of streptomycin and 50,000 IU of penicillin. May be stored two to three days at 41°F (5°C).

Prepare the glycerol-containing fraction by adding 14 percent glycerol to the above ex-

tender. Cool the semen in the non-glycerol fraction, and then add an equal volume of the glycerol-containing fraction. This will result in a final glycerol concentration of 7 percent.

The extended semen should then be allowed to set at 41°F (5°C) for two to three hours for equilibration before freezing. This step is believed necessary to condition the sperm cells and reduce subsequent damage during freezing.

***Commercial extenders***—There are various goat semen extenders in kit form on the market. These extenders may require the addition of distilled/ultrapure water, egg yolk, and/or glycerol based on directions of suppliers. Contact IMV International Corporation and Viam Pac for details.

**Packaging**—The cooled extended semen should be placed in straws (or glass ampules) for freezing. Straws holding 0.25 ml to 0.5 ml or glass ampules holding 0.5 ml to 1.0 ml are available and in use for frozen semen. The straws or ampules should be clearly labeled. There are printing machines made to do this. The name and code number of the buck and the collection code (date) should appear on the container. The extended semen is packaged into individual units by means of vacuum or pipet. Filled straws are sealed by ultrasound, plastic plugs, or powder plugs, depending upon the equipment used. Filled ampules are sealed by means of a flame applied to the tip.

**Freezing**—The goal in freezing semen is to decrease the temperature from 41° to −320°F (5° to −196°C) in gradual steps to avoid damaging delicate sperm cell membranes. This can be done by utilizing cryogenic

---

[6] P. Chemineau, et al. 1991. Training Manual on Artificial Insemination in Sheep and Goats. Publications Division, Food and Agriculture Organization (FAO) of the United Nations, Via delle Termedi Caracalla, 00100, Rome, Italy. p. 150.

nitrogen vapor or a dry ice and alcohol bath, as follows.

## Nitrogen Vapor Freezing Method

A widely used method for freezing semen is the nitrogen vapor method. With this method the straws or ampules of semen to be frozen are simply placed in a rack and positioned in the upper portion (vapor phase) of a wide-mouthed liquid nitrogen semen storage unit or one of the types used for storing cattle semen. Freezing at the desired rate is accomplished in about 5 minutes for straws and 30 minutes for ampules. The liquid nitrogen container must have at least 2 to 3 inches of $LN_2$ at the bottom. The semen is frozen by the vapor. It should not be placed directly in the liquid nitrogen during the freezing process. However, after the appropriate freezing period, the units should be submerged in liquid nitrogen.

## Dry Ice and Alcohol Freezing Method

The dry ice and alcohol method consists of adding dry ice gradually to an alcohol bath and checking temperatures so that freezing is at the following rate:

| | |
|---|---|
| 41° to 32°F (5° to 0°C) | 30 minutes |
| 32° to 23°F (0° to −5°C) | 10 minutes |
| 23° to 9°F (−5 to −13°C) | 5 minutes |
| 9° to 2°F (−13 to −17°C) | 3½ minutes |
| 2° to −110°F (−17° to −79°C) | 15½ minutes |

A temperature of −110°F (−79°C) is the lower limit available through the use of dry ice and alcohol. The present universal refrigerant is liquid nitrogen (−320°F [−196°C]).

If all processing steps have been properly carried out, semen frozen in nitrogen vapor or in a dry ice and alcohol mixture may be stored in the liquid nitrogen container for months, if desired, without material loss of fertility.

## Structure and Function— Female Reproductive Organs

Persons who expect to artificially inseminate goats or sheep should study the anatomy and physiology of the female reproductive tract in detail (Figure 28.7). Any of several books on animal reproduction will furnish this information. It is recommended that reproductive organs of slaughtered does and ewes also be studied so that the operator has a good mental image of the anatomical arrangement.

The essential organs of reproduction in the female are the *ovaries*, two in number, which produce the ova, or eggs, that unite with the sperm to form the new individual. The ovaries produce hormones responsible for estrus, maintenance of pregnancy, and finally parturition. The ovaries are influenced by the gonadotrophic hormones of the pituitary gland, located at the base of the brain. The *Fallopian tubes* (oviducts) convey the ova, when shed by the ovaries, to the uterus. Fertilization of an

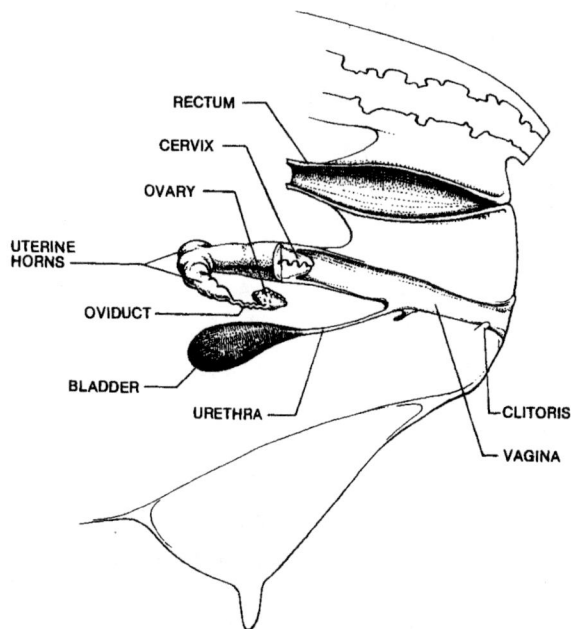

**Figure 28.7.** Diagrammatic view of reproductive organs of the ewe. (Those of the doe are quite similar.) (M. E. Ensminger. 1986. Sheep & Goat Science [5th Ed.]. Interstate Publishers, Inc., Danville, IL p. 352)

ovum, or egg, by the spermatozoon generally takes place in the upper portion of the Fallopian tube. The *uterus,* or womb, is a thick-walled, muscular organ with two branches, or horns. The growing fetus is carried in the uterus and expelled at the time of birth. The *cervix* is a thick-walled, muscular organ in the doe or ewe and is about an inch in length. It is sometimes called the *os uteri,* as it is the opening to the uterus. Semen is usually deposited in the cervix or the uterus during artificial insemination. During heat (estrus), the cervix usually relaxes slightly. During parturition, it expands greatly. The cervix opens posteriorly into the vagina. The *vagina,* which is an organ of copulation, extends from the cervix to the vulva. The *vestibule* of the vagina is common to both the reproductive tract and the urinary tract and is of greater diameter than the vagina. The vestibule is between the vagina proper and the vulva, or external opening of the genital tract.

## Insemination of the Doe

The breeding season for goats is mainly from September to January, although some may breed earlier or later. The limited breeding season makes heat detection of utmost importance. High conception results when breeding starts early in the fall, allowing ample time for return services. It is important to record any heat dates prior to breeding to know the estrous cycle of each doe.

**Detecting Heat**—The signs of heat are mainly changes in behavior. Most noticeable are frequent nervous bleating and an apparent twitching of the tail, particularly when in the presence of other goats. Decrease in milk flow and an inconsistent appetite may be observed. Swelling and change in color of the external genital organs are evident. There is a slight genital mucus discharge, which becomes whitish as the heat period progresses. The doe will attempt to familiarize with a buck when one is near. A doe showing one or more of these signs or actions should be considered in heat or coming into heat. The success of artificial breeding in goats is primarily determined by the owner's ability to observe heat signs.

Insemination may be carried out most easily if the doe is placed in a crate that stands 18 to 20 inches off the ground. If a crate is not available, the doe may stand on a table, with a stanchion or tie arranged.

Insemination may also be performed when an attendant lifts the doe by the rear quarters so that the feet are 10 to 12 inches off the floor (Figure 28.8).

**Thawing Semen**—In general, straws should be allowed to thaw in warm water (99°F [37°C]) for at least 30 seconds. However, *purchasers of frozen semen should use the thawing method recommended by the supplier.* Insemination guns with disposable sheaths are commercially available for use with 0.25-ml and 0.5-ml straws.

If ampules are used, frozen semen may be thawed in iced water (40°F [4°C]) or in water at 50° to 68°F (10° to 20°C). Let all of the ice on the ampule melt. When thawing is com-

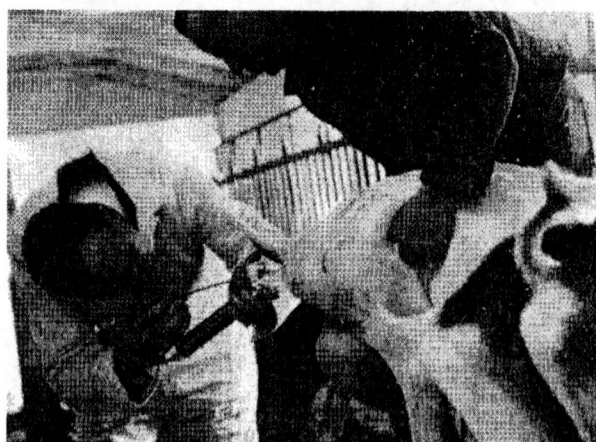

**Figure 28.8.** Inseminating the doe. An attendant lifts the rear quarters of the doe so that the feet are a few inches off the floor.

plete, remove the top of the ampule by using a file or ampule scribe, and draw the semen into the inseminating catheter. (*Note:* Some evidence shows that thawing the ampule at 99°F [37°C] in a small volume of water gives equally good results as the 50° to 68°F [10° to 20°C] method).

## Insemination Technique

Two insemination methods are available: (1) depositing semen in the cervix or the uterus by using a speculum (Figure 28.9) and (2) depositing semen in the vagina by simply introducing the insemination tube and expelling the semen. The latter method is known as "blind insemination" and is not recommended except for young does with which the use of a speculum is limited. Conception results are much lower by the "blind insemination" method than by the speculum method.

**Speculum Method**—The AI gun, insemination tube, or catheter with attached syringe or poly bulb should be loaded or filled and made ready for service. The straw system and

the AI gun are preferable. However, if ampules or other semen-packaging methods are used, it is recommended that plastic insemination tubes and poly bulbs be used. These items are disposable, inexpensive, and available at most AI supply houses.

When the doe is in position, either in the breeding rack with the hindquarters elevated or standing on the ground with the rear quarters lifted about 10 to 12 inches by an attendant, wipe the vulva clean with cotton gauze or a paper towel and apply a small amount of non-toxic lubricant to the vulva. While holding the doe's tail, slowly introduce the ¾-inch diameter speculum by gently rotating it and pushing it downward. By the aid of a headlight or penlight, gently move the speculum and locate the cervix (a small rosette-shaped structure with a central opening). (There is a commercially available speculum that has a light incorporated into its end, which facilitates finding the cervix and eliminates the need for a headlight or penlight.) When the cervix is located, introduce the AI gun or insemination tube about ½ to ¾ inch into the cervical canal. At the same time, holding the insemination tube in place, draw the speculum

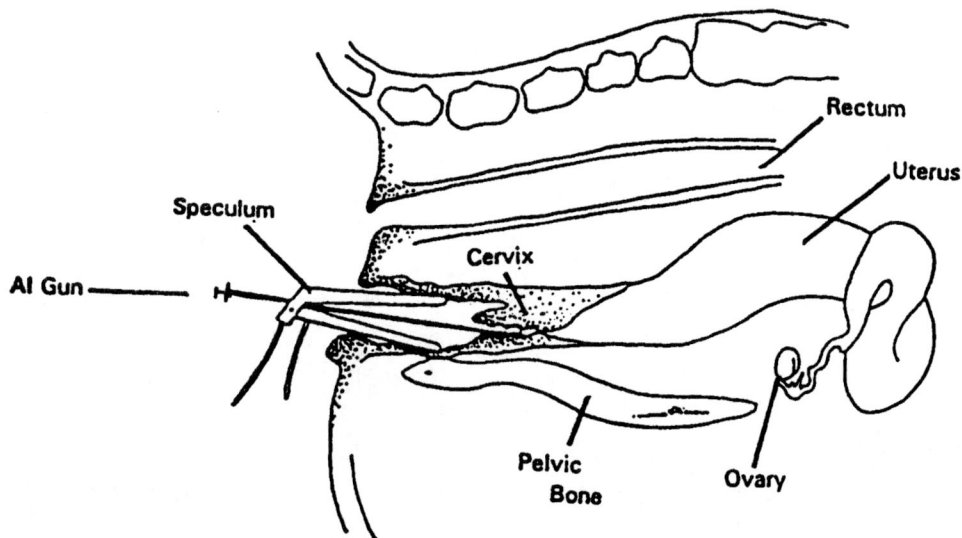

**Figure 28.9.** Schematic illustration of insemination in the doe by use of the speculum (duck-billed type) inserted into the vagina. Note the tip of the AI gun is placed midway through the cervical canal.

back about ¼ inch. Slowly expel the semen from the AI gun or insemination tube using gentle pressure on the plunger or poly bulb. When all the semen is expelled, withdraw the insemination tube and the speculum, but keep the doe's hindquarters elevated for another two or three minutes. This prevents loss of semen by expulsion of mucus from the cervix. The inseminated doe should be kept apart from the remainder of the herd until all signs of heat have disappeared.

**Blind Insemination**—For the insemination of virgin kids, a speculum ½ inch in diameter can be used and the same technique as outlined above followed. If it is apparent that the introduction of the smaller speculum will be difficult, the insemination tube containing the semen can be introduced into the vagina through the vulva. The tube should be directed as near as possible to the likely position of the cervix, and the semen expelled.

## Intrauterine Insemination

Some goat herd operators prefer intrauterine insemination. Using this method, the preparation of the doe in heat and the techniques for inserting the speculum and locating the cervix are the same as outlined above. The insemination tube is introduced into the cervical opening and gently worked through the cervix until the tube is barely past the last annular fold. The semen is slowly deposited into the uterus over a period of five seconds. In a young doe or in a doe not at the maximum stage of heat, difficulty will be encountered in passing the insemination tube through the cervix. Under these conditions it is best to deposit the semen in the mid-cervix. In many cases, the cervix of a mature doe in heat is not sufficiently relaxed to permit easy passage of the insemination tube. Forcing the tube through the cervix may cause injury to the delicate tissues, resulting in infection. Care must be taken to avoid such injuries. The AI gun for the straw system is generally smaller in diameter than plastic insemination tubes, and some types have a flexible tip that facilitates passage through the cervix.

## Stage of Heat to Breed

Insemination should be made during the last half of estrus or at 12-hour intervals as long as estrus lasts. The estrous cycle of the doe is about 18 to 21 days in length. Does remain in heat from about 24 to 48 hours, though the average is about 30 hours. If in doubt as to the time a doe came in heat, she should be inseminated two or three times at 6-hour intervals. (See Figure 28.10.)

**Conception Rate Expected**—It is not expected that artificial insemination in goats can exceed natural mating in efficiency. However, it should compare favorably, as does the comparison between natural and artificial insemination in cattle.

Results with liquid semen indicate that 65 to 75 percent of the does will settle on the first service. Figures for frozen semen indicate closely similar results. However, the ability of buck semen to withstand freezing varies widely, and results can be inconsistent. The solution is to utilize for frozen semen only those bucks that have demonstrated a desirable conception rate, Figure 28.11.

## Determining Pregnancy in Goats

It is generally assumed that does that fail to come into heat 22 to 24 days following breeding are pregnant. For a variety of reasons, there are some breeding failures. The result is often a long dry period for the doe, in addition to added breeding and feeding costs. If it can be determined some 22 to 24 days following breeding whether or not a doe is pregnant, loss of time and money can be avoided.

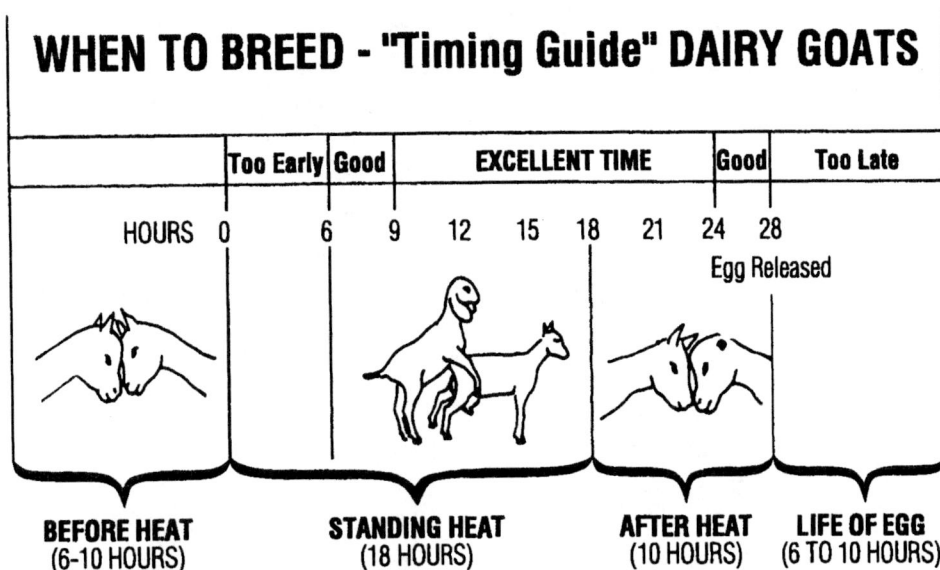

## WHEN TO BREED - "Timing Guide" DAIRY GOATS

| | Too Early | Good | EXCELLENT TIME | | | | Good | Too Late |

HOURS  0    6   9   12   15   18   21   24   28

Egg Released

BEFORE HEAT (6-10 HOURS)  STANDING HEAT (18 HOURS)  AFTER HEAT (10 HOURS)  LIFE OF EGG (6 TO 10 HOURS)

Determine your doe's heat cycle. It will vary with the season and from doe to doe.
AI is very successful in the standing-heat period as well as the after-heat period.

**Figure 28.10.** Timing guide for the artificial insemination of goats. (Dairy Goat Journal, August 1979, p. 20)

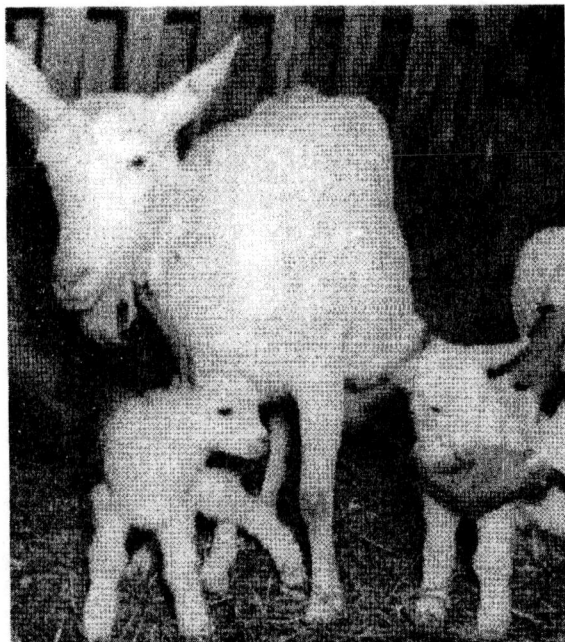

**Figure 28.11.** Twin kids born from a Saanen doe inseminated with frozen semen stored for 331 days after collection. (Courtesy, Dr. C. A. V. Barker, Ontario Veterinary College, Guelph, Ontario, Canada)

## The Milk Progesterone Test

The milk progesterone test for an early determination of non-pregnancy in cows and dairy goats is in general use worldwide. The test is made by measuring progesterone levels in milk samples collected from does 22 to 24 days after insemination. Preferably the milk samples collected are about the same volume as used for routine butterfat tests. The milk can be frozen until an assay is made, or it may be treated with preservatives. The assay of progesterone in the milk is made by radioimmunoassay. There are commercial laboratories conducting the test. However, on-farm test kits are also available (see Exercise 19).

**Accuracy of the Test**—In non-pregnant does with milk samples taken 22 to 24 days after insemination, results of the assay are nearly 100 percent accurate. For pregnant does, results are only about 75 to 80 percent accurate, since there can be pathological conditions of the reproductive tract, early embryonic death, and other abnormalities in reproduction that may confound the test interpretation. A higher correlation is probably not possible.

## Genetic Improvement Program

The dairy goat improvement program in the United States is administered through the National Dairy Herd Improvement (DHI) Program, and bucks are being sampled by the multiple-herd method. With an increasing number of daughters per buck, genetic measures of transmitting ability are being applied. USDA genetic evaluations list predicted transmitting abilities (PTA's) and reliability (Rel.) values or accuracy for traits of economic importance. Does are also evaluated for transmitting ability using the same measures applied to bucks. Does have a relatively low number of offspring; thus, it is difficult to obtain large numbers for genetic evaluation. In the present national improvement program, only the top

5 percent of does with recent kiddings are summarized.

An example of the summary used for bucks and does is shown in Table 28.1A and Table 28.1B, as reported by the USDA in July 2001. It will be noted (Table 28.1A) that the more tested daughters a buck has in multiple herds, the higher the reliability of the predicted transmitting ability. In the case of does, the more tested progeny with lactations, the higher the reliability of the proof.

Breed production averages in 2000 are shown in Table 28.2. As plus-progeny-proven bucks are used and the DHI testing program followed, production values should improve continually.

Table 28.3 lists state and national dairy goat herd statistics and production characteristics.

Goat breeders should contact their state dairy specialist, Agricultural Extension Service offices, and their state DHI association regarding participation in the National DHI Program.

**Table 28.1A.** Alpine USDA-DHIA Genetic Evaluations for Bucks with Recent Daughters for 2001[a]

| Registration Number | Name | Herds | Daus. | Lacts. | Rel. | Milk | Fat | | Prot. | | Pctile |
|---|---|---|---|---|---|---|---|---|---|---|---|
| | | | | | (%) | (lbs.) | (lbs.) | (%) | (lbs.) | (%) | |
| A180852680 | REDWOODHILLS ODYSSEY | 7 | 43 | 98 | 78 | 139 | 5.3 | 0.01 | 3.3 | −0.04 | 85 |
| A180879671 | SEMPERVIRENS BING CHERRY | 4 | 87 | 115 | 70 | 158 | 5.8 | 0.00 | 4.0 | −0.04 | 89 |
| A180602519 | SHAHENA'KO TC BRUT | 20 | 55 | 132 | 84 | 93 | 7.8 | 0.18 | 3.2 | 0.01 | 88 |
| A000916281 | STONEGATE HOLLI HALOGEN | 2 | 12 | 26 | 52 | 8 | 6.8 | 0.27 | 3.3 | 0.12 | 85 |
| A000982325 | SUNSHINE CONIT COUNTER | 1 | 38 | 49 | 57 | 230 | 6.4 | −0.08 | 4.2 | −0.11 | 90 |

Predicted Transmitting Abilities

[a]USDA-AIPL (2001).

320

**Table 28.1B.  Alpine USDA-DHIA Genetic Evaluations for Top 5% of Does with Recent Kiddings for July 2001[a]**

| Herd | Registration Number | Sire | Herds | Dau EQ | Lacts. | Predicted Transmitting Abilities | | | | | |
|---|---|---|---|---|---|---|---|---|---|---|---|
| | | | | | | Rel. | Milk | Fat | | Prot. | |
| | | | | | | (%) | (lbs.) | (lbs.) | (%) | (lbs.) | (%) |
| 21-03-5001 | 21CDJ0225 | 180974412 | 1 | 0.0 | 4 | 47 | 268 | 11.6 | 0.07 | 8.6 | 0.01 |
| 21-03-5001 | 21CDJ0276 | 180920015 | 1 | 0.0 | 2 | 49 | 335 | 10.4 | −0.07 | 7.6 | −0.10 |
| 21-10-5434 | 181065992 | 181033127 | 2 | 1.5 | 2 | 48 | 289 | 11.3 | 0.02 | 7.1 | −0.07 |
| 21-10-5454 | 16CDJ0120 | 180974412 | 1 | 1.5 | 4 | 56 | 354 | 8.0 | −0.18 | 8.3 | −0.10 |
| 21-10-5454 | 181049970 | 000720150 | 1 | 0.0 | 4 | 57 | 394 | 12.7 | −0.06 | 92 | −0.11 |

[a]USDA-AIPL (2001).


**Table 28.2.  ADGA Breed Averages—2000 Lactations[a]**

| Does 275-305 Days in Milk | N= | Avg. Age at Start of Lactation | Milk Lbs. | Range | Butterfat % | Protein % |
|---|---|---|---|---|---|---|
| Alpine | 883 | 3y0m | 2201 | 640-4686 | 3.4 | 2.9 |
| La Mancha | 281 | 3y1m | 2026 | 740-3975 | 4.0 | 3.3 |
| Nubian | 525 | 3y0m | 1783 | 560-5070 | 4.8 | 3.8 |
| Oberhasli | 77 | 2y7m | 1890 | 490-3450 | 3.5 | 2.9 |
| Saanen | 453 | 2y6m | 2383 | 810-5470 | 3.5 | 3.0 |
| Toggenburg | 359 | 3y0m | 2070 | 740-4230 | 3.3 | 2.8 |

[a]Based on 2000 ADGA DHIR Individual Doe Records.
Averages compiled by the ADGA Production Testing Committee.
**NOTE:** Protein averages include both true and crude protein for 2000.


Artificial insemination can play a major role in dairy goat improvement if several requirements are met, namely:

1. A continual supply of fertile buck semen, either fresh or frozen, must be available. This can be accomplished best if a syndicate of local or state dairy goat breeders cooperates in getting the potentially best bucks available used by AI in many herds.

2. There should be good cooperation between goat herd owners and a local AI business or its technician to provide service. No AI business can afford service for goats unless there is a sufficient volume of business to make it worthwhile.

3. Production testing of the progeny through the DHI association is essential and must be a vital part of any improvement program.

**Table 28.3.** Averages of Official DHI Goat Herds, by State, 2001[a]

| State | Herds | Doe-Years | Doe-Years per Herd | Milk (lb) | Fat (%) | Fat (lbs.) | Protein[b] Doe-years (%) | Protein (%) | Protein (lbs.) |
|---|---|---|---|---|---|---|---|---|---|
| Alabama | · | · | · | · | · | · | · | · | · |
| Alaska | · | · | · | · | · | · | · | · | · |
| Arizona | 4 | 27 | 7 | 1,877 | 3.77 | 71 | 77 | 3.28 | 68 |
| Arkansas | 5 | 82 | 17 | 1,614 | 3.63 | 59 | 100 | 2.94 | 47 |
| California | 48 | 1,356 | 29 | 2,065 | 3.55 | 73 | 97 | 3.00 | 62 |
| Colorado | 13 | 229 | 18 | 1,935 | 3.64 | 70 | 100 | 3.14 | 61 |
| Connecticut | 3 | 33 | 11 | 1,813 | 3.36 | 61 | 100 | 2.83 | 51 |
| Delaware | · | · | · | · | · | · | · | · | · |
| Florida | 6 | 59 | 10 | 1,375 | 3.62 | 50 | 70 | 3.26 | 47 |
| Georgia | 1 | 3 | 3 | 2,879 | 3.68 | 106 | 100 | 3.16 | 91 |
| Hawaii | · | · | · | · | · | · | · | · | · |
| Idaho | 7 | 180 | 26 | 1,836 | 3.50 | 64 | 100 | 2.89 | 53 |
| Illinois | 8 | 176 | 22 | 1,849 | 3.94 | 73 | 100 | 3.05 | 56 |
| Indiana | 16 | 374 | 24 | 1,430 | 3.69 | 53 | 100 | 2.99 | 43 |
| Iowa | 9 | 835 | 93 | 2,016 | 3.62 | 73 | 100 | 2.94 | 59 |
| Kansas | 10 | 111 | 11 | 1,786 | 3.97 | 71 | 90 | 3.02 | 56 |
| Kentucky | 3 | 55 | 19 | 1,704 | 4.17 | 71 | 100 | 3.48 | 59 |
| Louisiana | · | · | · | · | · | · | · | · | · |
| Maine | 15 | 175 | 12 | 1,392 | 3.52 | 49 | 100 | 3.05 | 43 |
| Maryland | 14 | 201 | 14 | 1,725 | 3.88 | 67 | 90 | 3.08 | 55 |
| Massachusetts | 6 | 41 | 7 | 1,861 | 3.94 | 73 | 100 | 3.01 | 56 |
| Michigan | 15 | 108 | 7 | 1,824 | 4.04 | 74 | 90 | 3.28 | 60 |
| Minnesota | 19 | 836 | 44 | 1,822 | 3.58 | 65 | 100 | 3.12 | 57 |
| Mississippi | 1 | 21 | 21 | 1,326 | 4.22 | 56 | 100 | 3.17 | 42 |
| Missouri | 6 | 73 | 12 | 2,143 | 4.30 | 92 | 100 | 3.40 | 73 |
| Montana | 2 | 29 | 15 | 1,244 | 3.54 | 44 | 100 | 3.28 | 41 |
| Nebraska | 2 | 64 | 32 | 2,122 | 3.45 | 73 | 100 | 2.92 | 62 |
| Nevada | 1 | 33 | 33 | 1,187 | 4.30 | 51 | 100 | 3.37 | 40 |
| New Hampshire | 6 | 95 | 16 | 1,319 | 4.19 | 55 | 100 | 3.23 | 43 |
| New Jersey | 5 | 40 | 8 | 1,810 | 4.16 | 75 | 100 | 3.00 | 54 |
| New Mexico | 2 | 14 | 7 | 1,765 | 4.04 | 71 | 100 | 3.60 | 63 |
| New York | 19 | 838 | 45 | 2,034 | 3.53 | 72 | 100 | 2.96 | 60 |
| North Carolina | 4 | 54 | 13 | 1,596 | 3.05 | 49 | 100 | 2.83 | 45 |
| North Dakota | 1 | 12 | 12 | 891 | 4.38 | 39 | 100 | 3.03 | 27 |
| Ohio | 20 | 990 | 50 | 1,538 | 3.74 | 57 | 96 | 3.00 | 47 |
| Oklahoma | 6 | 73 | 12 | 1,569 | 4.24 | 67 | 100 | 3.63 | 57 |
| Oregon | 56 | 727 | 13 | 1,707 | 3.87 | 66 | 90 | 3.07 | 53 |
| Pennsylvania | 23 | 610 | 27 | 1,811 | 3.70 | 67 | 100 | 3.04 | 55 |
| Puerto Rico | · | · | · | · | · | · | · | · | · |

| | | | | | | | | | |
|---|---|---|---|---|---|---|---|---|---|
| Rhode Island | · | · | · | · | · | · | · | · | · |
| South Carolina | 3 | 29 | 10 | 1,828 | 3.09 | 57 | 100 | 2.91 | 53 |
| South Dakota | · | · | · | · | · | · | · | · | · |
| Tennessee | 7 | 85 | 12 | 1,354 | 4.30 | 58 | 100 | 3.37 | 46 |
| Texas | 11 | 173 | 16 | 1,674 | 4.24 | 71 | 96 | 3.28 | 55 |
| Utah | 5 | 205 | 41 | 1,944 | 3.70 | 72 | 100 | 2.93 | 57 |
| Vermont | 3 | 255 | 85 | 1,495 | 4.05 | 61 | 100 | 3.04 | 45 |
| Virgin Islands | · | · | · | · | · | · | · | · | · |
| Virginia | 4 | 224 | 56 | 1,429 | 3.75 | 54 | 89 | 2.79 | 41 |
| Washington | 6 | 74 | 12 | 1,744 | 4.37 | 76 | 100 | 3.30 | 58 |
| West Virginia | 5 | 53 | 11 | 1,844 | 3.46 | 64 | 100 | 2.82 | 52 |
| Wisconsin | 32 | 1,769 | 56 | 1,707 | 3.78 | 65 | 90 | 3.01 | 55 |
| Wyoming | 10 | 82 | 8 | 1,529 | 3.77 | 58 | 82 | 3.06 | 46 |
| United States | 438 | 11,499 | 26 | 1,779 | 3.71 | 66 | 96 | 3.03 | 55 |

[a]USDA-AIPL (2001).

[b]Protein means are a mixture of true and crude protein.

## Artificial Insemination of Sheep

Artificial insemination of sheep is fairly limited in the United States. The larger sheep flocks are grazed on range land involving many acres, and the use of AI is not practical. However, there is some interest in the Midwest and the East, and in areas where flocks are smaller. Labor costs are a deterrent to the wide use of sheep AI in America, but it is used more extensively in some other countries, particularly Russia and Australia.

Some of the chief advantages of AI in sheep are (1) use of the best rams is increased, (2) genetic improvement is accelerated, (3) crossbreeding opportunities are more available, and (4) AI lowers ram costs.

The anatomy and physiology of goats and sheep are very similar. Consequently, the insemination techniques are similar. Refer to the preceding sections on dairy goat AI.

In general, to use AI in sheep, (1) the ewe flock should be confined and checked for heat twice daily, (2) teaser rams, either vasectomized or fitted with an apron with soft crayon applied, should be used to mark ewes in heat, and (3) sheep must be bred during their sexual season, which is usually in the fall of the year.

In some instances, heat synchronizing is utilized. The synchronizing agents listed in Appendix C are generally used. The estrus period of the ewe averages about 30 hours. Ovulation occurs in the last part of the estrus period, and the optimum time for insemination is about 12 to 15 hours after the beginning of estrus.

The average ram ejaculate is about 1.0 to 1.5 ml in volume and can contain from 1 to 3 billion sperm. Extenders for ram semen are the same as those listed for goat semen. The semen dilution rate is usually about 1:3, depending on the sperm concentration. The insemination dose can vary from 0.25 to 1.0 ml and should contain from 150 to 200 million viable sperm for cervical insemination, using liquid or frozen thawed semen, respectively. For laparoscopy insemination, about 20 million sperm per insemination seems to be adequate. Cervical insemination by means of a speculum, as described for the goat, is recommended. Intrauterine insemination through the cervix is more of a challenge due to the anatomical structure of the cervix. A fiber optic breeding device has been developed (Gourley

Scope) that facilitates deposition of semen into the uterus of the ewe (or other species) through the cervix. Several options are available, but training in use of the fiber optic device is required. Many operators use surgical means (laparoscopy) to introduce the semen directly into the uterine horns. This method requires less semen and results in a higher pregnancy rate than the cervical method.

However, the laparoscopy method requires skill and special equipment. One organization has offered a laparoscopic AI service for ewes at several locations throughout the central and western U.S. Refer to Chapter 15 of *Salamon's Artificial Insemination of Sheep and Goats*, listed in the references, for more specific information on sheep AI.

## QUESTIONS—DAIRY GOAT AI

1. Of what advantage is artificial insemination to the average dairy goat owner?
2. What can be done to make more production-proven bucks available through artificial insemination?
3. How is semen obtained from a buck? Which method is most widely used?
4. What extenders are generally used for buck semen in the liquid state? For frozen semen?
5. How is heat detected in the doe? What months of the year constitute the usual breeding season for dairy goats?
6. What are the steps to be carried out in inseminating a doe with frozen semen?

## QUESTIONS—SHEEP AI

1. Why isn't artificial insemination in sheep used more widely? What are its advantages and disadvantages?
2. How should the ewe herd be managed for the use of AI?
3. What are the two methods recommended for insemination in the ewe?
4. To what extent may ram semen be extended?
5. What is the gestation period for the ewe?
6. How successful is synchronization of estrus in sheep?

# REFERENCES

Chemineau, P., et al. 1991. Training Manual on Artificial Insemination in Sheep and Goats. Publications Division, Food and Agriculture Organization (FAO) of the United Nations, Via delle Termedi Caracalla, 00100, Rome, Italy. (Chs. in Part II.)

Evans, G., and W. M. C. Maxwell. 1987. Salamon's Artificial Insemination of Sheep and Goats. Butterworths, Sydney, Australia.

Extension Goat Handbook. 1984. Agr. Ext. Serv., USDA, Washington, DC.

Hafez, E. S. E. (Ed.). 1987. Reproduction in Farm Animals (5th Ed.). Lea & Febiger, Philadelphia. (Chs. 23, 25, 28.)

Herman, H. A. 1982. Artificial Insemination and Genetic Improvement of Dairy Goats. American Supply House, P.O. Box 1114, Columbia, MO 65205.

Proc. 3rd International Conf. on Goat Production and Disease. 1982. Dairy Goat Journal Publishing Co., P.O. Box 1808, Scottsdale, AZ 85252. (pp. 147, 469, and 537.)

Sorenson, A. M., Jr. 1979. Animal Reproduction: Principles and Practices. McGraw-Hill, New York.

Also current literature, Dairy Goat Journal, and the Farm Press.

# EXERCISE 29

# Artificial Insemination of Other Farm Animals and Additional Species

## OBJECT

To become familiar, with the use of artificial insemination for other farm animals and species.

## DISCUSSION

Artificial insemination and other biotechniques are being utilized today in the reproductive processes of most mammals. The greatest AI activity is in cattle, as described in the foregoing exercises. However, AI is also playing an important role in dairy goat breeding, swine production, and horse production. Poultry producers, especially turkey growers, utilize AI quite heavily to improve the fertility of hatching eggs. AI is widely used for laboratory animals and in programs to propagate endangered species in zoological park programs. Apiarists use AI for the fertilization of queen honey bees. There is a growing use of AI and *in vitro* fertilization in humans. The research and developments in these areas are steadily bringing forth new knowledge and techniques.

Follow progress for the listed farm animals and species as reported in the agricultural press, breeding journals, and scientific publications.

A brief review follows of AI in other farm animals and species.

## Artificial Insemination in Swine

Artificial insemination, with semen from progeny-tested boars, that transmit genetic characteristics for efficient growth and production of lean meat, is well established among global hog producers.

Swine AI has been widely used for some time in Russia, China, Japan, Europe Scandinavia, and in other countries and regions having large swine numbers. In North America, increasing numbers of hog producers are now using AI routinely. In the U.S. alone there has been an explosion in AI growth over the past decade. For example, less than 10 percent of sows were bred by AI in 1990 and by 2000, approximately 60 percent of sows were bred by AI. It is expected that by 2005, 80 percent of all litters farrowed in the U.S. will be the result of AI.[1]

The chief advantages of swine AI involving superior progeny-tested boars are:

1. Fewer boars are needed, and genetic improvements are made in the herd.

2. Housing and feeding costs are reduced when fewer boars are kept.

3. Risk of disease is greatly reduced because fewer purchased boars are added to the herd. (In fact, all boars could be housed away from the sow herd and AI used, thus reducing exposure to diseases.)

4. The number of boars and sows for sale that have superior genetics is increased.

---

[1] C. E. Kuster and G. C. Althouse. 2001. State of swine theriogenology. Proc. Ann. Conf. and Canine Symp.—Soc. for Theriogenology/ACT, Vancouver, B.C.

5. There is less risk of injury to the sows, the boar, and the people handling them when AI is used.

Currently there are approximately 115 boar collection centers in the U.S. that service close to 4 million sows. These include cooperative boar studs, commercial boar studs, commercial studs affiliated with an association, and boar studs owned by a swine production company. There are also numerous farms that collect their own boars, extend semen, and AI their own sows. Generally, swine AI service businesses sell fresh and some frozen semen, provide custom processing, on-site AI training, and sell AI supplies. Semen is sold throughout the United States and internationally. Examples of some active U.S. organizations include International Boar Semen, Eldora, Iowa, Swine Genetics International, Ltd., Cambridge, Iowa, and Lone Willow Genetics, Roanoke, Illinois. Several additional businesses are listed in advertising sections of the *National Hog Farmer* website under semen suppliers *(http:// inddustryclick.com/magazines.asp?magazine= 17&SiteID=5)*.

Links to Canadian swine AI centers can be found on the internet at *http://www. canswine.ca.*

**General Procedures for Swine AI—** The collection of semen from the boar may be accomplished by use of the artificial vagina (AV) or by the "gloved hand method." Since the average boar ejaculate contains from about 250 to 500 ml, collection methods must be geared to handle large semen volumes. The total number of sperm in an average ejaculate ranges from about 20 to 70 billion cells. The ejaculate consists of three fractions: (1) a pre-sperm fraction containing some gelatinous material, (2) the middle, or sperm-rich, fraction, and (3) a fraction low in sperm numbers with much gelatinous material. The middle, or sperm-rich, fraction is

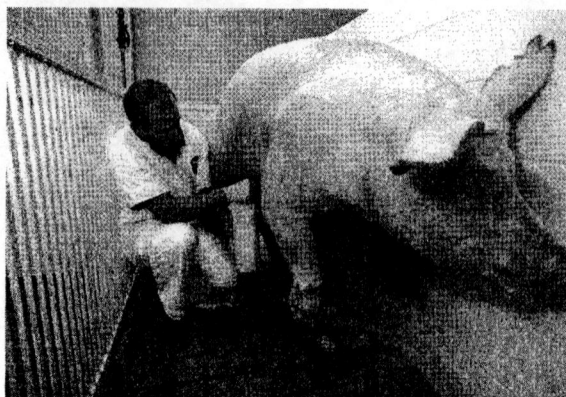

**Figure 29.1.** Collection of semen from the boar. (Courtesy Dr. Tim Safranski, Univ. Missouri, Columbia, MO)

used for AI service. The first and third fractions are often discarded.

A "dummy sow," or phantom, is used as a mount for the boar during semen collection (Figure 29.1). An artificial vagina (AV) similar to that used for bulls but somewhat shorter may be used for semen collection. With this method, the water in the AV should be at a temperature of 105°F (40°C), and the liner of the AV should be lubricated with K-Y jelly just prior to collection. The boar is allowed to tease the dummy mount, and if an estrus sow can be stationed nearby, this also will help to stimulate the boar. A 250 to 500-ml container fitted with a sterile cheesecloth or gauze cover will be used to hold the semen. The cheesecloth or gauze will separate out the gelatinous portion of the ejaculate. Then, as the boar mounts the dummy, the glans penis is directed into the AV. A great deal of pressure on the boar's penis is required to elicit ejaculation. The operator must squeeze the AV tightly during ejaculation, which usually requires several minutes or more to complete. Alternatively, an attached rubber air bulb can be used to produce the necessary AV pressure on the boar's penis. The middle fraction of the ejaculate is then evaluated and processed in accord with its intended use.

The "gloved hand method" is now preferred by most operators for collection of boar semen. The equipment needed is a latex or vinyl glove and a wide-mouth vacuum bottle with a sterile cheesecloth or gauze stretched over the top for use as a collection vessel. The boar is allowed to mount the dummy, and the gloved hand massages and squeezes the fluid from the prepuce. As the boar protrudes his penis, the spiral end is grasped and held firmly by the collector and directed to the side of the mount for collection. Pressure must be maintained throughout the collection period, or else the boar will dismount and end the process. The middle fraction of the ejaculate is used for insemination.

Most swine artificial insemination today involves the use of unfrozen liquid semen. The use of frozen semen has been limited due to its lower fertility. Generally, the fresh semen is extended and packaged in doses (bags, tubes, or bottles) containing 2.5 to 4 billion total sperm in a 70 to 100 ml. volume. The extended semen is stored and shipped at a temperature of about 16° to 18°C (~61° to 64°F). The extenders for boar semen are typically classified as short term, mid term, and long term (see Table 29.1). Although most semen is used within 3 days, some extenders allow for use up to 5 to 7 days without significant losses in fertility.

Researchers at the University of Minnesota reported success with frozen semen as early as 1971.[2] In those trials, extended

___

[2] E. F. Graham, et al. 1971. Fertility studies with frozen boar spermatozoa. The A.I. Digest 19:6.

## Table 29.1. Boar Semen Extenders and Length of Sperm Preservation[a]

| Arbitrary Classification | Name of Extender | Length of Sperm Preservation, Days (Maximum Number of Days) |
| --- | --- | --- |
| Short term | Beltsville Thawing Solution, BTS | 3 |
| | V.S.P. | 3 |
| | Modified BTS | 3 |
| Mid term | Modified Kiev/SpermAid | 3 to 5 |
| | Modena | 3 to 5 |
| | VITAL® | 4 to 5 |
| | Merck III™/Kiev/EDTA | 4 to 6 |
| Long term | Modified Modena | 5 to 7 |
| | MR-A | 6 to 7 |
| | Androhep® | 6 to 7 |
| | Androhep lite™ | 6 |
| | Androhep PLUS™ | 7 |
| | X-CELL™ | 7 |
| | ACROMAX | 7 to 8 |
| Very long term | Mulberry III* | 7 to 14 |

*This product has not been field tested in the United States. The product is marketed by a company in Belgium called V.M.D.n.v. The advertisement does not include any data on reproductive performance.

[a]D. G. Levis. 2000. Boar semen extenders:purpose, types and function of ingredients. Midwest Boar Stud Conference. W. Lafayette, IN. April 13-14.

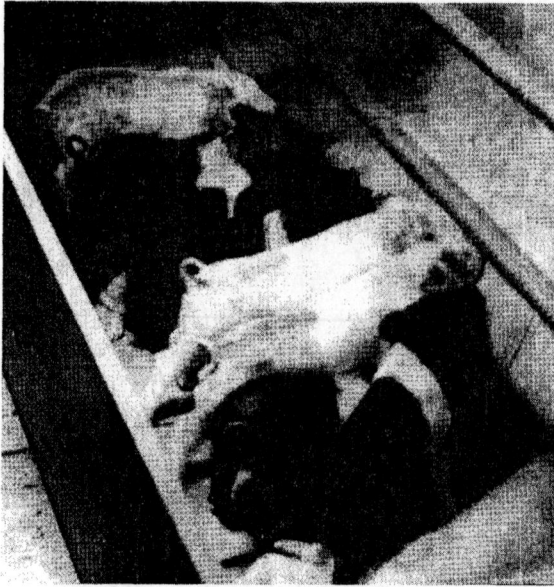

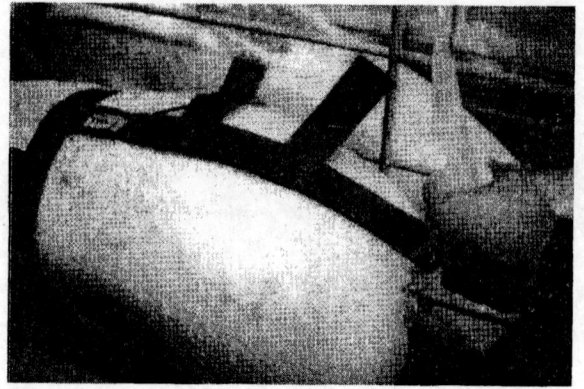

**Figure 29.3.** Artificial insemination of swine with the use of a breeding belt/strap. B. A. Didion. 2000. Technical aspects of swine AI. Proc. 18th Tech. Conf. on Artificial Insemination and Reproduction. NAAB. p. 69.

**Figure 29.2.** One of the first litters of pigs resulting from the use of frozen boar semen. (Courtesy, E. F. Graham, University of Minnesota, St. Paul)

semen (see reference for extender formula) was frozen in pellet form. A total of 98 sows were inseminated once using 35 to 90 ml of the thawed semen containing 2.5 billion live sperm. Fertility ranged from 15 to 45 percent, and the pregnant sows averaged 7.7 pigs per litter, Figure 29.2. Most extenders used for freezing boar semen include sugars, proteins or lipoproteins, buffers, and low concentrations of glycerol.[3] Various thawing solutions are used, and inseminations are performed around the time of ovulation. Frozen semen generally contains higher numbers of sperm than unfrozen liquid semen, and inseminate volumes range from 50 to 80 ml.[4] However, additional research is needed to improve fertility of frozen boar semen before widespread application is plausible. Although claims of breakthroughs with frozen semen are occa-

[3] V. G. Pursel. 1979. Advances in preservation of swine spermatozoa. In: H. W. Hawk (Ed.). Animal Reproduction. BARC Symp. No. 3. Allanheld, Osmun & Co., Montclair, NJ. p. 145.
[4] Ibid.

sionally heard, little new information has been reported in the scientific literature.

The determination of sperm cell concentration and calculations for extension rates for boar semen are similar to the procedures followed for bull semen (Exercise 13). Appropriate antibiotics should be used in all extending fluids, typically at the same rate as for bull semen. Many commercial extender mixes contain antibiotics.

Insemination is carried out by means of a catheter with a spiral end that simulates the shape of the boar's glans penis. After sanitary insertion of the catheter into the sow's or gilt's reproductive tract, the catheter tip is placed against the cervical opening and gently turned counterclockwise to enter the cervix. When the catheter is in place, the cervix will contract and hold the catheter tip. Females are normally inseminated twice after detection of estrus. Semen contained in an attached plastic dispensing bottle, bag, or tube is then slowly deposited into the reproductive tract. Typically, 70 to 100 ml of extended semen is used per insemination. In recent years, breeding belts have become popular as they simulate a "more natural delivery" of sperm into the female reproductive tract, and they allow technicians to inseminate more than one sow at a time. The breeding belt is a harness with straps which accommodates attachment of the inseminating rod and semen dose to the female (see Figure 29.3). The estrous cycle of the sow is normally 19 to 23 days in length. The duration of estrus averages about 60 hours in sows and 44 hours in gilts. Inseminations are made on the first day and the second day of heat. Liquid semen processed and stored at ~61° to 64°F (16° to 18°C) has given best results when used on day 1 or day 2 after collection. In general, fertility decreases after day 3.

## Artificial Insemination in Horses

The current number of horses in the United States has been estimated to be between 5.2 and 10 million head.[5] However, actual figures are difficult to determine, because there is no census of the horse population. The horses are largely pleasure animals, and the number is increasing. The purebred breeds are enjoying their greatest growth ever. Artificial insemination can be a convenience to the owner of one to several horses or ponies. It can also be a means of making improvement in horses by the greater use of the best stallions. In recent years, the use of liquid-cooled, transported semen has become common, with good fertility results. Encouraging results also have been obtained with frozen semen. However, the fertility level has been lower than with either fresh or cooled unfrozen liquid semen. However, with continual research, important developments in horse artificial insemination lie ahead.

Through the years, fertility in horses has been lower than in other farm animals. In the days of horse-drawn vehicles and implements, the foal crop on farms averaged only about 60 percent. Even today only about 70 percent of

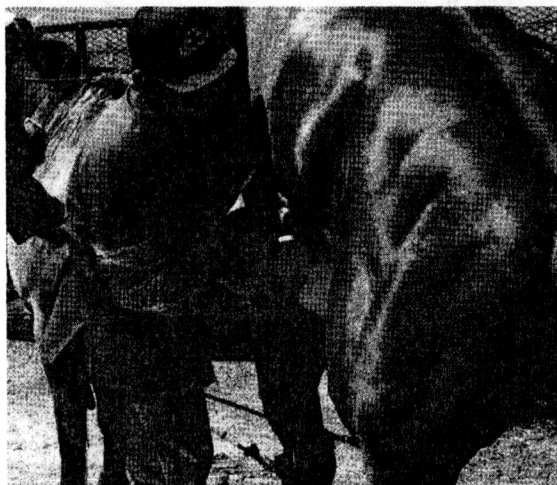

**Figure 29.4.** Collection of semen from the stallion. (Courtesy, Colorado State University)

mares, under the best of care, deliver foals each year.

Semen for artificial insemination is collected by means of the stallion model artificial vagina (Figure 29.4). The stallion model AV is considerably larger than the one used for the bull, and various types are available (e.g., Missouri, Colorado, Hanover, HarVet).[6] After it is assembled and warm water added, it is lubricated and a collection receptacle attached. Some models are fitted with a nylon filter that catches the gel fraction of the ejaculate before it becomes mixed with the sperm-rich fraction. The typical ejaculate volume is about 50 ml but can range from 40 to over 150 ml. The sperm concentration ranges from 30 million to 800 million per milliliter, with a total of about 6 to 10 billion sperm per ejaculate. Customarily, horse breeding farms and racing stables use fresh semen to inseminate mares. Several mares may be inseminated with fresh extended liquid semen from the same ejaculate.

[5] A. Borton. 1990. Introduction. In: J. W. Evans, et al. (Eds.). The Horse (2nd Ed.). W. H. Freeman, New York. p. 3.

[6] J. P. Hurtgen. 1998. Semen collection in stallions: a variety of methods for obtaining semen. Proc. Stallion Symp. ACT/SFT/AAEP. p. 27.

The semen may be extended from one to several times, depending upon sperm concentration and quality. Numerous extenders have been used for the extension and storage of stallion semen. Most have included egg yolk, milk, milk byproducts, or chemicals to regulate osmolarity and/or pH.[7] A satisfactory extender that is easy to prepare is the Non-fat Dried Milk Solids (NFDMS)—glucose formulation presented in Table 29.2. Various commercial extenders are also available. Extenders should be prepared on the day of semen collection. It is recommended that mares be inseminated with 500 million motile sperm, normally contained in anywhere from 10 to 100 ml. of extender. The extended unfrozen stallion semen may be stored at temperatures ranging from 41° to 68°F (5° to 20°C) and is normally used during a 24- to 48-hour period. However, it should be noted that individual stallions vary widely in their spermatozoa tolerance to cooling temperatures.

Various equine breed registries now allow the use of semen that has been stored and transported, thereby eliminating the requirement that the mare and the stallion be located on the same farm or ranch when the insemination is performed. However, certain registries still do not allow transported *frozen* semen.

Detailed procedures for the processing and use of frozen stallion semen have been described by Pickett, et al.,[8] and by Amann and Pickett.[9] For semen packaged in 0.5-, 2.5-, 4.0-, or 5.0-ml plastic straws, centrifugation of the semen is routinely performed to increase sperm cell concentration and allow removal of seminal plasma, which may sometimes be deleterious to sperm viability. Examples of centrifugation media are listed in Table 29.3. After gentle centrifugation at 400× g for 15 minutes, the concentrated sperm are resuspended in a freezing extender, such as lactose—EDTA—egg yolk (Table 29.4). Freezing extenders consisting of mixtures of skim milk and egg yolk or other components and glycerol also have been used successfully. Extended semen is filled into the labeled straws and then frozen in liquid nitrogen vapor. Some organizations use a programmable freezer. Pelleted frozen semen also has been used; however, there have been concerns about identification and possible contamination. Semen should be packaged at a concentration that will yield a minimum of 150 to 200 million progressively motile sperm after thawing.[10] Semen in straws should be rapidly

---

[7] B. W. Pickett, et al. 1987. Procedures for Collection, Evaluation and Utilization of Stallion Semen for Artificial Insemination. Animal Reproduction Laboratory Bull. No. 3. Colorado State Univ., Ft. Collins.

**Table 29.2.** **Composition of Non-fat Dried Milk Solids—Glucose Extender[a]**

| Ingredients | Quantity |
|---|---|
| Sanalac (instant non-fat dry milk) (g) | 2.4 |
| Glucose monohydrate (g) | 4.9 |
| Sodium bicarbonate (7.5% solution) (ml) | 2.0 |
| Gentamicin sulfate (reagent grade) (ml) | 2.0 |
| Distilled water (ml) | 92.0 |
| Osmolality (mOsm/kg)[b] | 375.0 ±2.0 |
| pH[b] | 6.99 ±.02 |

The liquids should be mixed before adding powder; otherwise, the acidity of gentamicin will curdle the milk powder.

[a]B. W. Pickett, et al. 1987. Procedures for Collection, Evaluation and Utilization of Stallion Semen for Artificial Insemination. Animal Reproduction Laboratory Bull. No. 3. Colorado State Univ., Ft. Collins. p. 65.
[b]Mean± SEM.

---

[8] Ibid.
[9] R. P. Amann and B. W. Pickett. 1984. An Overview of Frozen Equine Semen: Procedures for Thawing and Insemination of Frozen Equine Spermatozoa. Special Series No. 33. Colorado State Univ., Ft. Collins.
[10] Ibid.

**Table 29.3.** Composition of the Citrate-EDTA Centrifugation Medium and the Glucose-EDTA Solution Used During Centrifugation and for Preparation of Freezing Extender[a]

| Component | Citrate-EDTA[b] | Glucose-EDTA[b] |
|---|---|---|
| Glucose | 1.5 | 59.985 |
| Sodium citrate, dihydrate (g) | 25.95 | 3.7 |
| Disodium EDTA (g) | 3.699 | 3.699 |
| Sodium bicarbonate (g) | 1.2 | 1.2 |
| Polymyxin B sulfate (IU) | | $10.0^6$ |
| pH | 6.89 | 6.59 |
| mOsm/kg | 290.0 | 409.0 |

[a]B. W. Pickett, et al. 1987. Procedures for Collection, Evaluation and Utilization of Stallion Semen for Artificial Insemination. Animal Reproduction Laboratory Bull. No. 3. Colorado State Univ., Ft. Collins. p. 81.

[b]Dilute to 1,000 ml with deionized water.

**Table 29.4.** Composition of Lactose—EDTA—Egg Yolk Freezing Extender[a]

| | |
|---|---|
| Lactose solution (11% w/v) (ml) | 50.0 |
| Glucose—EDTA solution (Table 29.3) (ml) | 25.0 |
| Egg yolk (ml) | 20.0 |
| Glycerol (ml) | 5.0 |
| Equex STM (ml) | 0.5 |

[a]B. W. Pickett, et al. 1987. Procedures for Collection, Evaluation and Utilization of Stallion Semen for Artificial Insemination. Animal Reproduction Laboratory Bull. No. 3. Colorado State Univ., Ft. Collins. p. 81.

thawed in hot or warm water. Various temperatures and thawing times have been recommended.

The estrous cycle of the mare is quite variable, ranging from 10 to 37 days but averaging about 21 to 23 days. Heat usually lasts 4 to 7 days. Ovulation commonly occurs 24 to 36 hours before the end of heat. The mare should be inseminated about two days before the end to one day after the end of the heat period. Figure 29.5 shows the reproductive organs of the mare. It has been customary to breed mares at least twice (daily or every other day starting on day 2 or 3 of estrus) during the heat period, as the time of the ovulation is quite variable. However, this strategy depends on the availability and cost of the semen. More intensive management of the mare, including the use of transrectal ultrasound or palpation to determine approaching ovulation (presence of a 35-mm follicle) and the subsequent use of ovulatory drugs, may enhance efficiency of semen usage for maximum conception rate.

Procedures for inseminating the mare are the same whether using unfrozen liquid semen or frozen-thawed semen. For liquid semen, a syringe attached to a plastic disposable horse-breeding tube is frequently utilized. For frozen-thawed semen in straws, an insemination gun similar to one for cattle is used. Prior to insemination, the mare's buttocks and external genitalia should be cleaned and disinfected. A clean paper towel is used to wipe the lips of the vulva prior to entry. A disposable shoulder-length plastic

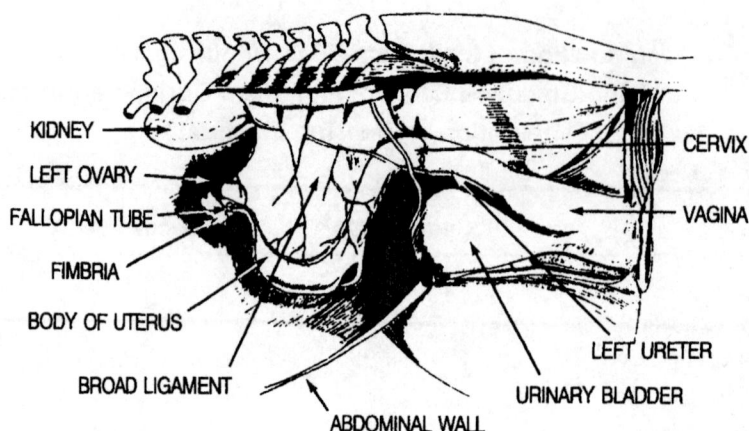

**Figure 29.5.** Reproductive organs of the mare.

insemination glove that has been sanitized is put on the arm and lubricated. With the fingers of the gloved hand placed around the end of the insemination tube or gun, the hand and insemination tube or gun are gently inserted into the mare's vagina and directed forward until the cervix is contacted. The index finger is then passed through the cervical canal, which is normally open during estrus. The tip of the insemination tube or syringe is guided along the inserted index finger and passed through the cervix into the body of the uterus. Then the semen is slowly expelled into the body of the uterus. After deposition of semen, the inseminating tube or gun and hand are withdrawn.

A wide range in fertility of frozen stallion semen has been reported in the literature (i.e., 8 to 66 percent one-cycle pregnancy rates[11]). Generally, results have not consistently equaled fertility using unfrozen liquid semen. However, for certain stallions, acceptable pregnancy rates are quite possible with frozen semen (Figure 29.6). It is obvious, though, that additional research to improve methods for cryopreserving stallion semen is needed.

*Note:* The regulations for using artificial insemination vary among the horse recording (registry) organizations. If registered animals are involved, the horse owner should contact the proper recording organization before proceeding.

## Artificial Insemination in Dogs

Some of the earliest success with artificial insemination was work done with dogs by the Italian Spallanzani in 1780. In recent years, artificial insemination in dogs has been used with unextended fresh semen or semen extended in heated milk, egg yolk–citrate, egg yolk–tris, and lactose–egg yolk formulations. Commercially available extenders are commonly used.

In 1969, Seager[12] was the first to report successful pregnancies resulting from frozen dog semen (that had been stored for nine months) (Figure 29.7).

---

[11] P. R. Loomis. 1999. Artificial insemination of horses: where is it going? Proc. Ann. Conf. and Semen Cryopreservation/AI Symp. Society for Theriogenology/ACT, Nashville, TN. p. 325.

[12] S. W. J. Seager. 1969. Successful pregnancies utilizing frozen dog semen. The A.I. Digest 17:6.

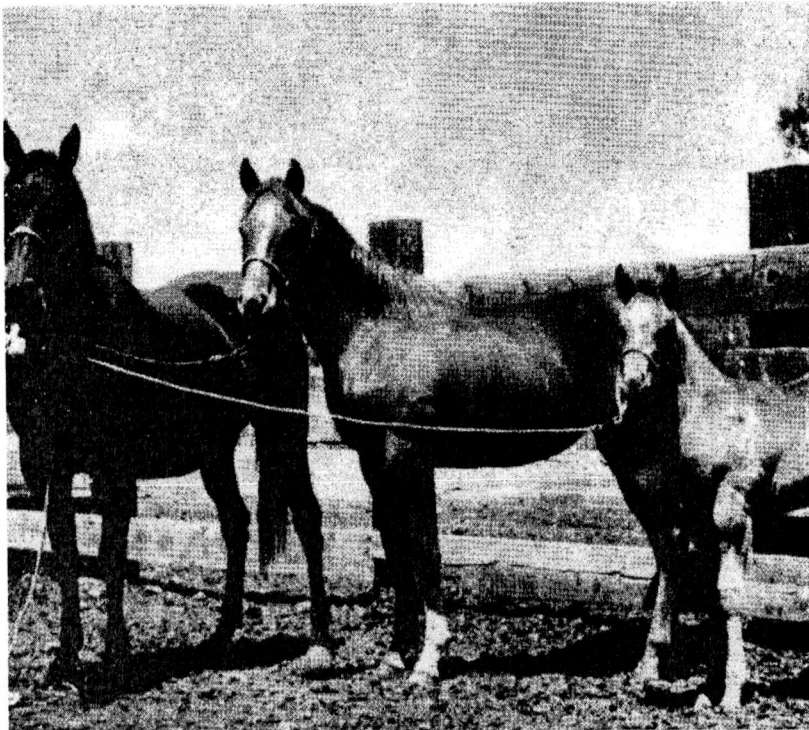

**Figure 29.6.** A mare with her colts, born a year apart and both resulting from the use of frozen stallion semen. (Courtesy, ABS Global, DeForest, WI)

Semen collection from the dog is accomplished by digital manipulation of the penis or by use of an artificial vagina. Normal seminal characteristics for the dog are outlined by the Society for Theriogenology.[13] In general, the procedures for semen extension, evaluation, cooling, and freezing are similar to those followed for the bull. Frozen semen is typically packaged in 0.25- or 0.5-ml plastic straws. Vaginal cytology of the female is normally monitored to determine the correct time for breeding. During estrus, the bitch is inseminated one or more times. A syringe attached to a plastic insemination tube or an insemina-tion gun for straws is used to deposit semen into the cervix. Intrauterine insemination is generally conducted surgically.

The artificial insemination of dogs is now fairly common, utilizing fresh extended liquid semen and, in many cases, frozen semen. Veterinarians and dog fanciers find these developments helpful for special matings. Anyone planning to use AI for registered dogs should obtain information on the regulations and procedures required by the American Kennel Club, 5580 Centerview Dr., Raleigh, NC 27606 *(http://www.akc.org/registration/policies/).*

---

[13] B. J. Purswell, et al. 1992. Guidelines for Using the Canine Breeding Soundness Evaluation Form. Theriogenology Handbook, SA-C1. Society for Theriogenology, Hastings, NE.

## Artificial Insemination in Poultry

Artificial insemination is used to improve the hatchability of chicken and turkey eggs. It

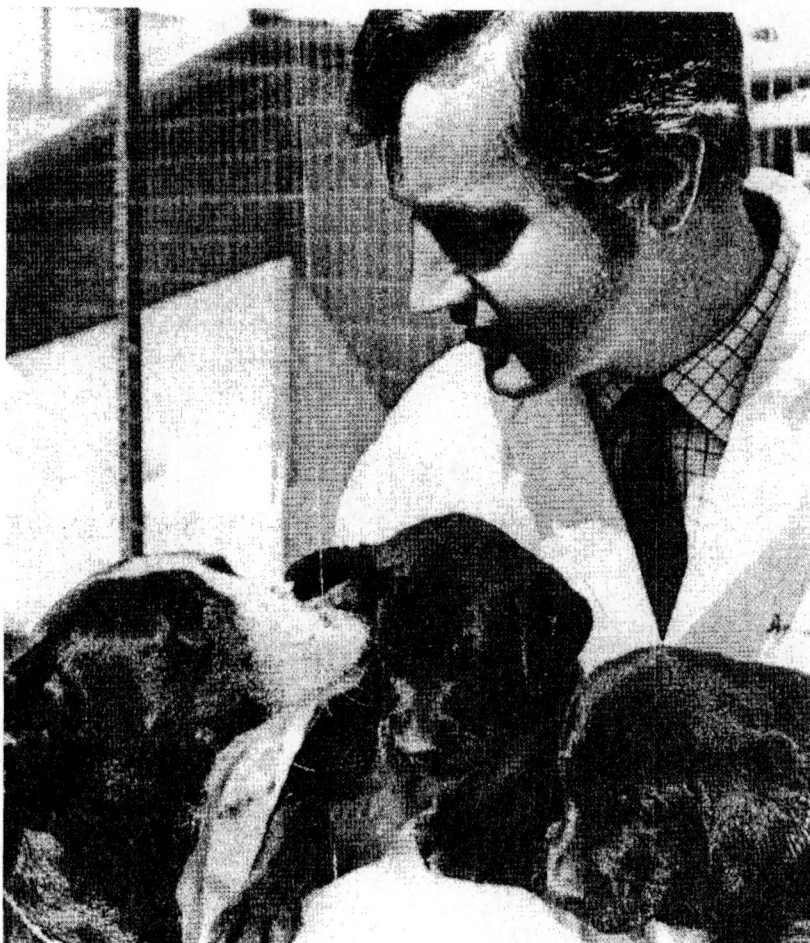

**Figure 29.7.** Dr. Seager holds two puppies that were among the first to result from the use of frozen semen. The protective mother looks on.

also overcomes problems associated with physical incompatibility and reduces the spread of reproductive diseases. AI is widely used for turkey hens producing hatching eggs, and it is used to a lesser extent for chickens. However, it is likely that the increased selection pressure for breast conformation and white meat yield in broilers will result in greater use of AI in chickens.

Inseminating turkey hens at two-week intervals maintains the desired high fertility of hatching eggs. Many turkey producers maintain a flock of males. However, the establishment of turkey "stud farms" is now taking place, allowing producers to keep fewer toms and purchase semen. Semen in poultry is collected by the abdominal massage technique (Figure 29.8) and is often used in the fresh state. However, most turkey producers extend the semen by use of a medium consisting of a buffered salt solution, glucose, milk, and antibiotics (see Hafez [Ref.], pp. 393–396). The average ejaculate volume is about 0.25 to 0.5 ml and is usually sufficient for 20 hens. Extended semen (normally containing 100 to 200 million sperm) is deposited in the hen's vagina by means of a multidose syringe fitted with a disposable tip or a poultry insemination tube (Figure 29.9). Turkey hens are usually inseminated at one- to two-week intervals during the laying season. Techniques for the freezing of poultry

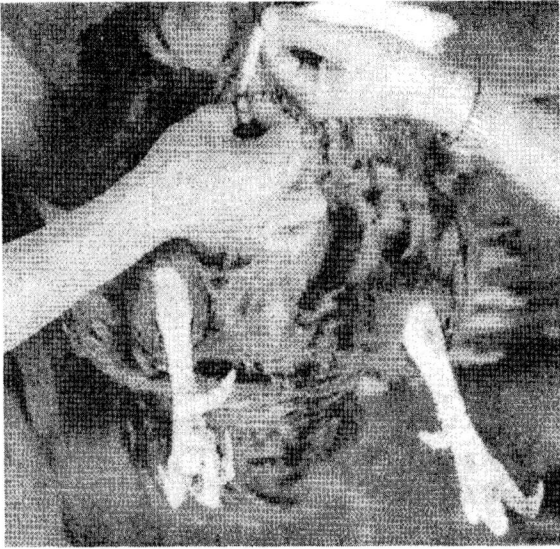

**Figure 29.8.** Manual collection of poultry semen. (Courtesy, Dr. Y. Nishikawa, Japan)

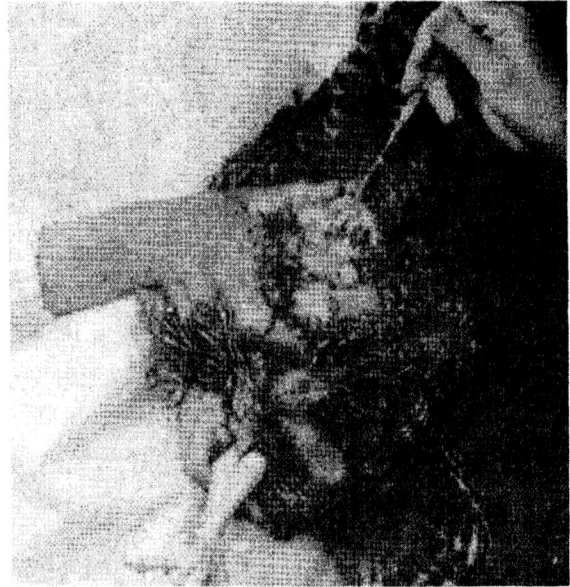

**Figure 29.9.** Deposition of semen for poultry AI. (Courtesy, Dr. Y. Nishikawa, Japan)

semen have been developed; however, hatchability is lower for frozen-thawed semen. Commercial applications of frozen bird semen have included the selective breeding of certain genetic lines and the preserving of endangered bird species.

## Nondomestic Species

In recent years there has been considerable interest by zoological parks in the banking of frozen semen and the use of artificial insemination and embryo transfer in certain non-domestic species. As numbers of exotic wild species continue to decline, the captive propagation of the species can be facilitated by using these reproductive techniques. Artificial insemination of these species, using fresh or frozen-thawed semen, can increase the breeding potential of genetically superior animals, expand the gene pool without the risk and expense of maintaining and transporting sires, and allow utilization of males unable to mate naturally.[14] Organized strategies to investigate the basic reproductive and endocrine characteristics of these species, improve their reproductive efficiency through fertility evaluation, and propagate them through use of artificial insemination are ongoing. As an example, a major breakthrough occurred in November 1999 when the world's first elephant calf resulting from artificial insemination was born in Springfield, MO.[15]

[14] J. Howard, et al. 1986. Semen collection, analysis and cryopreservation in nondomestic mammals. In: D. A. Morrow (Ed.). Current Therapy in Theriogenology 2. W. B. Saunders Company, Philadelphia. p. 1047.

[15] M. McCarry. 2000. Scientific breakthroughs lead to success after 25 yrs; future 'suddenly brighter.' The White Tops. Vol. 73. No. 1. p. 2.

# QUESTIONS

1. Is artificial insemination of swine widely practiced in the United States? Explain. What if any are the limiting factors?

2. How is semen collected from the boar?

3. Which fraction of the boar ejaculate is utilized for artificial insemination?

4. What equipment is used and what procedures are followed in inseminating the sow?

5. Is artificial insemination of horses in general use? Explain.

6. What is the average fertility (foaling rate) of well-managed mares? Is artificial insemination used by horse breeding farms and racing stables? If so, what are the advantages?

7. When should the mare be inseminated during the heat period?

8. Describe the procedures followed when inseminating the mare.

9. When is artificial insemination used for dogs? What are the advantages?

10. Why is artificial insemination widely used for laying turkey hens? Is frozen semen utilized in poultry operations? Explain.

# REFERENCES

Almond, G. et al. 1994. The Swine AI Book. p. 1-108.

Flowers, W. L. 1996. An update on swine AI. Proc. 16th Tech. Conf. on Artificial Insemination and Reproduction. NAAB. p. 88.

Gill, S. P. et al. 1999. Poultry artificial insemination: procedures, current status and future needs. Proc. Ann. Conf. and Semen Cryopreservation & AI Symp., Soc. for Theriogenology/ACT, Nashville, TN. p. 353.

Hafez, E. S. E. (Ed.). 1987. Reproduction in Farm Animals (5th Ed.). Lea & Febiger, Philadelphia. (Chs. 15, 16, 17, 18, 23, 28.)

Held, J. P. 1999. Canine artificial insemination: where are we? Proc. Ann. Conf. and Semen Cryopreservation and AI Symp., Soc. for Theriogenology/ACT, Nashville, TN. p. 347.

Knox, R. V. 2000. Semen processing, extending and storage for artificial insemination in swine. Midwest Boar Stud Conference. W. Lafayette, Indiana. April 13-14.

Singleton, W. L. 2001. State of the art in artificial insemination of pigs in the United States. Therio. 56: 1305.

Sorenson, A. M., Jr. 1979. Animal Reproduction: Principles and Practices. McGraw-Hill, New York. pp. 167, 169.

# Appendices

# APPENDIX A

# NAAB Uniform Coding System for Identifying Semen

### National Association of Animal Breeders
### Columbia, Missouri

The purpose of the NAAB Uniform Coding System for Identifying Semen is to provide a unique designation for each bull that includes: 1) identification of the source of the semen (the organization that processed the semen), 2) identification of the breed of the bull, and 3) a code number identifying each respective bull within breed within each AI organization.

It is recognized that the registry identification (ID) number for each bull is a unique number. However, it does not identify the source of the semen and in some cases is not readily recognizable by the breed. Experience has proven that individual herd owners, managers, and technicians prefer to use a more familiar code instead of the registry ID number when identifying a sire used. The NAAB Uniform Code will in many cases be seven to ten characters, which is equally as long as a registry ID number. However, since different segments of the Uniform Code have specific meanings, the entire code is much easier to remember and more acceptable by people in the field than is the registry ID number. In addition, by eliminating all blanks and leading zeros, the NAAB Uniform Code, when written, will often be shorter than most registry ID numbers.

The NAAB Uniform Code was originally developed for use by commercial AI organizations for identification of semen as it is exchanged and sold throughout the industry. In addition, the AI requirements of the Purebred Dairy Cattle Association require a code identifying the source of dairy sire semen on each individual unit. Certified Semen Services (CSS) also requires all participating AI businesses to label each breeding unit of semen produced by them with the elements of the NAAB Uniform Code. Logically, there are other needs for a code number identifying the source of semen. It would not be feasible to print a different code number for each of these and other purposes on each unit of semen, in view of space availability and unnecessary duplication.

Incomplete sire identification by registry ID number in Dairy Herd Improvement (DHI) records has for years been a concern because of the significant loss of records that otherwise would be available for sire evaluation. Many herd owners and managers use NAAB Uniform bull code numbers instead of registry ID when completing production record forms. Thus, it is logical that the Uniform Code be a unique designation that can be uniformly converted to the correct registry ID number by use of a cross-reference listing of each bull (i.e., the bull's Uniform Code number cross-referenced to his registry ID number). For this purpose, the entire NAAB Uniform Code, including AI center (stud) and breed identification and individual bull number, is necessary for the number to be unique for each bull. This system is being employed by the Dairy Record Processing Centers, and there is little doubt that such a system will be useful in beef performance record programs.

The NAAB Uniform Code for Identifying Semen consists of a maximum of 10 characters according to the following combination scheme:

| | |
|---|---|
| *AI center (stud) code* | Indicates the semen producing organization (stud) that collected and processed the semen. AI center (stud) code numbers are assigned by the NAAB to its member organizations and other semen producing organizations where warranted. It is comprised of one or more numeric characters. [Maximum of three characters.] |
| *Breed code* | Indicates the breed of bull. Dairy breed codes are two alphabetic characters and consistent with |

codes designated by USDA for the DHI program. Changes in dairy breed codes should be made only upon mutual agreement of the NAAB, USDA, and DHI computing centers. Beef breed codes are two alphabetic characters and are assigned by NAAB in conjunction with Agriculture Canada and the Canadian AI industry. [Maximum of two characters.]

*Bull code*    Indicates the respective bull's number assigned by the AI organization collecting and processing the semen. Bull codes should be numeric codes with a maximum of five characters from 1 to 99999. All leading zeros and blanks should be omitted. If a bull is transferred to a second AI organization for collection, a different code number should be assigned to the same bull. Since the AI center code is different for each organization, it is not necessary to retain the same individual bull code when a bull is moved to a different AI center (stud). [Maximum of five characters.]

Examples:

**1HO777**

1   = Stud code for Genex Cooperative/CRI
HO = Breed code for Holstein
777 = Bull code for Coastal Cleitus Andrew, Registry ID No. USA2110495

**109SM284**

109 = Stud code for Reproduction Enterprises, Inc.
SM  = Breed code for Simmental
284 = Bull code for Black Knight US, Registry ID No. 1138189

# APPENDIX B

# NAAB Uniform Breed Codes

## DAIRY BREEDS

| Breed | Code | Breed | Code |
|---|---|---|---|
| AMERICAN LINEBACK | LD | HOLSTEIN | HO |
| AYRSHIRE | AY | JERSEY | JE |
| BROWN SWISS | BS | RED & WHITE | WW |
| GUERNSEY | GU | SHORTHORN (Milking) | MS |

## BEEF, DUAL PURPOSE, LESSER DAIRY, OTHER BREEDS

| Breed | Code | Breed | Code |
|---|---|---|---|
| AFRICANDER | AF | DEXTER | DR |
| ANGUS | AN | DUTCH BELTED | DL |
| ANKINA | AK | ERINGER | ER |
| ANKOLE-WATUSI | AW | FLAMAND | FA |
| AMERICAN BREED | AE | FLORIDA CRACKER | FC |
| AMERIFAX | AM | FRIBOURG | FR |
| BARZONA | BA | GALLOWAY | GA |
| BEEFALO | BE | GELBRAY | GE |
| BEEF FRIESIAN | BF | GELBVIEH | GV |
| BEEFMASTER | BM | GRAUVIEH | GI |
| BELGIAN BLUE | BB | GRONINGEN | GR |
| BELTED GALLOWAY | BG | GUZERA | GZ |
| BLONDE d'AQUITAINE | BD | GYR (or Gir) | GY |
| BONSMARA | NS | HAYS CONVERTER | HC |
| BRAFORD | BO | HEREFORD (Horned) | HH |
| BRAHMAN | BR | HEREFORD (Polled) | HP |
| BRAHMOUSIN | BI | HIGHLAND (Scotch) | SH |
| BRALER | BL | HYBRID (Alberta) | HY |
| BRANGUS | BN | INDU BRAZIL | IB |
| BRAUNVIEH | BU | KOBE (Wagyu) | KB |
| BRITISH WHITE | BW | LIMOUSIN | LM |
| BROWN SWISS (Beef) | SB | LINCOLN RED | LR |
| BUELINGO | BQ | LOWLINE (Loala) | LO |
| CANADIENNE | CN | LUING | LU |
| CHARBRAY | CB | MAINE-ANJOU | MA |
| CHAROLAIS | CH | MASHONA | MH |
| CHI-ANGUS | CG | MANDALONG SPECIAL | ML |
| CHIANINA | CA | MARCHIGIANA | MR |
| CHI-MAINE | CM | MAREMMANA | ME |
| DANISH RED & WHITE | RW | MEXICAN CORRIENTE | MC |
| DEVON | DE | MUESE-RHINE-ISSEL | MI |

| Breed | Code | Breed | Code |
|---|---|---|---|
| MURRAH | MU | SANTA GERTRUDIS | SG |
| MURRAY GREY | MG | SENEPOL | SE |
| NELLORE | NE | SHORTHORN (Beef Scotch) | SS |
| NORMANDE | NM | SHORTHORN (Polled) | SP |
| NORWEGIAN RED | NR | SHORTHORN (Illwarra) | IS |
| PARTHENAISE | PA | SIMBRAH | SI |
| PIEDMONTESE | PI | SIMMENTAL | SM |
| PINZGAUER | PZ | SOUTH DEVON | DS |
| RANGER | RA | SUSSEX | SX |
| RED ANGUS | AR | TABAPUA | TB |
| RED BRAHMAN | RR | TARENTAISE | TA |
| RED BRANGUS | RB | TAURINDICUS | TN |
| RED DANE | RD | TEXAS LONGHORN | TL |
| RED POLL | RP | TULI | TI |
| ROMAGNOLA | RN | WELSH BLACK | WB |
| ROMOSINUANO | RS | WEST FLEMISH RED | WF |
| ROTBUNTE | RO | WHITE PARK | WP |
| SAHIWAL | SW | CROSSBREEDS (TWINNER) | XT |
| SALERS | SA | CROSSBREEDS | XX |

# APPENDIX C

# Manufacturers/Suppliers of AI and ET Equipment and Related Products

## ARTIFICIAL VAGINAS: CASINGS, LINERS, CONES, ETC.

**Alliance Rubber, Inc.**
P.O. Box 599
Franklin, KY 42134

**Breeders Equipment Co.**
P.O. Box 177
Flourtown, PA 19031
*(AV casings)*

**Crown Rubber Co.**
6000 N. 60th St.
Milwaukee, WI 53218

**Richard Ela Co.**
744 Williamson
Madison, WI 53703
*(AV casings)*

**Fournier Rubber**
1341 Norton Ave.
Columbus, OH 43212
*(AV casings)*

**C. R. Freeman and Co., Ltd.**
49 St. Mary's Gate
Nottingham, England

**Gates Rubber Co.**
P.O. Box 5887
Denver, CO 80217
*(AV casings)*

**IMV International Corporation**
11725 95th Avenue North
Maple Grove, MN 55369
http://www.imvusa.com

**Nasco International, Inc.**
901 Janesville Ave.
Fort Atkinson, WI 53538
http://www.enasco.com/prod/Home

**Raven Corp.**
237 South St.
Newark, NJ 07114

## JACKETS FOR ARTIFICIAL VAGINAS

**American Breeders Service**
P.O. Box 459
DeForest, WI 53532
*(Plastic AV covers)*

**Hawkeye Breeders Service**
4535 N.W. First St.
Des Moines, IA 50313

**Shoes and Gloves**
400 E. Wilson Bridge Rd.
Worthington, OH 43085

**Welco Custom Trim**
704 W. Buffalo St.
Ithaca, NY 14850

## COLLECTION VIALS AND GLASSWARE

**American Scientific Products**
P.O. Box 41515
Minneapolis, MN 55441

**Cole-Palmer Instrument Co.**
7425 N. Oak Park Ave.
Chicago, IL 60648

**Curtin-Matheson Scientific**
2218 University Ave. S.E.
Minneapolis, MN 55414

**Fisher Scientific Products**
2170 Martin Ave.
Santa Clara, CA 95050

**Kontes of Illinois**
1916 Greenleaf St.
Evanston, IL 60204

**Miles Laboratory**
P.O. Box 91701
Chicago, IL 60693

**Arthur H. Thomas Co.**
Vine St. at Third
P.O. Box 779
Philadelphia, PA 19105

**VWR Scientific**
P.O. Box 39396
Denver, CO 80239

## DISPOSABLE GLOVES, BOOTS, PLASTIC STRAWS, POLYBULBS

**Atlantis Plastics**
P.O. Box 4309
Mankato, MN 56002
http://www.atlantisplastics.com

**Continental Plastic Corp.**
P.O. Box "C"
Delavan, WI 53115
http://www.continentalplastic.com

**Cryo-Vet Intl.**
721 Ballentine Rd.
Menomonie, WI 54751
email: *cryovet@win.bright.net*

**IMV International Corporation**
11725 95th Avenue North
Maple Grove, MN 55369
http://www.imvusa.com

**Minitube of America**
P.O. Box 93018
Verona, WI 53953
http://minitube.com/main.html

**Nasco International, Inc.**
901 Janesville Ave.
Fort Atkinson, WI 53538
http://www.enasco.com/prod/Home

**National Poly Products**
7954 Chesshire Ct.
Maple Grove, MN 55369

**Reproduction Resources**
10015 Green St.
Hebron, IL 60034
email: *reprores@eddinc.net*

## ALUMINUM CANISTERS, AMPULE RACKS, PLASTIC GOBLETS, VIALS, IDENTIFICATION TABS, AI KITS

**Brooklyn Tool, Inc.**
7875 Ranchers Rd.
Fridley, MN 55432

**Caprine Supply**
P.O. Box Y
33001 W. 83rd St.
De Soto, KS 66018
http://www.caprinesupply.com

**Continental Plastic Corp.**
P.O. Box "C"
Delavan, WI 53115
http://www.continentalplastic.com

**IMV International Corporation**
11725 95th Avenue North
Maple Grove, MN 55369
http://www.imvusa.com

**Nasco International, Inc.**
901 Janesville Ave.
Fort Atkinson, WI 53538
http://www.enasco.com/prod/Home

**Reproduction Resources**
10015 Green St.
Hebron, IL 60034
email: *reprores@eddinc.net*

**Shur-Bend Mfg. Co., Inc.**
5709 - 29th Ave. N.
Minneapolis, MN 55422

## CRYOGENIC REFRIGERATORS

**Chart-MVE**
3505 County Rd 42 West
Burnsville, MN 55306
http://www.mve-inc.com/
p-cryobiologicalmarket.html

**Cryogenic Services, Inc.**
I-575 & Airport Dr., P.O. Box 1312
Canton, GA 30114

**Cryo Port**
2713 Bonnie Beach Pl.
Los Angeles, CA 90023
http://www.cryoport.com

**IMV International Corp.**
11725 95th Avenue North
Maple Grove, MN 55369
http://www.imvusa.com
*(L'air Liquide cryogenic equipment)*

**International Cryogenics, Inc.**
4040 Championship Dr.
Indianapolis, IN 46268
http://www.intlcryo.com

**Nasco International, Inc.**
901 Janesville Ave.
Fort Atkinson, WI 53538
http://www.enasco.com/prod/Home

**Taylor-Wharton**
Cryogenic Equipment Division
4075 Hamilton Blvd.
Theodore, AL 36590-0568
http://www.taylor-wharton.com

**T.S. Scientific**
P.O. Box 198
Perkasie, PA 18944


# EMBRYO TRANSFER EQUIPMENT AND SUPPLIES

**A.B. Technology, Inc.**
WSU Research & Tech. Park
N.E. 1345 Terreview Dr.
Pullman, WA 99163
http://www.abtechnology.com

**Agtech, Inc.**
P.O. Box 1222
Manhattan, KS 66502
http://www.agtechinc.com

**Continental Plastic Corp.**
P.O. Box "C"
Delavan, WI 53115
http://www.continentalplastic.com

**Cryo-Med**
49659 Leona Dr.
Mt. Clemens, MI 48045

**EM-TEX Supply Co., Inc.**
2741 S. Great SW Parkway
Grand Prairie, TX 75051

**GIBCO**
3175 Staley Rd.
Grand Island, NY 14072

**IMV International Corporation**
11725 95th Avenue North
Maple Grove, MN 55369
http://www.imvusa.com

**Micromanipulator Microscope Co., Inc.**
1120 Industrial Ave.
Escondido, CA 92025

**Minitube of America**
P.O. Box 93018
Verona, WI 53953
http://minitube.com/main.html

**Nasco International, Inc.**
901 Janesville Ave.
Fort Atkinson, WI 53538
http://www.enasco.com/prod/Home

**PETS**
27221 Garden Valley Rd.
Tyler, TX 75702

**Reproduction Resources**
10015 Green St.
Hebron, IL 60034
email: *reprores@eddinc.net*

**Stoelting**
620 Wheat Lane
Wood Dale, IL 60191
http://www.stoeltingco.com

**T.S. Scientific**
P.O. Box 198
Perkasie, PA 18944

**Thermo Sonics, Inc.**
P.O. Box 318
Quakertown, PA 18951

**Veterinary Concepts**
100 McKay Ave.
Spring Valley, WI 54767

## HEAT DETECTION AIDS AND SUPPLIES

**Automated Process Control**
616 Ridgewood Rd.
P.O. Box 1024
Ridgeland, MS 39158
*(Electronic estrus detectors)*

**DENNO International, Inc.**
6082 Westgate Dr.
Orlando, FL 32811
*(Bovine ovulation detectors)*

**Estrotec, Inc.**
10015 Green St.
Hebron, IL 60034
*(Estrotector™)*

**KAMAR, Inc.**
56 Evergreen St.
Portland, ME 04103
*(Heat mount detection pads)*

**Nasco International, Inc.**
901 Janesville Ave.
Fort Atkinson, WI 53538
http://www.enasco.com/prod/Home

**Omni Glow Corp.**
http://www.bovinebeacon.com
*(Bovine Beacon standing heat activators)*

**Pen-O-Block**
5009 Vernon Rd.
Tallahassee, FL 32301
*(For detector bulls)*


## ESTRUS/OVULATION SYNCHRONIZATION MATERIALS AND PROGRAMS

**Agtech, Inc.**
P.O. Box 1222
Manhattan, KS 66502
http://www.agtechinc.com

**Ft. Dodge Animal Health**
9401 Indian Creek Pkwy
Overland Park, KS 66210
*(Bovilene®)*
*(Factrel®)*

**Intervet, Inc.**
Millsboro, DE 19966
http://www.intervetusa.com/
*(Fertagyl®)*

**Merial Ltd.**
3239 Satellite Blvd.
Duluth, GA 30096
http://www.merial.com
*(Synchro-Mate B®)*
*(Cystorelin)*

**Pharmacia Animal Health**
7000 Portage Rd.
Kalamazoo, MI 49001
http://www.pharmaciaah.com/
*(CIDR®)*
*(Lutalyse®)*
*(MGA®, feed additive approved for suppression of estrus in feedlot heifers)*

**Schering-Plough Animal Health Corp.**
2000 Galloping Hill Rd.
Kenilworth, NJ 07033
http://www.schering-plough.com/
*(Estrumate®)*


## BULL-HANDLING SUPPLIES:

## COLLARS, SNAPS, SWIVELS, RINGS, STALL MATS, ETC.

**Baron Mfg. Co.**
2035 W. Charleston
Chicago, IL 60647

**Adolfo Betancur**
4743 Coral Dr.
Baton Rouge, LA 70814
*(Stall mats)*

**Bylers Harness Shop**
Rt. 4
Mercer, PA 16137

**Calburn Co.**
P.O. Box 147
Whitewater, WI 53109

**Covert Mfg. Co.**
P.O. Box 778
Troy, NY 12181

**Crentzburg, Inc.**
Box 7
Paradise, PA 17562

**Humane Equipment Co.**
805 Monroe St.
Baraboo, WI 53913

**Linear Rubber Products**
6525 - 50th Ave.
Kenosha, WI 53140
*(Rubber mats)*

**Millers Harness Shop**
10700 U.S. 42
Plain City, OH 43064

**Nasco International, Inc.**
901 Janesville Ave.
Fort Atkinson, WI 53538
http://www.enasco.com/prod/Home

**Planks Harness Shop**
Rt. 1
Broadhead, WI 53520

**Raber Bros.**
10899 Converse Rd.
Plain City, OH 43064
*(Tilt tables)*

**Shanks Machine Co.**
1704 E. 18th St.
P.O. Box 562
Sterling, IL 61081
*(Tilt tables for large animals)*

**Sisco Co.**
1943 Crows Landing Rd.
Modesto, CA 95352

**Slotteos Shoe Repair**
506 W. State St.
Ithaca, NY 14850

## INSULATED SHIPPING CONTAINERS

**Hamilton Research, Inc.**
P.O. Box 2099
S. Hamilton, MA 01982
http://www.equitainer.com

**Polyfoam Packers Corp.**
2320 S. Foster Ave.
Wheeling, IL 60090-6572
http://www.polyfoam.com

## DISINFECTANTS, GERMICIDAL DETERGENTS

**Alcide Corporation**
One Willard Rd.
Norwalk, CT 06851
http://www.alcide.com
*(LD disinfectant, Exspor®)*

**Ft. Dodge Laboratories**
9401 Indian Creek Pkwy
Overland Park, KS 66210
*(Nolvasan®)*

**Pharmacia Animal Health**
7000 Portage Rd.
Kalamazoo, MI 49001
http://www.pharmaciaah.com/
*(Roccal D®)*

**Provet Companies**
P.O. Box 2286
Loves Park, IL 61131
*(Procidal 40+™)*

**Steris Corp.**
5960 Heisley Rd.
Mentor, OH 44060
http://www.steris.com
*(One-Stroke Environ®)*
*(LPH®)*

## MICROSCOPES, SPECTROPHOTO-METERS, STAGE WARMERS, COMPUTERIZED SEMEN ANALYZERS

**American Optical**
Scientific Instrument Division
Buffalo, NY 14215

**Animal Reproduction Systems**
14395 Ramona Ave.
Chino, CA 91710
http://www.arssales.com

**Bausch & Lomb**
Scientific Optical Prod. Div.
1400 N. Goodman St.
Rochester, NY 14602

**Bunton Instrument Co.**
615 S. Stonestreet Ave.
Rockville, MD 20850

**CRYO Resources, Ltd.**
701 Seventh Ave.
New York, NY 10036
*(Cell Soft System)*

**Frank Fryer Co.**
60 E. Main St.
Carpentersville, IL 60110
*(Microscopes, heating stage)*

**Hamilton-Thorn Research**
30-A Cherry Hill Dr.
Danvers, MA 01923
*(HTM computerized semen analyzer)*

**Leeds Precision Instruments, Inc.**
801 Boone Ave.
Minneapolis, MN 55427
*(Microscopes)*

**E. Leitz, Inc.**
Rockleigh, NJ 07647

**Minitube of America**
P.O. Box 93018
Verona, WI 53953
http://minitube.com/main.html
*(SM-CMA computerized motility analyzer)*

**Motion Analysis Corp.**
90 Stony Cir.
Santa Rosa, CA 95401
*(Expert Vision System)*

**Nikon, Inc., Instrument Div.**
623 Stewart Ave.
Garden City, NY 11530

**Research Instrument Mfg.**
Rt. 2
Guelph, Ontario, Canada
*(Warm stage)*

**Rocky Mountain Microscope Corp.**
440 Link Lane
Fort Collins, CO 80524
*(Microscopes, heating stage)*

**Carl Zeiss, Inc.**
444 - 5th Ave.
New York, NY 10018

## SEMEN EXTENDERS/ANTIBIOTICS

**Continental Plastic Corp.**
P.O. Box "C"

Delavan, WI 53115
http://www.continentalplastic.com

**Elanco Animal Health**
500 E. 96th St.
Indianapolis, IN 46240
http://www.elanco.com
*(Tylosin)*

**Griffin Riddle Co.**
519 Morgan Mill Rd.
Monroe, NC 28110
*(Tylosin)*

**IMV International Corporation**
11725 95th Avenue North
Maple Grove, MN 55369
http://www.imvusa.com

**Minitube of America**
P.O. Box 93018
Verona, WI 53953
http://minitube.com/main.html

**Pharmacia Animal Health**
7000 Portage Rd.
Kalamazoo, MI 49001
http://www.pharmaciaah.com/
*(Linco-Spectin®)*

**Sigma-Aldrich Chemicals**
P.O. Box 14508
St. Louis, MO 63178
http://sigmaaldrich.com
*(Gentamicin)*

**VIAM-PAC, Inc.**
1026 280th St.
Glenwood City, WI 54103
email: *hgraham@baldwin-telecom.net*

*Note:* This appendix does not constitute a complete listing of AI and ET suppliers. A detailed laboratory buyer's guide can be obtained from American Laboratory, P.O. Box 485, Arlington, MA 02174-9982. Herd operators should check with their semen suppliers when equipment or products relative to artificial insemination are needed. Most AI businesses either carry supplies or can order them for patrons.

# APPENDIX D

# U.S. Businesses That Sell Semen and AI Service and, in Some Cases, Provide Custom Freezing and Embryo Transfer

REGULAR MEMBERS[1]—NAAB

## ABS GLOBAL

P.O. Box 459
(1525 River Rd.)
DeForest, WI 53532
Tel: 608/846-3721
Fax: 608/846-6444 or 6446
Ian Biggs, President & CEO
http://www.absglobal.com

## ACCELERATED GENETICS

E10890 Penny Ln.
Baraboo, WI 53913
Tel: 608/356-8357
Fax: 608/356-4387
Roger Ripley, Gen. Manager

## ACCELERATED—PRODUCTION FACILITY

Rt. 2, Box 50
Westby, WI 54667
Tel: 608/634-3111
Fax: 608/634-2295
http://www.accelgen.com

## ALTA GENETICS—USA

P.O. Box 437
(N8350 High Rd.)
Watertown, WI 53094
Tel: 920/261-5065
Fax: 920/262-8025
Dean Hermsdorff, Manager
http://www.altagenetics.com

## ALTA GENETICS—Secondary Location

ALTA-CALIFORNIA
P.O. Box 669
(20421 Geer Ave.)
Hilmar, CA 95324
Tel: 209/632-5836
Fax: 209/632-6499
Mike Hobby, Manager
Lab: Tracy, CA Tel: 209/833-3975

## ANDROGENICS

P.O. Box 183
(11240 26 Mile Rd.)
Oakdale, CA 95361-0183
Tel: 209/833-3975
Fax: 209/847-5711
Michael J. Miller, Owner/Manager

## CENTRAL VALLEY DAIRY BREEDERS

P.O. Box 1375
(11116 Sierra Rd.)
Oakdale, CA 95361
Tel: 209/847-4797
Fax: 209/847-5874
Larry Gerber, Jack Lerch, Managers

## CVDB—Secondary Location

32077 Road 144
Visalia, CA 93277
Tel: 559/798-2290
Fax: 559/798-0103
Joe Berry, Owner/President

---

[1] Regular members of the National Association of Animal Breeders, Inc., as published in 2002. All of the NAAB members participate in the CSS program.

## COOPERATIVE RESOURCES INT'L (CRI)

P.O. Box 469
(100 MBC Dr.)
Shawano, WI 54166
Tel: 715/526-2141
Fax: 715/526-3219
Doug Wilson, Chief Executive Officer
http://www.crinet.com

## GENEX COOP., INC.—HEADQUARTERS

P.O. Box 469
(100 MBC Dr.)
Shawano, WI 54166
Tel: 715/526-2141
Fax: 715/526-3219

## GENEX—Secondary Locations

GENEX CUSTOM COLLECTION
SERVICES—ALABAMA
200 Valhalla SE
Ft. Payne, AL 35967
Bobby Fair, Manager
Tel: 256/845-2530
Fax: 256/845-7201
Jill McConnell, Facilities Manager

GENEX COOP, INC.
2288 Gourrier Ave.
Baton, Rouge, LA 70808
Tel: 225/388-3292
Fax: 225/388-4239
Bobby Fair, Manager

GENEX COOP., INC.
8134 E. State Hwy C
Strafford, MO 65757
Tel: 417/736-2125
Fax: 417/736-3312
Steve Trantham, Manager

GENEX—HAWKEYE-WEST
3642 South 56th St. West
Billings, MT 59101
Tel: 406/656-9034
Fax: 406/656-9870
Scott Spickard, Manager

GENEX COOP., INC.
P.O. Box 5518
(391 Pinetree Rd.)
Ithaca, NY 14850-5518
Tel: 607/272-2011
Fax: 607/272-3928
Gordon Nickerson, Manager

GENEX COOP., INC.
P.O. Box 607
(752 E. State Rd. 18)
Tiffin, OH 44883
Tel: 419/447-6262
Fax: 419/447-6084
Mike Landers, Production Manager

## COTTAGE FARM GENETICS

971 Old Bells Rd.
Jackson, TN 38305
Tel: 731/664-7400
Fax: 731/664-6258
Wesley Klipfel, Manager

## ELGIN BREEDING SERVICE

P.O. Box 68
(Webberville Rd.)
Elgin, TX 78621
Tel: 512/285-2712
Fax: 512/285-9673
Brad Cardwell, Owner/Manager

## EBS/WEST—Secondary Location

Box 696
(Hwy. 48 S. at Nogal Rd.)
Capitan, NM 88316
Tel: 505/354-2929
Fax: 505/354-2942
Sherrie Huddleston, Manager

## GREAT PLAINS BREEDERS SERVICE/TAURUS

Box 468,
(N. Hwy. 83)
Shamrock, TX 79079
Tel: 806/256-5414
Fax: 806/256-3517
Jim Bob Nall, Owner/Manager

## HAWKEYE BREEDERS SERVICE

3257 Old Portland Rd.
Adel, IA 50003
Tel: 515/993-4711 or 4712
Fax: 515/993-4176
Lloyd Jungmann, President/Manager
http://www.hawkeyebreeders.com

## HAWKEYE—Secondary Location

Dakota Sire Service
40275 257th St.
Mitchell, SD 57301

605/996-9100
John Weston, Manager

## HIGH PLAINS GENETICS RESEARCH

HC 80, Box 835-10
Piedmont, SD 57769
Tel: 605/787-4808
Fax: 605/787-7127
Dr. Merlin Gebauer, Manager

## INTERGLOBE GENETICS

14814 N. 1500 E. Airport Rd.
Pontiac, IL 61764
Tel: 815/844-3733
Fax: 815/844-3552
William J. Nolan, Gen. Manager

## JLG ENTERPRISES

P.O. Box 1375
(11116 Sierra Rd.)
Oakdale, CA 95361
Tel: 209/847-4797
Fax: 209/847-5874
Larry Gerber, Jack Lerch, Managers

## K.A.B.S.U.

1401 College Ave. - KSU
Manhattan, KS 66502
Tel: 785/539-3554
Fax: 785/537-4265
Dr. Tom Taul, Manager
http://www.vet.ksu.edu/index/htm

## NEBRASKA BULL SERVICE, LLC

HC 30, Box 97
McCook, NE 69001
Tel: 308/345-2900
Fax: 308/345-2632
Brian Schafer, Manager

## REPRODUCTION ENTERPRISES, INC.

908 N. Prairie Rd.
Stillwater, OK 74074
Tel: 405/377-8037
Fax: 405/377-4541
Les Hutchens, Owner/Manager
http://www.reprod-ent.com

## ROCKY MTN. SIRE SERVICE

1616 Manila Rd.
Bennett, CO 80102
Tel: 303/644-3246

Fax: 303/644-3554
David M. Lewis, Owner/Manager

## SELECT SIRES, INC.

11740 U.S. 42
Plain City, OH 43064
Tel: 614/873-4683
Fax: 614/873-5751
Dave Thorbahn, Gen. Manager
http://www.selectsires.com

## SELECT SIRES—Secondary Location

21 Sire Power Drive
Tunkhannock, PA 18657-9604
Tel: 570/836-3168
Fax: 570/836-1490
Wayne Dudley, Manager

## TAURUS SERVICE, INC.

P.O. Box 164
(Grist Flat Rd.)
Mehoopany, PA 18629
Tel: 570/833-5513 or 5123
Fax: 570/833-2690
Richard W. Witter, Gen. Manager
http://www.taurus-service.com

## ULTIMATE GENETICS

P.O. Box 314
Wheelock, TX 77882
Tel: 979/828-2248
Fax: 979/828-2251
Cary Crow, Manager
http://www.ultimategenetics.com

The following organizations are not NAAB members; however, they participate in Certified Semen Services:

## COLORADO STATE UNIV.

3801 W. Rampart Rd.
CSU Foothills Research Campus
Ft. Collins, CO 80523
Tel: 970/491-4764
Fax: 970/491-4374
Dr. Jim Graham, Dir. Of Science
http://xyinc.com

## FRONTIER GENETICS

80756 Hickey Lane
Hermiston, OR 97838
Tel: 541/567-2930

Fax: 541/567-7982
Dr. Don Peter, Owner/Manager

## GREAT LAKES SIRE SERVICE

723 Himebaugh Rd.
Bronson, MI 49028
Tel: 616/489-9888
Earl Souva, Owner/Manager

## HOFFMAN AI BREEDERS

1950 S. Hwy 89-91
Logan, UT 84321
Tel: 435/753-7883
Fax: 435/753-2951
Lance Moore, President
Doug Coombs, VP, Manager
http://www.hoffmanaibreeders.com

## NICHOLS CRYO-GENETICS

8827 NE 29th
Ankeny, IA 50021
Tel: 515/965-1551
Fax: 515/964-2268
Marvin Nichols, Manager

## NOKOTA GENETICS

6921 Hwy 83 N
Minot, ND 58703-0241
Tel: 701/838-9389
Fax: 701/839-3078
Randy Graham, Manager

## NORTH AMERICAN BREEDERS

P.O. Box 228
Berryville, VA 22611
Tel: 540/955-3647
Tim Schofield, Manager

## PRAIRIE STATE/SELECT SIRES

41W 394 US Hwy 20
Hampshire, IL 60140
Tel: 847/464-5281
Fax: 847/464-4088
Mike Goggin, Manager

## PRAIRIE STATE/SELECT SIRES—
### Secondary Location

201 Park, Box 321
Cornell, IL 61319

## ROBERTS CATTLE SERVICES

6028 Victoria Lane
Billings, MT 59106
Tel: 406/652-3900
Fax: 406/652-1663
Art Roberts, Owner/Manager

## SIRE TECHNOLOGY

5001 County Line Rd.
Springfield, OH 45502
Tel: 937/399-1201
Fax: 360/323-2197
Bob Adams, Owner/Manager
http://www.siretech.com

## SOUTHEASTERN SEMEN SERVICES

16878 45th St.
Wellborn, FL 32094
Tel: 386/963-5916
Fax: 386/963-4319
Scott Randell, Owner/Manager

## VOGLER SEMEN CENTRE LAB, INC.

27104 Church Rd.
Ashland, NE 68003
Tel.: 402/944-2584
Fax: 402/944-2758
Lloyd Vogler, Manager

# CSS International Participating Organizations

## ALTA GENETICS

R.R. 2
Balzac, Alberta, Canada T0M 0E0
Tel: 403/226-0666
Fax: 403/226-4259
Lutz Goedde, Chief Executive Officer
http://www.altagenetics.com

## ALTA EUROPE

Semen Collection Centre
Dijksterweg 51
9977 TD Klein Huisjes

The Netherlands
Tel: 011 315 9552 6661
Fax: 011 315 9552 6667
Focko P. Zwanenburg, Veterinarian

## RAB AUSTRALIA

PMB 6003
Albury, NSW 2640
Australia
Tel: 011 61 2 6026 2226
Fax: 011 61 2 6026 2387

Warwick Ashby, Chief Executive Officer
http://www.rab.com.au

## TOTAL LIVESTOCK GENETICS

P.O. Box 105
Camperdown, Victoria 3260
Australia
Tel: 011 03 5593 2016
Fax: 011 03 5593 2630
Dr. Shane Ashworth, Owner/Manager
http://www.tlg.com.au

# APPENDIX E

# Gestation Table for Cattle

# Gestation Table for Cattle[1]

| Date of Service (JAN) | Due to Calve | Date of Service (FEB) | Due to Calve | Date of Service (MAR) | Due to Calve | Date of Service (APR) | Due to Calve | Date of Service (MAY) | Due to Calve | Date of Service (JUN) | Due to Calve | Date of Service (JUL) | Due to Calve | Date of Service (AUG) | Due to Calve | Date of Service (SEPT) | Due to Calve | Date of Service (OCT) | Due to Calve | Date of Service (NOV) | Due to Calve | Date of Service (DEC) | Due to Calve |
|---|---|---|---|---|---|---|---|---|---|---|---|---|---|---|---|---|---|---|---|---|---|---|---|
| 1 | OCT 10 | 1 | NOV 10 | 1 | DEC 8 | 1 | JAN 8 | 1 | FEB 7 | 1 | MAR 10 | 1 | APR 9 | 1 | MAY 10 | 1 | JUN 10 | 1 | JUL 10 | 1 | AUG 10 | 1 | SEPT 9 |
| 2 | 11 | 2 | 11 | 2 | 9 | 2 | 9 | 2 | 8 | 2 | 11 | 2 | 10 | 2 | 11 | 2 | 11 | 2 | 11 | 2 | 11 | 2 | 10 |
| 3 | 12 | 3 | 12 | 3 | 10 | 3 | 10 | 3 | 9 | 3 | 12 | 3 | 11 | 3 | 12 | 3 | 12 | 3 | 12 | 3 | 12 | 3 | 11 |
| 4 | 13 | 4 | 13 | 4 | 11 | 4 | 11 | 4 | 10 | 4 | 13 | 4 | 12 | 4 | 13 | 4 | 13 | 4 | 13 | 4 | 13 | 4 | 12 |
| 5 | 14 | 5 | 14 | 5 | 12 | 5 | 12 | 5 | 11 | 5 | 14 | 5 | 13 | 5 | 14 | 5 | 14 | 5 | 14 | 5 | 14 | 5 | 13 |
| 6 | 15 | 6 | 15 | 6 | 13 | 6 | 13 | 6 | 12 | 6 | 15 | 6 | 14 | 6 | 15 | 6 | 15 | 6 | 15 | 6 | 15 | 6 | 14 |
| 7 | 16 | 7 | 16 | 7 | 14 | 7 | 14 | 7 | 13 | 7 | 16 | 7 | 15 | 7 | 16 | 7 | 16 | 7 | 16 | 7 | 16 | 7 | 15 |
| 8 | 17 | 8 | 17 | 8 | 15 | 8 | 15 | 8 | 14 | 8 | 17 | 8 | 16 | 8 | 17 | 8 | 17 | 8 | 17 | 8 | 17 | 8 | 16 |
| 9 | 18 | 9 | 18 | 9 | 16 | 9 | 16 | 9 | 15 | 9 | 18 | 9 | 17 | 9 | 18 | 9 | 18 | 9 | 18 | 9 | 18 | 9 | 17 |
| 10 | 19 | 10 | 19 | 10 | 17 | 10 | 17 | 10 | 16 | 10 | 19 | 10 | 18 | 10 | 19 | 10 | 19 | 10 | 19 | 10 | 19 | 10 | 18 |
| 11 | 20 | 11 | 20 | 11 | 18 | 11 | 18 | 11 | 17 | 11 | 20 | 11 | 19 | 11 | 20 | 11 | 20 | 11 | 20 | 11 | 20 | 11 | 19 |
| 12 | 21 | 12 | 21 | 12 | 19 | 12 | 19 | 12 | 18 | 12 | 21 | 12 | 20 | 12 | 21 | 12 | 21 | 12 | 21 | 12 | 21 | 12 | 20 |
| 13 | 22 | 13 | 22 | 13 | 20 | 13 | 20 | 13 | 19 | 13 | 22 | 13 | 21 | 13 | 22 | 13 | 22 | 13 | 22 | 13 | 22 | 13 | 21 |
| 14 | 23 | 14 | 23 | 14 | 21 | 14 | 21 | 14 | 20 | 14 | 23 | 14 | 22 | 14 | 23 | 14 | 23 | 14 | 23 | 14 | 23 | 14 | 22 |
| 15 | 24 | 15 | 24 | 15 | 22 | 15 | 22 | 15 | 21 | 15 | 24 | 15 | 23 | 15 | 24 | 15 | 24 | 15 | 24 | 15 | 24 | 15 | 23 |
| 16 | 25 | 16 | 25 | 16 | 23 | 16 | 23 | 16 | 22 | 16 | 25 | 16 | 24 | 16 | 25 | 16 | 25 | 16 | 25 | 16 | 25 | 16 | 24 |
| 17 | 26 | 17 | 26 | 17 | 24 | 17 | 24 | 17 | 23 | 17 | 26 | 17 | 25 | 17 | 26 | 17 | 26 | 17 | 26 | 17 | 26 | 17 | 25 |
| 18 | 27 | 18 | 27 | 18 | 25 | 18 | 25 | 18 | 24 | 18 | 27 | 18 | 26 | 18 | 27 | 18 | 27 | 18 | 27 | 18 | 27 | 18 | 26 |
| 19 | 28 | 19 | 28 | 19 | 26 | 19 | 26 | 19 | 25 | 19 | 28 | 19 | 27 | 19 | 28 | 19 | 28 | 19 | 28 | 19 | 28 | 19 | 27 |
| 20 | 29 | 20 | 29 | 20 | 27 | 20 | 27 | 20 | 26 | 20 | 29 | 20 | 28 | 20 | 29 | 20 | 29 | 20 | 29 | 20 | 29 | 20 | 28 |
| 21 | 30 | 21 | 30 | 21 | 28 | 21 | 28 | 21 | 27 | 21 | 30 | 21 | 29 | 21 | 30 | 21 | 30 | 21 | 30 | 21 | 30 | 21 | 29 |
| 22 | 31 | 22 | DEC 1 | 22 | 29 | 22 | 29 | 22 | 28 | 22 | 31 | 22 | 30 | 22 | 31 | 22 | JUL 1 | 22 | 31 | 22 | 31 | 22 | 30 |
| 23 | NOV 1 | 23 | 2 | 23 | 30 | 23 | 30 | 23 | MAR 1 | 23 | APR 1 | 23 | MAY 1 | 23 | JUN 1 | 23 | 2 | 23 | AUG 1 | 23 | SEPT 1 | 23 | OCT 1 |
| 24 | 2 | 24 | 3 | 24 | 31 | 24 | 31 | 24 | 2 | 24 | 2 | 24 | 2 | 24 | 2 | 24 | 3 | 24 | 2 | 24 | 2 | 24 | 2 |
| 25 | 3 | 25 | 4 | 25 | JAN 1 | 25 | FEB 1 | 25 | 3 | 25 | 3 | 25 | 3 | 25 | 3 | 25 | 4 | 25 | 3 | 25 | 3 | 25 | 3 |
| 26 | 4 | 26 | 5 | 26 | 2 | 26 | 2 | 26 | 4 | 26 | 4 | 26 | 4 | 26 | 4 | 26 | 5 | 26 | 4 | 26 | 4 | 26 | 4 |
| 27 | 5 | 27 | 6 | 27 | 3 | 27 | 3 | 27 | 5 | 27 | 5 | 27 | 5 | 27 | 5 | 27 | 6 | 27 | 5 | 27 | 5 | 27 | 5 |
| 28 | 6 | 28 | 7 | 28 | 4 | 28 | 4 | 28 | 6 | 28 | 6 | 28 | 6 | 28 | 6 | 28 | 7 | 28 | 6 | 28 | 6 | 28 | 6 |
| 29 | 7 | 29 | 8 | 29 | 5 | 29 | 5 | 29 | 7 | 29 | 7 | 29 | 7 | 29 | 7 | 29 | 8 | 29 | 7 | 29 | 7 | 29 | 7 |
| 30 | 8 | ... | ... | 30 | 6 | 30 | 6 | 30 | 8 | 30 | 8 | 30 | 8 | 30 | 8 | 30 | 9 | 30 | 8 | 30 | 8 | 30 | 8 |
| 31 | 9 | ... | ... | 31 | 7 | ... | ... | 31 | 9 | ... | ... | 31 | 9 | 31 | 9 | ... | ... | 31 | 9 | ... | ... | 31 | 9 |

[1] The average length of gestation for cattle ranges from 270 to 290 days, with an average of about 280 days. The above table indicates a gestation length of 282 days. Holsteins generally have a gestation of one or two days less than the other breeds. Bull calves are carried one to two days longer than heifers. Twins or multi-birth calves may be born one to two weeks earlier than single-birth calves.

# Stud Code Numbers Assigned

National Association of Animal Breeders
P.O. Box 1033
Columbia, Missouri 65205

| Stud Code | Organization and Address | Date Assigned |
|---|---|---|
| 1. | Noba, Inc./21st Century Genetics/Genex Cooperative, subsidiaries of Cooperative Resources International, P.O. Box 469, Shawano, WI 54166 Tel: 715/526-2141; Fax:715/526-3219 (formerly assigned to Noba, Inc.) | 01/01/95 |
| 2. | COBA/Select Sires, 1224 Alton Darby Rd., Columbus, OH 43228 Tel: 614/878-5333; Fax: 614/870-2622 | |
| 3. | Genex Cooperative, P.O. Box 5518, Ithaca, NY 14852-5518 Tel: 607/272-2011; Fax:607/272-3928 (formerly assigned to Eastern AI Coop) | 12/15/73 |
| 4. | Northstar/Select Sires, Inc., P.O. Box 23157, E. Lansing MI 48909-3157 Tel: 517/351-3180 (formerly assigned to MABC/SS) | |
| 5. | KABA/Select Sires, 1930 Herr Lane, Louisville, KY 40222 Tel: 502/425-1868 | |
| 6. | Prairie State Breeders/Select Sires, 41W 394 US Hwy 20, Hampshire, IL 60140 Tel: 847/464-5281; Fax: 847/464-4088 (formerly assigned to Illinois Brdng. Coop.) | |
| 7. | Select Sires, Inc. 11740 U.S. 42, Plain City, OH 43064 Tel: 614/873-4683; Fax: 614/873-5751 | 12/12/73 |
| 8. | Genex Cooperative, P.O. Box 5518, Ithaca, NY 14852 Tel: 607/272-2011; Fax: 607/272-3928 (formerly assigned to Federated Genetics, formerly assigned to Louisiana Animal Breeders Coop) | 11/01/85 |
| 9. | Sire Power, Inc., 21 Sire Power Dr., Tunkhannock, PA 18657 Tel: 570/836-3168; Fax: 570/836-1490 | 11/03/69 |
| 10. | Mississippi Animal Breeders Cooperative, Drawer BA, State College, MS 39762 | |
| 11. | Alta Genetics—USA, P.O. Box 437, N8350 High Rd., Watertown, WI 53094 Tel: 920/261-5065; Fax: 920/262-8025 (formerly assigned to Landmark Genetics, formerly assigned to Carnation/Genetics) | 11/01/72 |
| 12. | Cache Valley Breeding Association, 1950 N. Main, Logan, UT 84321 Tel: 801/752-2022 | |
| 13. | All West Breeders, P.O. Box 507, Burlington, WA 98233 Tel: 360/757-6093 | |
| 14. | Accelerated Genetics, Rt 2, Box 50, Westby, WI 54667 Tel: 608/356-8357; Fax: 608/356-4387 (formerly assigned to Tri-State Breeders Coop) | |

15. Genex Cooperative, 1575 Apollo Drive, Lancaster, PA 17601
    Tel: 717/569-0413 (formerly assigned to Atlantic Breeders Service)

16. Kansas Artificial Breeding Service Unit, 1401 College Ave., KSU, Manhattan,
    KS 66502 Tel: 785/539-3554; Fax: 785/537-4265

17. Minnesota Valley Breeders Association, P.O. Box 500,
    New Prague, MN 56071

18. East Tennessee Artificial Breeders Assn., Route 10, Tipton Station Rd.,
    Knoxville, TN 37020 Tel: 615/577-4892

19. Virginia/North Carolina/Select Sires, P.O. Box 370, Rocky Mount,          11/02/65
    VA 42151 Tel: 703/483-5123

20. Union Régionale des Coopératies d'Elevage de l'Ouest (URCEO) 50, rue
    Brizeux, Loudeac, France Tel: 96 28 25 83                                 05/18/95
    (formerly assigned to Tennessee Artificial Breeding [11/16/65] Franklin, TN
    24151 Tel: 615/790-9914)

21. 21st Century Genetics, P.O. Box 469, Shawano, WI 54166                     05/09/67
    Tel: 715/526-2141; Fax: 715/526-3219 (formerly assigned to Midwest
    Breeders Coop.)

22. Fry's Reproductive Center, 191 Fry Rd., Rose Bud, AR 72137                 11/15/87
    Tel: 501/556-5080; Fax:501/556-4771 (formerly assigned to Norwood
    Breeding Center;Codding-Noba)

23. Excelsior Farms, 7401 Hamner Rd, Corona, CA 91720 Tel: 909/737-2343;      01/29/69
    Fax:909/737-2344

24. Genetics, Hughson, CA (sold to Carnation 11/1/72) Tel: 209/883-4001

25. Sire Power, Inc. Custom Service, 21 Sire Power Dr., Tunkhannock, PA 18657, 03/20/95
    (formerly assigned to NEBA, Rt. 2, Tunkhannock, PA 18657, 09/16/68)

26. East Central Breeders Assn., Box 191, Waupun, WI 53963                     09/22/69
    Tel: 414/324-3505

27. Herdsman, Inc., Box 391, Putnam, CT 06260                                  11/07/69

28. Alta Genetics, Canadian AI Division, RR #2, Balzac, Alberta, Canada        05/04/70
    T0M 0E0 Tel: 403/226-0666; Fax: 403/226-4259 (formerly assigned to
    Western Breeders Service, Ltd.)

29. ABS Global, Inc. , P.O. Box 459, DeForest, WI 53532 Tel: 608/846-3721;     05/27/70
    Fax:608/846-6444 or 6446 (formerly assigned to American Breeders
    Service)

30. Genetic Engineering, Inc., P.O. Box 33554, Northglenn, CO 80233            11/12/80
    Tel: 303/457-1311

31. Golden State Breeders, 18907 E. Lone Tree Rd., Escalon CA 95320            08/29/70
    Tel: 209/838-7891 (formerly assigned to The Bull Bank)

32. Larry Moore Ranch, Inc., Suamico, WI 54173                                 10/06/70

33. Excelsior Farms Custom Freezing Service, 7401 Hamner Ave., Corona,         12/29/78
    CA 91720 Tel: 909/737-2343; Fax:909/737-2344

34. Nokota Genetics, Rt. 1, Box 143, Minot, ND 58701 Tel:701/838-9389;         10/28/82
    Fax:701/839-3078

35. Spring Creek Ranch, 380 Collierville-Arlington Rd., Collierville, TN 38017    10/28/82
Tel: 901/853-7660

36. North American Breeders, Inc., Rt. 1, Box 228, Berryville, VA 22611    12/01/70
Tel: 540/955-3647

37. 21st Century Genetics, PO Box 500, New Prague, MN    06/04/91

38. Big Beef Hybrids, Box 248, Stillwater, MN 55082[1]    03/05/71

39. Westgen, Box 40, Milner, BC, Canada V0X 1T0 Tel: 604/530-1144;    04/29/71
Fax:604/534-3036 (formerly assigned to British Columbia AI Centre)

40. Curtiss Breeding Industries, Cary, IL 60013 (formerly assigned to Curtiss    07/26/71
Breeding Service)

41. Sire Management Services, LLC, 355 Highway 26 East, Elko, GA 31025    12/17/96
Tel: 912/987-2171; Fax: 912/987-4431 (formerly assigned to Noba-Georgia,
formerly assigned to D & D Bull Motel)

42. Southwest A.I. Custom Freezing Center, Rt. 1, Box 50-A Ponder, TX 76259    11/10/71

43. International Genes, Inc., 2120 Argonne Dr., Minneapolis MN 54421*    03/01/72

44. Central Valley Dairy Breeders, 32077 Road 144, Visalia, CA 93277    06/08/93
Tel: 209/798-2290; Fax: 209/798-0103 (formerly assigned to Adohr Dairy
Farms, Box 88, Camarillo, CA 93010)

45. Artificial Insemination Program of Puerto Rico, Box 726, Dorado, PR 00646    01/30/74
(Select Sires, Columbus, OH 7/5/72)

46. Wye Plantation, Queenstown, MD 21658    08/15/72

47. Genex Coop., 2288 Gourrier Ave, Baton Rouge, LA 70803    11/01/85
Tel: 225/388-3292; Fax:225/388-4239 (formerly assigned to Louisiana
Animal Breeders Coop.,formerly assigned to Pioneer Beef Cattle Co.)

48. Genex Custom Collection Services—Alabama, 200 Valhalla SE, Ft. Payne,    02/21/02
AL 35967 Tel: 256/845-2530; Fax: 256/845-7201 (formerly 21st Century
Custom Service, Shawano, WI 54166) (formerly assigned to Midwest Breeders
Custom Service)

49. 21st Century Genetics Custom Freezing Service, Rt. 3, Box 295-100,    11/25/85
Strafford, MO 65757 Tel: 417/736-2125 (formerly assigned to Maryland
Artificial Brdng Coop.)

50. Sire Power Custom Freezing Service (formerly assigned to West Virginia
Artificial Breeders Cooperative, Box 555, Frederick, MD 21701, 11/30/74)

51. Ontario Swine Association, P.O. Box 457, Woodstock,Ont., Canada    12/31/75
N4S 7Y7 Tel: 519/539-5636 (Codding Cattle Research—inactive)

52. Colorado State University, Animal Reproduction Laboratory, Ft. Collins,
CO 80521 Tel: 970/491-4764; Fax: 970/491-4374    01/30/74

53. General Genetics, 13811 Cypress, Sand Lake, MI 49343 Tel: 616/636-5032    01/30/74

54. Hawkeye Breeders Service, 3257 Old Portland Road, Adel, IA 50003    01/30/74
Tel: 515/993-4711;Fax:515/993-4176

55. International Cryo Biological Service, Inc., 1935 W. Country Rd., B-2,    01/30/74
St. Paul, MN 55113*

56. Ultimate Genetics, P.O. Box 314, Wheelock, TX 77882 Tel: 979/828-2248; Fax: 979/828-2251 (formerly Medina Valley A.I. Lab) — 01/30/74

57. New Breeds Industries, Box 959, Manhattan, KS 66502 Tel: 913/537-2914 — 01/30/74

58. Pioneer Beef Cattle Co., Box 37, Johnston, IA 50323* — 10/01/72

59. Rocky Mountain Sire Service, 1616 Manilla Road, Bennett, CO 80102 Tel: 303/644-3246; Fax:303/644-3554 (formerly assigned to Ankony Shadow Isle; Premier Breeding Center)

60. Al Rose Breeding Service, 517 W. Granada Ct., Ontario, CA 91672 Tel: 714/947-0309 — 01/30/74

61. Soligenics Frozen Semen Service, 584 Thompsonville Rd., Suffield, CT 06078 — 01/30/74

62. Southeastern Frozen Semen Service, 3522 New Berlin, Box 26088, Jacksonville, FL 32218 — 01/30/74

63. Topline A.I. Service, Inc., Rt. 10, Galyon Lane, Knoxville, TN 37920* — 01/30/74

64. West Tennessee Artificial Breeding Assn., Box 38, Yorkville, TN 38389 — 01/30/74

65. Roy Selover Co. Livestock Enterprises, 924 Elm St., Modesto, CA 95351 — 01/30/74

66. BOV Imports, Inc., 205 Livestock Exchg. Bldg., Denver, CO 80216 — 01/30/74

67. Canadian Stock Breeders Service, Ltd., Box 98, Winterburn, ALB Canada — 01/30/74

68. Chilliwack Artificial Insemination Centre, 10119 Kent Rd., Chilliwack, British Columbia, Canada* — 01/30/74

69. Nova Scotia Animal Breeders Coop. Ltd., Rt. 1, Truro, NS, Canada — 01/30/74

70. Eastern Breeders, Inc., Box 2000 Kemptville, Ontario, Canada K0G 1J0 Tel: 613/258-5944; Fax:613/258-3719 — 01/30/74

71. Gencor, Rt. 5, Guelph, Ont, Canada, N1H 6J2 Tel: 519/821-2150 (formerly assigned to United Breeders, Inc.) — 01/30/74

72. Gencor, Rt. 5, Guelph, Ont, Canada, N1H 6J2 Tel: 519/821-2150 (formerly assigned to Western Ontario Breeders, Inc.) — 01/30/74

73. Quebec Artificial Breeding Centre (CIAQ), C.P. 518, St. Hyacinthe Quebec, Canada J2S 7B8 Tel: 514/774-1141; Fax:514/774-9318 — 01/30/74

74. Universal Genetics, Ltd., P.O. Box 910, Cardston, Alberta Canada T0K 0K0 Tel: 403/653-4437 (formerly assigned to Universal Semen Service, Ltd.) — 01/30/74

75. High Plains Genetics Research, Inc., HC80, Box 835-10, Piedmont Rt., Piedmont, SD 57769 Tel: 605/787-4808; Fax:605/787-7127 (formerly assigned to Y Tex Corp) — 10/27/83

76. Taurus-Service Inc., P.O. Box 164, Mehoopany, PA 18629 Tel: 570/833-5513; Fax:570/833-2690 — 03/22/74

77. Pan American Breeders, 702 E 18th St., Greeley, CO 80631 — 04/08/74

78. Genex Cooperative Custom Semen Service, P.O. Box 5518 Ithaca, NY 14851 Tel: 607/272-2011; Fax: 607/272-3928 — 05/02/74

| 79. | Northeast Frozen Semen Service, P.O. Box 153, Lafayette, NC 13084 | 06/21/74 |
|---|---|---|
| 80. | Steele's Semen Service, Box 2, Dimock, PA 18816 | 07/03/74 |
| 81. | Hybrid Vigor, Inc., Buffalo Valley, TN 38548 | 07/16/74 |
| 82. | North Carolina State University, P.O. Box 5127, Raleigh, NC 27607 | 07/05/74 |
| 83. | Illini Sire Service, 201 Park St., Cornell, Il 61319 Tel: 815/358-2897 (formerly assigned to Bovine Cryogenics, Inc.) | 07/05/74 |
| 84. | Landmark Genetics Custom Freezing Business, Box 939, Hughson, CA 95326 Tel: 209/883-4001 (formerly assigned to Carnation/Genetics) | 07/16/74 |
| 85. | Tri-State Breeders Coop Custom Freezing Business, Westby, WI 54467 Tel: 608/356-8357 | 07/16/74 |
| 86. | Ozark Bull Center, Rt 4, Box 223, Ava, MO 65608 Tel:417/683-3894 | 07/30/74 |
| 87. | Arizona Bull Center Custom Semen Freezing Service, 14217 N. 51st Ave., Glendale, AZ 85306 | 07/30/74 |
| 88. | Frontier Genetics, 80756 Hickey Ln., Hermiston, OR 97838 Tel: 541/567-2930; Fax: 541/567-7982 (formerly assigned to Oasis Genetics, International Breeders Service, and Gibson's Custom Collection Service) | 02/10/97 |
| 89. | New Brunswick Central A.I. Coop. Ltd., Box 1567, Fredericton, New Brunswick, Canada E3B 5G2 Tel: 506/454-3327 | 08/20/74 |
| 90. | Genex—Hawkeye West, 3642 Dustin Dr., Rt. 9, Billings, MT 59101 Tel: 406/656-9034; Fax:406/656-9870 (formerly assigned to Hawkeye West, Big Sky Genetics) | 08/13/92 |
| 91. | Dependa-Bull Services, R.D. 2, Verona, NY 14378 Tel 315/829-2250 | 10/03/74 |
| 92. | A.I. International, Ltd., Rt. 2, Box 136-E, Philomath, OR 97370* | 10/03/74 |
| 93. | Smith Livestock Service, Box 775, Roundup, MT 59072 | 11/04/74 |
| 94. | St. Jacobs ABC, RR. #1, Elmira, Ontario, Canada N3B 2Z1 Tel: 519/664-1616 | 12/02/74 |
| 95. | Canadian Genetics, Ltd., Box 6, Yorkton, Sask. Canada S3N 2V6 (formerly assigned to Sask. Artificial Brdrs. Coop. Ltd.) | 12/02/74 |
| 96. | Hualalai Ranch & Vet. Clinic Reproduction Lab., Rt. 1 Box 394, Holualoa, HI 96725 Tel: 808/325-7112 | 12/06/74 |
| 97. | Holland Genetics v.o.f., P.O. Box 5073, Arnhem, The Netherlands Tel: 31.26.3864100; Fax: 31.26.3864122 (formerly assigned to Bovine Test Center) | 09/22/97 |
| 98. | Cattle Reproduction, Inc., 4527 88th St., Omaha, NE 68127 | |
| 99. | Hoffman A.I. Breeders, 1950 S. Hwy 89-91, Logan, UT 84321 Tel: 435/753-7883 (formerly assigned to Hi Country AI) | 03/12/85 |
| 100. | JLG Enterprises, Inc., P.O. Box 1375, Oakdale, CA 95361 Tel: 209/847-4797; Fax:209/874-5874 (formerly assigned to JLG Custom Freezing Service) | 04/22/75 |
| 101. | Johansen's Custom Collecting and Freezing Service, Rt. 3, Box 3144, Nampa, ID 83650* | 04/22/75 |

| | | |
|---|---|---|
| 102. | Agro Brothers Ltd., Rt. 2, Hamilton, Ontario, Canada | 04/22/75 |
| 103. | Treasure Valley Breeding Service, P.O. Box 615, Meridan, ID 83642 | 06/06/75 |
| 104. | Newk's Semen Processing, Rt. 1, Mt. Vernon, MO 65712 | 02/14/76 |
| 105. | AI Breeding Service, 3668 Summerhill, Carson City, NV 89701 | 06/22/76 |
| 106. | Nebraska Bull Service, HC 30, Box 97, McCook, NE 69001 Tel: 308/345-2900; Fax: 308/345-2632 | 02/14/77 |
| 107. | A A Breeders Service, P.O. Box 161, Fayette, IA 52142 | 03/10/77 |
| 108. | Minnesota Valley Breeders Assn. Custom Collection Service New Prague, MN 56071 Tel: 612/758-4443 | 05/02/77 |
| 109. | Reproduction Enterprises, Rt. 1, Box 645, Stillwater, OK 74074 Tel: 405/377-8037; Fax: 405/377-4541 | 12/19/77 |
| 110. | Western Herd Sires/Delta G, P.O. Box 1807, Turlock, CA 95380 Tel: 209/667-2323 | 01/03/78 |
| 111. | Longview Marketing Inc., P.O. Box 297, Mead, CO 80542 | 03/02/79 |
| 112. | Ministry of Agriculture & Fisheries, Livestock Development Div., Old Harbour P.O., Bodles, Jamaica, West Indies | 02/14/78 |
| 113. | Center Insemination Porcine du Quebec, C.P. 220, St. Lambert de Levis, Beauce Nord, Quebec, Canada G0S 2W0 | 04/25/78 |
| 114. | Independent Breeders Service, P.O. Box 3608, Aidrie, Alberta, Canada T4B 2B8 Tel: 403/946-5667; Fax: 403/946-5721 | 08/31/78 |
| 115. | Alberta Swine Breeding Center, RR #2, Leduc, Alberta, Canada T0E 2X2 | 04/04/79 |
| 116. | Bainbrook Dairy Goat AI Center, Milgrove, Ontario, Canada | 04/04/79 |
| 117. | International Agricultural Services, Inc., 320 Judah St., San Francisco, CA 94122 Tel: 415/664-4636 | 06/13/80 |
| 118. | Superior Genetics, PO Box 189, Shandon, OH 45063 Tel: 513/738-3885 (formerly assigned to Ohio Breeders Supply, 2864 Chapel Rd., Okeana, OH 45053-12/24/80) | 12/24/80 |
| 119. | Southern Genetic Services, Rt. 1, Box 63-B, Poteau, OK 74953 Tel: 918/647-8145 (formerly assigned to Southeastern OK Reprod. Services) | 10/23/81 |
| 120. | Zimmerman Custom Freezing, 131 Red Well Road, New Holland, PA 17557 Tel: 717/299-4885 (formerly Better Life Research, Inc.) | 08/11/83 |
| 121. | Advanced Genetics, Inc., R.F.D. 2, Leesburg, ID 46538 Tel: 219/453-3602 | 09/19/83 |
| 122. | Network Genetics, P.O. Box 669, Hilmar, CA 95324 Tel: 209/632-5836; Fax: 209/632-6499 (formerly assigned to Spermco, Inc. 10/27/83) | 06/01/95 |
| 123. | J. N. Farnham Custom Freezing Service, 8338 W. Glenrosa Ave. Phoenix, AZ 85037 | 01/14/84 |
| 124. | Texas Breeders Service, Inc., P.O. Box 1635, San Marcos, TX 78667 Tel: 512/357-6162 (formerly assigned to Genetic Resources) | 02/06/84 |
| 125. | Southeastern Reproduction Center, Rt. 3, Box 216, Graceville, FL 32440 Tel: 904/263-6983 | 04/19/84 |

| 126. | Price's Embryo Genetics, 1601 E. 2nd St., Rosewell, NM 88201<br>Tel: 505/622-2181 | 04/24/84 |
|---|---|---|
| 127. | Palouse Embryonics, N.W. 2105 Friel, Pullman, WA 99163 | 06/25/84 |
| 128. | CryovaTech International, Inc., Rt. 5, Box 48, Hwy 35 N. River Falls, WI 54022 Tel: 715/425-6661 | 09/07/84 |
| 129. | Vogler Semen Centre Lab, Inc., 27104 Church Rd., Ashland, NE 68003<br>Tel: 402/944-2584; Fax: 402/944-2758 (formerly assigned to Semen Centre) | 09/11/84 |
| 130. | National Breeding Company, 27765 Case Rd., Wauconda, IL 60084<br>Tel: 312/526-8310 | 11/21/84 |
| 131. | Majestic Bovines, P.O. Box 166, Elberta, UT 84626 Tel: 801/667-3333 | 01/29/85 |
| 132. | Leprechaun Genetics, 18116 Garden Valley Rd., Marengo IL 60152<br>Tel: 815/568-8398 | 04/09/85 |
| 133. | Dr. Barry Hays, DVM, P.O. Box 877, Shelbyville, KY 40065<br>Tel: 502/633-4338 | 05/20/85 |
| 134. | Kentucky Bovine Services, Rt. 6, Box 2 T J Rd., Leitchfield, KY 42654 | 06/26/85 |
| 135. | Southern Genetics, P.O. Box 141, Shady Dale, GA 31085<br>Tel: 404/468-2188 | 07/01/85 |
| 136. | DJR Collection Service, P.O. Box 446, Irrigon, OR 97844 Tel: 503/922-4342 | 08/13/85 |
| 137. | Nichols Cryo-Genetics, 8827 NE 29th, Ankeny, IA 50021 Tel: 515/965-1551;<br>Fax: 515/964-2268 (formerly assigned to Iowa State University) | 07/12/99 |
| 138. | Interglobe Genetics, Route 1 Box 293, Airport Road, Pontiac, IL 61764<br>Tel: 815/844-3733; Fax: 815/844-3552 | 11/12/85 |
| 139. | Progressive Genetics, P.O. Box 1378, Bartow, FL 33830 | 12/26/85 |
| 140. | Sire Technology International, 5001 County Line Rd.,Springfield, OH 45502<br>Tel: 937/399-1201; Fax: 360/323-2197 | 03/07/86 |
| 141. | Granada Sire Services, Inc., P.O. Box 99, Wheelock, TX 77882<br>Tel: 409/828-5156 | 03/24/86 |
| 142. | Sire Services, 6248 Ramona St., Rancho Cucamonga, CA 91701 | 04/28/86 |
| 143. | Purebred Embryos Company, Inc. 3927 Green Valley Dr. Bryan, TX 77802<br>Tel: 409/822-5922 | 08/11/86 |
| 144. | Custom Cryogenics, P.O. Box 1122, Oakdale, CA 95361 Tel: 209/847-7112 | 09/12/86 |
| 145. | Powell Genetic Services, RR 2, Box 107, Howard, SD 57349 | 03/09/87 |
| 146. | Premier Veterinary Services, P.O. Box 607, Shelbyville, KY 40065 | 04/20/87 |
| 147. | Androgenics, 11240 26 Mile Rd., Oakdale, CA 95361 Tel: 209/8471101 | 12/16/87 |
| 148. | Greater Northern Genetics Int'l, Ltd., RR2, Box 13A, Kathryn, ND 58049<br>Tel: 701/762-4469 | 02/08/88 |
| 149. | Rocky Mountain Bovine Reproduction Center, 13601 N. Washington St.,<br>Denver, CO 80233 Tel: 970/522-9011 | 02/10/88 |
| 150. | Equine Veterinary Services, P.O. Box 1097, Half Moon Bay, CA 94019<br>Tel: 715/726-2305 | 02/17/88 |

| 151. | Trans World Genetics, N124 Willow Rd., Sheboygan Falls, WI 53085<br>Tel: 920/893-8844; Fax: 920/892-4282 (Formerly Complete Sire<br>Services, Inc.) | 05/02/88 |
| 152. | Apex Genetics, Rt. 4, Box 342-D, Hwy 55 E, Apex, NC 27502<br>Tel: 919/362-8878 | 05/03/88 |
| 153. | Southeastern Semen Services, Inc., 16878 45th Rd., Wellborn, FL 32094<br>Tel: 386/963-5916 | 12/08/88 |
| 154. | EBS/West, Box 696, Capitan, NM 88316 505/354-2929<br>(EBS, Box 68, Elgin, TX 78621 Tel: 512/285-2712; Fax:512/285-9673) | 07/13/89<br>(01/11/90) |
| 155. | Clarks Custom Collection, W1211-178 Riverview Dr., Sullivan, WI 53178 | 08/25/89 |
| 156. | Cottage Farm Genetics, 971 Old Bells Rd., Jackson, TN 38305<br>Tel: 731/664-7400; Fax: 731/664-6258 | 01/20/90 |
| 157. | Great Plains Breeders Service/Taurus, Box 468, Shamrock, TX 79079<br>Tel: 806/256-5414; Fax: 806/256-3517 | 06/18/90 |
| 158. | Galaxie Genetics Reproductive Center, Inc., 4173 Lyman Dr. Hilliard,<br>OH 43026 Tel: 614/857-1221 | 06/22/90 |
| 159. | Special Sires, Inc., 131 Zook Mill Rd, POB 487, Brownstown, PA 17508<br>Tel: 717/399-6445 | 08/07/90 |
| 160. | Genetics Australia Cooperative Society Limited, P.O. Box 195, Bacchus<br>Marsh, Victoria 3340, Australia Tel: 61 3 5367 3888 (formerly Victorian<br>Artificial Breeders Coop. Society) | 01/14/98 |
| 161. | Excel Breeders Int'l., Box 2353, Bismarck, ND 58502-2353<br>Tel: 701/663-0724 (formerly assigned to Western Breeders International) | 09/25/91 |
| 162. | C.O.F.A. (Cooperativa di Fecondazione Artificiale), Corso Campi 46, 26100<br>Cremona, Italy Tel: 39 372 460320 | 11/05/92 |
| 163. | Ambreed, NZ Ltd., PO Box 176, Hamilton, New Zealand Tel: (64) 78275058 | 11/09/92 |
| 164. | Kvægavlsforeningen Fyn, Orbækvej 276, Odense SØ 5220 Denmark<br>Tel: 45 66 15 73 33 | 11/17/92 |
| 165. | Hampshire Cattle Breeder's Society, AI Centre, Lyndhurst, Hampshire,<br>SO43 7NN, England Tel: 0703-283606 | 12/07/92 |
| 166. | Pecplan Bradesco Inseminação Artificial LTDA, Cidade De Deus - Villa Yara,<br>Osasco, São Paulo 06029-900, Brazil Tel: (55) 11 704 57 44 | 12/09/92 |
| 167. | Animal Fertility Service, 80034 Kenzie Rd., Covington, LA 70433<br>Tel: 504/893-3839 | 03/19/93 |
| 168. | Double D Genetics, HCR 67, Box 30E, Kenedy, TX 78119<br>Tel: 210/583-9967 | 05/03/93 |
| 169. | Centre d'insemination Ovine du Québec (C.I.O.Q.), 198 Ave. Industrielle,<br>C.P. 1539, LaPocatiere, Quebec, Canada. Tel: 418/856-5422 | 05/20/93 |
| 170. | Holland Genetics, POB 5073, 6802 FB Arnhem, The Netherlands<br>Tel: 312 6386410 | 03/31/94 |
| 171. | Zuid-Oost Genetics, PO Box 79, 7240 AB, Lochem, The Netherlands<br>Tel: 31 0573-38100 | 03/31/94 |

172.  Coop 'Land Van Cuijk,' Dr. Moonsweg 5, 5437 BG, Beers, The Netherlands          03/31/94
      Tel: 31 8850-12754

173.  Tyrestation Skaerup, Helleskovvej 3A, 7480 Vildbjerg, Denmark                   08/12/94
      Tel: 45 97 13 23 82

174.  Osnabrucker Herdbuch, Fockinghausen, 49324 Melle, Germany                       08/19/94
      Tel: +49-5422-9870

175.  South Texas Breeding Service, HCR 67, Box STBS, Kenedy, TX 78119                12/15/94
      Tel: 210/583-3496; Fax: 830/583-3518

176.  Haliba, Route D'Obourg, 65, 7000 Mons Belgium, Tel: 65.36.23.02                 12/16/94

177.  C.I.A. Linllalux, Rue des Champs Elysées 18, B5590 Ciney, Belgium              12/16/94
      Tel: 32.83.215795

178.  Roberts Cattle Services, Inc., 6028 Victoria Lane, Billings, MT 59106           02/02/95
      Tel: 406/652-3900

179.  Great Lakes Sire Service, 723 Himebaugh Rd., Bronson, MI 49028                  03/09/95
      Tel: 616/489-9888

180.  Ouest Genetique Elevage Reproduction (OGER), LA Bussierie, BP80 Blain,          05/18/95
      44130 France. Tel: 40 79 02 74

181.  Rocky Ridge Cattle Services, Box 181, Evans Ranch of Rocky Ridge,               07/24/95
      Raynesford, MT 59469 Tel: 406/738-4316

182.  Holstein Genetique France, 3595 Route de Tournai, 59500 Douai, France           09/11/95
      Tel: (33)27.99.29.29; Fax: (33)27.88.09.27

183.  Union Nord-Ouest Genetique (UNOG), Bosc Berenger, 76680 Saint Saens,            12/08/95
      France Tel: 0033 35 34 52 81; Fax: 0033 35 32 35 39

184.  Rinder-Union West e. G., Schiffahrter Damm 235A, Muenster, Germany              12/21/95
      Tel: 49 2 51 92 88 2 58; Fax: 49 2 51 92 88 2 36

185.  VOSt-OV, Besamungstation Georgsheil, Am Bahndamm 4, 2664                        02/20/96
      Südbrookmerland, Germany, Tel:0491/8004-9; Fax: 0491/8004-22

186.  Holbrook Artificial Breeders, Byng St., Holbrook, NSW 2644, Australia           02/27/96
      Tel: 6160 362 374; Fax: 6160 362 615

187.  Total Livestock Genetics, Pty Ltd, PO Box 105, Camperdown, Victoria 3260,       03/08/96
      Australia Tel: 011 03 5593 2016; Fax: 011 03 5593 2630

188.  Belmont Breeders, Box 391, Intercourse, PA 17534 Tel: 717/808-4907;             05/30/96
      Fax: 717/768-8553

189.  Reproductive Progress, 175 Gibbons Place, Athens, GA 30605                      06/07/96
      Tel: 706/546-7005 (no fax)

190.  Livestock Improvement Corporation, Ltd., CNR Ruakura/Morrinsville Rds.          09/10/96
      Private Bag 3016, Hamilton, New Zealand, Tel:64-7-856-0700;
      Fax:64-7-856-2428

191.  Central Wisconsin Semen Freezing Service, Box 36, 406 Chestnut St.,             10/31/96
      Spencer, WI 54479-0036 Tel: 715/659-4992

192.  France Embryon, B.P. 24, 42210 Montrond-Les-Bains, France                       12/20/96
      Tel:(033)77 36 34 44; Fax:(033)77 36 34 49

193. Columbia Animal Hospital, 1409 Hwy 98 E, Columbia, MS 39425          07/10/97
Tel: 601/736-3041; Fax: 601/731-2320

194. Gene-Pool Ltd, (Genbank Kft.) P.O. Box 24, Mezohegyes, Hungary 5820          08/08/97
Tel: (36)60-484-550; Fax: (36)60-484-550

195. AltaPon, Antumerweg 5, 9893 TA Garnwerd, The Netherlands          08/15/97
Tel: +31(0)594 621777; Fax: +31(0)594 621459

196. Swiss Federation for Artificial Insemination/AI Center Muelligen,          09/12/97
SVKB—Besamungsstation, Muelligan, AG CH-5200, Switzerland
Tel: 41 56 225 13 33; Fax: 41 56 225 26 18

197. Swiss Federation for Artificial Insemination/AI Center Buetschwil, St. Gallen,          09/12/97
CH-9606, Switzerland Tel: 41 71 983 23 11; Fax: 41 71 983 39 70

198. INTERMIZOO S.p.A., Corso Australia 67, Padova, Italy 35126          03/19/98
Tel: 49 872 4757; Fax: 49 872 4868

199. Ente Lombardo Potenziamento Zootecnico S.p.A., Centro Tori, 26829          03/26/98
Zorlesco, Italy Tel: 0377 831236; Fax: 0377 89635

200. Semex Alliance, 130 Stone Rd West, Guelph, Ontario N1G 3Z2 Canada          05/28/97
Tel: 519/821-5060; Fax: 519/821-7225 (partners include BCAI, CIAQ,
EBI, Gencor)

201. AI Station Lithor, Agrovysocina a.s., Horni ulice 30, Zdar nad Sazavou          02/12/98
Czech Rep. 591 01 Tel: 0042 0617 420 289; Fax: 00420 617 420 289

202. Saxonian Cattle Breeders Association, Winterbergstrasse 98, Dresden          04/03/98
Sachsen, 01237, Germany, Tel: 49 351 2527300; Fax: 49 351 2527306

203. Genetic Resources Int'l., 22575 State Hwy 6 South, Navasota, TX 77868          04/03/98
Tel: 409/870-3960; Fax: 409/870-3963 (formerly Technological Advances
in Farm Animals (TAFA), 1715 Laura Ln., College Station, TX 77840)

204. Excalibur Sires, 1815 Summit Drive NE, Rochester, MN 55906          04/24/98
Tel: 507/282-7451; Fax: 507/280-4400

205. Hunters Bamawm Bull Farm & Semen Collections (HBBS), RMB 3810,          05/05/98
Rochester, Victoria 3561, Australia Tel: 011 61 35 486 2287;
Fax: 011 61 35 486 2443

206. Consorzio Incremento Zootecnico SRL, Via Maremmana 1/A/C, La Serra          05/07/98
(PI) 56020, Italy Tel: 011 39 571 460355; Fax: 011 39 571 460259

207. Rinderbesamungs-Genossenschaft Memmingen, Memmington, Germany          07/17/98
87700 Tel: 00498331-63026; Fax: 00498331-61579

208. National Livestock Cooperatives Federation Dairy Cattle Improvment          10/14/98
Center #38 4 Wondang-Dong, G-Yang Si, Kyunggi-Do 411-030, Korea
Tel: 344/965-9588; Fax: 344/963-4559

209. Rinderzucht M-V GmbH, Am Bullenberg 1, 17348 Woldegk, D-Germany          10/20/98
Tel: 03963/25590; Fax: 03963/25592

210. SemenItaly, S.r.1., Via Cadiane, n° 181-41100 Saliceta S. Giuliano, Modena,          11/30/98
Italy Tel: 059-51-1611; Fax: 059-51-4697

211. Emtech Genetics Saskatchewan, Ltd., Box 148, Hague, Sask. Canada          01/04/99
S0K 1X0 Tel: 306/225-2261; Fax: 306/225-4412

| | | |
|---|---|---|
| 212. | Alpenseme—Federazione Prov. Le Allevatori—Trento, Via Castello, n° 10, Toss, Di Ton, Italy Tel: 0641-657602; Fax: 0641-657930 | 05/19/99 |
| 213. | Agire, BP 32, Versun, 14790 France Tel: 33 023 180 7192; Fax: 33 023 180 1709 | 06/29/99 |
| 214. | Interselection Normande, 38, rue de la mérillière, 61300 L'Aigle, France Tel: 02 33 84 48 79 4884; Fax: 02 33 84 48 90 | 06/29/99 |
| 215. | Plemenari Brno, Osvobodiletu, Zlin 1370, Czech Republic Tel: 011 420 5 412 15400; Fax: 011 420 621 322303 | 11/04/99 |
| 216. | Rosethyme Farm, 8 Henry St., Poughkeepsie, NY 12601 Tel: 914/485-3165 | 01/06/00 |
| 217. | Jura-Betail, Route De Lons-Le-Saunier, 39570, France Tel: 03 84 482 277; Fax: 03 84 482 575 | 08/02/00 |
| 218. | Genetica 2000 S.R.L., Via Masaccio, 11 - Mancasale, Reggio Emilia, 42010, Italy Tel: 39-0522-271262; Fax: 39-0522-271264 | 08/21/00 |
| 219. | Centro Provinciale Per La Fecondazione Artificiale, Via Leopoldo Pilla 28 Curatone, Mantova 46010, Italy Tel: 39-0376-349027; Fax: 39-0376-349365 | 08/21/00 |
| 220. | Cooperative Agricole D'Insemination Artificielle de Crehen, B.P. 19, 22130 Plancoet - France Tel: 33/26 5950 05; Fax: 33/26 5950 25 | 06/26/95 |
| 221. | RAB Australia Pty. Ltd., Private Mail Bag 6003, Auburn, NSW 2640 Australia Tel: 011 61 2 6026 2226; Fax: 011 61 2 6026 2387 | 08/28/00 |
| 222. | KI Samen B.V., Lorbaan 27, Grashoek, 5085, The Netherlands Tel: 31-77-3071592; Fax: 31-77-3077133 | 02/28/97 |
| 223. | Genoservis, J.Jaburkove 1, 779 74, Olomouc, Czech Republic Tel: 420-68-411005; Fax: 420-68-5413387 | 09/19/00 |
| 224. | Cogent, Woodhouse Farm, Aldford, Chester, Cheshire CH3 6JD, UK Tel: 44 1244 622000; Fax: 44 1244 620373 | 09/27/00 |
| 225. | Natural-SRO, Hradistko pod Mednikem 252 09, Czech Republic Tel: 01142 02 9941348; Fax: 01142 02 9941550 | 11/03/00 |
| 226. | Rinderzucht Schleswig-Holstein eG, Rendsburger Str. 178, Neumünster 24573 Germany Tel: (49) 4321 90530; Fax: (49) 4321 905396 | 01/15/01 |
| 227. | Collecta-Bull Services, 249 Layton Road, Stanfordville, NY 12581 Tel: 845/868-7145; Fax: 845/868-1490 | 02/12/01 |
| 228. | AI Center Viking Genetics, Landbovej 4, 6650 Brørup, Denmark Tel: 0045 7538 4500; Fax: 0045 7538 1015 | 02/26/01 |
| 229. | Circle J Custom Collecting, 10919 Hwy 42, Newton, WI 53063 Tel: 920/693-8883; Fax: 920/693-8883 | 09/07/01 |
| 230. | Rinderzuchtverband Sachsen-Anhalt eG, Bahnhofstraße 32, Stendal, Germany Tel: (0049) 03931/6964-0; Fax: (0049) 03931/212932 | 05/09/02 |
| 231. | RPN Rinderproduktion Niedersachsen Gmbh Bremen-Hanover, Verden (Aller), Niedersachsen 27283, Germany Tel: 04231/672-0; Fax: 04231/672-80 | 05/09/02 |
| 232. | RBB Rinderproduktion, Berlin-Brandenburg GmbH, Ketziner Str 12, Schmergow, Brandenburg 14550, Germany Tel: 033207/533-0; Fax: 033207/533-10 | 05/09/02 |

233.     Weser-EMS-Union eG, Feldlinie 2A, BAD Zwischenahn 26160, Germany     05/09/03 Tel: 01149-4403-932640; Fax: 01149-4403-932642

234.     Landesverband Thüromger Rinderzüchter Zucht-und Absatzgenossenschaft e.G.,    05/09/02 Stotternheimer Str. 19, Erfurt, Thüringen 99087, Germany Tel: 0361/77974-0; Fax: 0361/77974-44

235.     Aberekin, S.A., Barrio de Arteaga no. 25, 48160 Derio-Vizcaya, Spain     05/20/02 Tel: 34 94 454 15 77; Fax: 34 94 454 08 78

236.     A.I. Center Taurus, Ebeltoftvej 16, Drastrup, Randers 8900, Denmark     06/19/02 Tel: 45 87 95 94 00; Fax: 45 87 95 94 01

237.     ORIgen, Inc., 100 N. 27th, Suite 230, Billings, MT 59101-2054     10/07/02 Tel: 406/867-4436; Fax: 406/867-4437

238.     Global Genetics and Biologicals, 4011 SH 47, Bryan, TX 77807     11/20/02 Tel: 979/822-4000; Fax: 979/822-4022

239.     Besamungsverein Neustadt a.d. Aisch e.V., Karl Eibl-Str. 17-27 Neustadt    12/19/02 a.d. Aisch, Bavaria D-91413, Germany Tel: 49 09161 7870; Fax: 49 09161 787250

240.     GENSUR Ltda., Nueva York 1610, Montevideo, NA 11800, Uruguay     12/19/02 Tel: 598 2 9290260; Fax: 598 2 9246655

241.     USDA ARID Goat Breeding and Research Center, Highway 1, Yeghegnadzor,    01/02/03 Vayots Dzor Marz, Armenia Tel: +3741-28-26-97; Fax: +3741-58-79-28

---

*Do not have written release. Could not make contact by mail or telephone.

# CSS Guidelines for
# Artificial Insemination Center (AIC)
# Management Practices

## GENERAL WELFARE

The AI industry recognizes an ethical obligation and also an economic and genetic need to practice excellent husbandry methods. From an operational standpoint, the role of a genetically superior bull is to produce quantities of fertile spermatozoa for transmitting superior traits. To maximize the superior bull's potential, AI centers make significant investments in labor, feed, and facilities to provide optimal care for the bulls. Nutritionally correct rations and attention to individual health to reduce physical stress are provided. The AI industry recognizes that sound animal husbandry practices may increase the longevity and productivity of these bulls.

Bulls are housed in clean, well-lit, ventilated buildings or outside in facilities that protect them from inclement conditions. Social interaction both visually and vocally is permitted by housing design. Bulls are raised and cared for by dedicated employees.

Human safety and animal safety are two prominent concerns underlying the management practices of AI centers. By virtue of their size and disposition, bulls may be considered one of the more dangerous males of the domestic species. Therefore, management procedures are designed to protect human life as well as to provide for bull welfare.

## TRANSPORTATION

Bulls normally first come under the care of AIC personnel when they are transported from the farm or ranch of origin to the AIC facilities. During transit it is recommended that adequate protection be provided from adverse environmental conditions. Procedures intended to minimize stress or in-jury of bulls should be followed during their transport to and from the facilities of an AIC or between the facilities of the AIC. Individuals transporting bulls must be knowledgeable in the basic care of bulls. The transporting vehicle must be safe and allow for adequate space and ventilation for the bulls. During extended trips, the animals must be examined periodically for evidence of injury or illness. Veterinary care for bulls in transit should be provided as necessary. Feed and water are to be provided in accordance with good husbandry practices. Care is observed in loading and unloading of the animals. Animals are transported to the AIC in clean and disinfected livestock trailers.

## DISEASE SURVEILLANCE

The addition of new animals (bulls, mount animals) to a herd presents an opportunity for infectious disease to enter the resident population. Procedures necessary to prevent the introduction of potential diseases into the AIC must be followed.

The "Certified Semen Services (CSS) Minimum Requirements for Disease Control of Semen Produced for AI" provides a minimum industry standard for AIC health management. These requirements include testing and examination of bulls prior to their entry, during an isolation period and semiannually throughout their residency at the AIC.

Animals that do not satisfactorily meet the pre-entry and isolation health testing requirements pose a potential threat to the health of the resident herd and shall be denied admittance. However, successful completion of the isolation health testing protocol will allow animals to finally enter the resident herd where they will continue to undergo continuous surveillance testing semiannually or as specified by CSS. Mount animals are required to undergo the same health testing regimen as bulls.

# SIRE HYGIENE AND HANDLING

Sire hygiene and handling refer to the conditions and practices necessary to establish and maintain the health of animals.

Each AIC follows established procedures to insure sanitation and avoid transmission of potentially infectious material. Once a bull has been accepted, the primary objective is to maintain its optimal health and safety. Normally, young bulls are identified, receive a veterinary examination, and are treated to prevent specific diseases after arrival at the isolation facility.

Isolation premises should be washed and disinfected prior to the admittance of each new group of animals. Animals exhibiting any signs of illness upon arrival or during the isolation period need to be removed to a separate area.

Internal surfaces of the housing and pens allow for effective cleaning and disinfection.

In the semen laboratory and AV preparation area, the counter tops and equipment should be routinely washed and disinfected.

The walls and concrete flooring of the collection area are cleaned and disinfected on a regular schedule. Non-concrete flooring should be routinely misted with an appropriate disinfectant.

Visitors coming onto the AI center premises should be required to wear protective footwear to avoid transmitting potential organism to the AIC animals.

Within a facility, bulls are moved from one area to another for semen collection, facility cleaning, and to maintain bull hygiene. Bulls may be led by handlers in alleyways, or at other times, a series of gates and pens create a passageway for trained dogs to "move" the bulls. Mechanical devices also may be used to "walk" the bull, either for exercise or movement within a facility.

Physical restraint of a mature bull is required for health tests, veterinary examination, and proper hoof care. Generally, bulls are restrained in locking stanchions or haltered.

# ENVIRONMENT AND FACILITIES

Bulls are adaptable to a wide range of environmental conditions. Basic criteria for a satisfactory environment include physical comfort, disease control, access to adequate nutrition, and safety for bulls and handlers.

A variety of indoor or outdoor housing systems are used to provide for the needs of bulls. The type of housing system used will vary based on geographic location, age, and collection status of the bulls. The housing system selected should be considered acceptable if the basic needs of the animals are met satisfactorily.

Each bull should have adequate space and a dry area to lie down comfortably. In "tie stall" facilities bulls may be tethered, which allows the bull to lay down, stand, have limited movement, and to eat and drink unhindered. Stalls should be cleaned regularly, and suitable bedding materials should be used.

Cattle can tolerate a wide range of ambient temperatures; however, housing should be designed to protect bulls from extreme heat or cold. Bulls housed outdoors should have access to shelter for protection from sun and severe weather. Enclosed structures should be properly ventilated or air conditioned to help provide a comfortable environment. Ventilation can be provided actively by mechanical systems or passively with windows and vents, depending on the building design.

Internal surfaces of the housing and pens should allow for effective cleansing and disinfection. Also, to avoid injury, internal surfaces and fittings of buildings and pens should not have sharp edges or projections. Various paints and/or preservatives which may be toxic should not be used on surfaces with which the animals come into contact.

It is recommended that provisions be made for the segregation of sick or injured animals.

The essential mechanical equipment of the facilities, such as waterers, ventilator fans, heating and lighting units, fire-extinguishers, alarm systems, etc. should be inspected regularly to ensure they are in proper working condition. All electrical installations should be inaccessible to cattle and properly grounded.

The facilities and management procedures should provide safety for bulls and handlers. Fences should be designed in a way to contain bulls effectively. Bulls housed in groups should be dehorned to limit the potential for injury to other bulls. Handling procedures intended to provide control of the bull should be employed when bulls are moved. The facilities should be designed and lighted to permit effective visual inspection of the bulls. Facilities can be adequately adapted for the comfort of older animals with age-related physical conditions by adding heat lamps, extra bedding, larger stalls, and so forth.

In general, performance of the bulls should be the primary indicator of the adequacy of the environment.

## FEEDING AND WATERING

Bulls should be fed a nutritionally balanced ration. This may be based on National Research Council (NRC) guidelines or adjusted per professional consultation. The feed ingredients should be of good quality; feed ingredients may vary among AI centers depending on availability and types of regionally grown feed commodities. Bulls may be fed once or several times daily.

Clean and good quality water must be readily available. Water heaters need to be provided in cold climates to prevent freezing.

## VETERINARY AND PROFESSIONAL CARE

For bulls to achieve and maintain their optimum growth and semen production potential, they must remain in good health and physical condition. Various preventive medicine programs are conducted to maintain the health of bulls.

Bulls are regularly observed by trained and experienced personnel, as well as veterinarians, for clinical health problems or lameness. When a clinical abnormality, illness, or lameness is observed, the bull is evaluated and appropriate action taken. Veterinarians, licensed in their respective states, diagnose and treat disease or injury when such problems occur.

A major component of preventive medicine programs at AI centers is the semiannual (or annual for some diseases) surveillance testing for numerous bovine diseases. Regular testing provides increased assurance that seminal transmission of specific bovine disease agents will not occur. Testing procedures and specimen collections are conducted professionally so that accurate test results are obtained.

Preventive medicine by specific vaccination programs may also be practiced in an AIC; however, the bovine diseases prevented by vaccination may be selectively chosen. High-security isolation can be provided as a substitute for some vaccinations.

Inherent in any genetic advancement or preventive medicine program is the accurate identification of all animals. Bulls are identified by their registration certificate, which is unique to each animal by its color markings, or ear tattoo. When a bull is accepted into an AIC, it is thereafter designated by a unique sire code number per the NAAB Uniform Coding System. The management of an AIC will identify each bull by its NAAB stud code number by applying either an eartag, tattoo, neck tag, or leg band. Ear tagging can be accomplished quickly and safely with various commercially available applicator products. Some ear taggers are disinfected between each animal; others are designed that do not have direct contact with the animal's ear tissue when the tag is applied.

To make handling and leading of the bulls safe for barn personnel, nose rings are applied to most bulls. Trained and experienced barn personnel can safely and quickly insert a bull nose ring when the bull is appropriately restrained and the proper tools are used. Sedation or analgesia may be appropriate for some animals, and adequate healing time is provided.

Hoof care is an important segment of a complete bull health program. Facilities in which hoof examinations can be conducted, along with appropriate hoof exam and trimming equipment, should be available. Trained AIC personnel may then attend to bulls exhibiting lameness or provide preventive hoof care examination. Alternatively, the AIC should be able to transport a bull to a facility where hoof care can be conducted or call in a professional hoof care specialist. Dehorning may be regularly conducted in some AIC management programs. Dehorning bulls of horned breeds provides increased safety to bull handlers and also to other bulls when bulls are maintained in group housing. However, there are situations when it is not practical or appropriate to dehorn bulls. For example, AICs may prefer bulls to be horned when bulls are tethered in individual stalls. There are also selected breed considerations or simply age situations wherein it is not practical to dehorn bulls. These differences must be recognized. When dehorning is conducted at an AIC, procedures should be performed according to standard accepted veterinary surgical procedures, including administration of local anesthesia.

Within the scope of usual AIC management, castration is obviously not a frequently performed procedure. However, there are circumstances when castration is required. One example would be to further utilize an otherwise healthy but inferior bull as a mount animal. While castration is not always required in this situation, it is an acceptable option available to AIC management. Other situations for unilateral or bilateral castration include diagnostic or therapeutic reasons pertinent toward the study or treatment of specific genital problems. When castration is conducted, it is performed according to standard accepted veterinary surgical procedures, including sedation or anesthesia.

## SEMINAL COLLECTION

Seminal collection from bulls is basically a simple procedure. However, because of the nature of the AI industry, seminal collections must be accomplished under established guidelines and policies regarding health and cleanliness of bulls, and safety for bull handlers. In addition to operating under these guidelines and policies above, all seminal collections must meet certain quantitative and qualitative standards. To achieve these criteria, certain methods and procedures are followed for handling the bulls.

Normally, the collection of semen is best accomplished by a work team consisting of the semen collector, bull handler, and may include a mount handler. These individuals work together to provide for and control the appropriate stimulus situation(s) for the bull.

*Semen collector*  Manages the artificial vagina and performs the actual collection of semen. This person usually is the leader of the team and determines when the bull is properly prepared and when the seminal collection can be taken safely. In addition, the collector must insure that procedures are hygienic and that semen is identified accurately.

*Bull handler*  Handles the bull using a lead rope. This person must be responsible for keeping the bull under control and safely away from other persons and bulls in the collection arena. This person is also responsible for appropriate mount animal restraint unless the animal is managed by a separate handler.

*Mount handler*  Handles the mount animal using a lead rope or halter. This person is responsible for keeping the mount animal under control while the bull is being prepared for collection.

## Seminal Collection Procedure

Seminal collection procedures normally include: sexual stimulation, sexual preparation, and collection of the semen.

**Sexual Stimulation**—Providing a stimulus situation which elicits mounting behavior in the bull is termed sexual stimulation. The stimulation process starts by exposing the bull to a mount animal in a collection environment. The presence of other animals in this environment and various visual, olfactory, and auditory stimuli, sexually arouse the bull. When the bull is sexually aroused, he will have an erection of the penis and will want to mount other bulls and/or a mount animal. (A mount animal is another bull or steer whose purpose is to sexually stimulate the bull and stand in a sturdy position as the bull mounts him, as if in a natural breeding situation). Cows are not excluded as mount animals, but their use is not advocated. Depending upon the libido of the bull and the frequency of collection, the stimulation may be accomplished in a matter of minutes or it may take much longer.

**Sexual Preparation**—Sexual preparation is the intentional prolongation of sexual stimulation. It is achieved through a series of false mounts (allowing the bull to mount, but not ejaculate) and restraint, and ultimately results in an increase in the quantity and quality of sperm ejaculated. The type of preparation varies widely depending upon the libido and physical condition of the bull.

For all false mounts, the semen collector should be at the bull's side to hold the sheath aside so the penis does not come in contact with the rear quarters of the mount animal. This preventive action reduces the chance of contaminating the penis and also serves to prevent possible injury. Due to physical and health conditions, especially rear limb and spinal disabilities, some bulls may need to be limited in the number of false mounts allowed. The seminal collection procedure for such bulls should be under the direction of a professional livestock person or a veterinarian.

**Collection of Semen**—The collector should work with the bull throughout the preparation procedure and determine the optimum time for seminal collection. Typically, the seminal collection is performed immediately after the false mounting regime is completed.

The semen is collected through the use of an artificial vagina (AV). This device is made to simulate the natural breeding situation as much as possible. Intromission and ejaculation into the AV are performed by the bull in a manner nearly identical to natural mating. Since the final ejaculation cascade results from tactile stimuli to the bull's glans penis, the temperature, turgidity, and lubrication of the AV are important to successful sperm harvest. AV water temperatures between (104°F (40°C) and 140°F (60°C)) are common. A sterile and non-spermicidal lubricant applied to the upper one-third of the AV liner will improve the response of the bull and minimize penile abrasions. Normally the AIC will provide AVs of different length and diameter to accommodate differences among bulls. The AV is equipped in such a way that the semen drains into a collection vial. After the collection has been completed, the vial is removed, properly labeled, and prepared for processing.

To prevent potential transmission of disease-producing agents during semen collection, the hindquarters of the mount animal must be effectively and thoroughly disinfected between successively mounting bulls. In addition, AV equipment is thoroughly cleansed and disinfected or sterilized prior to each use. A separate AV or AV liner must be used for each ejaculate.

## THE SEMINAL COLLECTION FACILITIES

Seminal collection from bulls should be performed using the proper facilities and equipment. The safety of the personnel and animals are of utmost importance.

## Seminal Collection Arena

It is recommended the collection arena consist of an area large enough to accommodate the safe semen collection from one or more bulls. The size of the arena should be such that the individual bulls and mount animals can be led throughout the area without interfering with one another.

It is important that the collection area provide good "footing" for the bull and mount animal to prevent slipping and subsequent injury. Concrete should be avoided unless surfaces are grooved.

The passageway leading from the bull housing area to the collection arena should be equipped with a sturdy guard rail to allow the bull handlers to separate themselves from the bull. The railing is generally placed near the center of a walkway so that it allows the bull to be led on one side of the rail while the bull handler(s) walk on the opposite side of the rail. It is recommended the railing be built in 7- to 14-foot lengths with each length being separated by a gap or a safety man-pass of approximately 14 inches. This safety man-pass provides the bull handlers the opportunity to switch from one side of the railing to the other should the need arise. The 14 inch man-pass is of such size that the bull handler can easily pass through while a large bull cannot. It is also recommended that similar safety equipment and precautions be applied to the collection arena.

## ALTERNATIVE MEANS OF SEMINAL COLLECTION

The use of electro-ejaculation as an alternative seminal collection method should be limited to those circumstances when the temperament or physical condition of a bull renders collection of semen by AV unsafe or impossible. If this method is applied in other situations, it should be employed only after a diligent effort to harvest spermatozoa using the AV has failed, including systematic trial of different teaser animals and collection sites. Casual substitution of this method for diligent collection room management is not recommended.

In situations where bulls display shyness of collection personnel, collection accompanied by use of a blindfold should be attempted before resorting to electro-ejaculation. This approach should be tried repeatedly before use of electro-ejaculation. Complete physical and behavioral evaluation are essential before electro-ejaculation is considered.

The practice of electro-ejaculation of young bulls that have failed to demonstrate normal libido is not recommended. Electro-ejaculation should not be used to compensate for congenital abnormalities of the reproductive organs that make intromission and/or normal ejaculation impossible.

Collection of semen by this method can be accomplished in a humane and safe manner providing consideration is given to the equipment employed, the site and method of restraint, and the training of the operator of the electro-ejaculator.

The electro-ejaculators used in CSS-approved AICs should be of the solid-state, low-amperage type with complete grounding of the electronics. Current output should not exceed one ampere at maximum power. Machines must be regularly maintained, with particular attention to possible short circuits. The use of rectal probes with ventrally oriented electrodes, hand-held, or finger electrodes are advocated to minimize extraneous skeletal muscle stimulation.

The restraint chute selected for electro-ejaculation should provide lateral immobilization. Ventral support may be provided for bulls affected with posterior paresis using leather straps or belts between both the thoracic and pelvic limbs and fastened securely to the chute frame. Chemical tranquillization can be employed prior to electro-ejaculation, but the drug and dosage utilized should be selected by the attending AIC veterinarian and administered under his/her supervision. Positive conditioning such as brushing or even feeding may relax the animal; any abusive treatment of the bull must not be tolerated.

Proper training of machine operators must involve the supervision by an experienced machine operator and/or veterinarian. The operator must be completely familiar with the instrument's controls, the chute, and the bull. The controls must always be checked to verify that the electrical output is nil before the electrodes are inserted into the bull's rectum. Clearing of fecal material from the rectum with a sleeved arm and use of a non-irritating lubricant are essential. Care must be taken to dilate the anus and rectum gently, not forcibly, and if a rectal probe is used, it must be inserted slowly so the rectal lining is not injured.

Consideration must be given to the temperament, physical condition, and response of the bull when determining whether to collect semen by this method. Considerable individual variation in response can be expected, and operators must terminate stimulation if the animal becomes fractious, loses its footing, or is in distress. Slow, methodical increases of power at the lower amperage levels usually produce ejaculation well below the maximum output of the machine. Stimulation frequency and level may also be minimized by a period of precollection sexual preparation of some bulls, either by massage of the pelvic genitalia or active preparation with a teaser animal. Following alternative collection procedures, the probes and electrodes must be thoroughly cleaned and disinfected prior to next use.

Seminal collection by ampullar massage is another alternative collection method. This method has proven to be less consistent in harvesting semen of acceptable quality and should be employed only by an individual experienced in the methodology.

AIC management must support and foster humane considerations in the management of bulls, including the recommendations of technical staff regarding the unsuitability of particular sires for collection by electro-ejaculation. Livestock handlers in daily contact with the bulls are often the most astute judges of the temperament and physical response of bulls, and their evaluations of the response of individual bulls to electro-ejaculation should be solicited and heeded.

Certified Semen Services
P.O. Box 1033
Columbia, MO 65205-1033
Tel: 573/445-4406
Fax: 573/446-2279
E-mail: naab-css@naab-css.org
Website: www.naab-css.org

# APPENDIX H

# The Breeder's Guide to Certified Semen Services

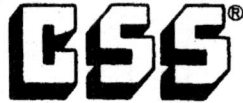

**CSS**®

## WHAT CSS IS

Certified Semen Services (CSS) is a wholly-owned subsidiary of the National Association of Animal Breeders, the trade association for the Artificial Insemination industry. Formed in 1976, CSS is an objective auditing service developed by responsible AI industry leaders through NAAB. CSS provides industry self-regulation.

CSS was developed by the AI industry to provide services to participating AI businesses to enhance the national AI program through uniform standards for sire health testing and semen identification.

## WHO PARTICIPATES IN CSS

Not all AI businesses do. Only those businesses which enter into a contract with CSS are eligible to carry the CSS logo in their advertising and on their semen packages. All semen suppliers are not equal. Some choose to have their health and identification procedures audited by CSS, others do not.

Any AI business engaged in collection and processing of livestock semen may participate in the CSS program upon entering into an "Agreement for Semen Identification and Sire Health Auditing Service."

Distributors who purchase semen for resale directly from a CSS-approved producing organization are also eligible to participate in CSS as an "Exclusive Distributor" and as such are allowed to use the CSS Exclusive Distributor logo.

## HOW IT WORKS

AI businesses entering into an agreement with CSS are audited at least once a year. During this audit, the CSS Service Director determines whether Certified Semen Services is in compliance with minimum requirements and agreement provisions.

The CSS Service Director makes at least one visit annually to each participating AI business to review procedures and records related to identification and health testing of bulls and semen from the time of sire procurement to semen sale. Each AI business uses internal controls to assure accurate identification of semen and health testing of bulls.

A complete report of this review is provided to the president and manager of the AI business audited. This report outlines in detail the procedures followed and recommends pertinent changes.

## SIRE HEALTH

Through CSS audits, participating AI businesses maintain efficient and reliable sire health testing programs. CSS requirements call for minimum testing for six diseases. Also reviewed are sanitation and isolation procedures for bulls and mount animals.

A primary and long-recognized advantage of AI is as an aid to avoid or prevent recurrence of certain diseases which affect reproduction in livestock.

Dairy and beef producers should be aware that a number of diseases may be transmitted through frozen semen. For example, leptospirosis may be shed in semen if the genital organs of the bull are infected. However, transmission via commercially frozen semen is highly unlikely. Diseases such as tuberculosis, brucellosis, campylobacteriosis (vibriosis), and trichomoniasis, under certain circumstances, have been found to be transmitted by AI when semen originated from diseased bulls. It has also been demonstrated that bulls persistently infected with BVD virus (early in fetal life) consistently shed virus into semen. If AI is to aid in disease prevention, the semen must be from a bull that is free of these diseases.

During the last 45 years in the U.S., there have been no prominent instances reported of a major disease being transmitted through AI. In practice, this is a direct result of the conscious voluntary effort of the AI industry to test for diseases which may be transmitted through frozen bovine semen.

The CSS Minimum Requirements for Disease Control of Semen Produced for AI (CSS Minimum Requirements) outline specific testing procedures for bulls and mount animals during three distinct periods: before entering isolation (pre-entry to isolation), during isolation, and for bulls housed in a central location after completing isolation (resident herd). Specific diseases tested for in the CSS Sire Health Program are: tuberculosis, brucellosis, leptospirosis (5 serotypes), BVD virus, campylobacteriosis (vibriosis), and trichomoniasis.

Intervals between tests and the number of tests to be conducted vary with each disease and are outlined in the "CSS Minimum Requirements for Disease Control of Semen Produced for AI" document. Testing intervals for resident bulls are designed to provide reasonable assurance that bulls, while in active AI service, are continuously free of diseases described in the CSS Sire Health Program.

In addition, CSS Minimum Requirements deal with general sanitary conditions and specify the use of antibiotics in semen processing. An important point to remember is that treating semen with antibiotics prior to freezing does not preclude the necessity for a complete health testing program.

## IDENTIFICATION

**Procedures for identifying semen are reviewed in detail to diminish the chance of semen from one bull being identified as that of another.**

The CSS program ensures checks and double checks of semen identification at all points and departments including: the bull's arrival at the facility, collection, evaluation and extension of the semen, packaging, inventory and shipping, as well as point of sale. Tools for identification include blood typing/DNA profiling, registration papers, records of sire procurement, breeding receipts, and sales invoices, as well as the registry ID number and name of bull, the collection code, breed code, the AI cen-

ter code assigned by NAAB, and bull number assigned by the processing organization.

## MAKING IT WORK FOR YOU

**To ensure the semen you use meets CSS identification and health testing requirements, look for the CSS logo in semen advertising and on semen packages. Buy only semen packages carrying the CSS logo.**

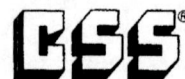

CSS recognizes there is semen produced which does not meet its minimum requirements. Therefore, the CSS Sire Health and Semen Identification Program is designed to make a distinction between semen from bulls meeting the CSS requirements and semen from bulls not meeting the requirements. In the CSS program, only semen packages containing semen from bulls meeting the requirements may have the registered CSS logo placed on them.

Use of the CSS logo in advertising by each individual AI business is based on the "all or none" principle. The CSS logo may be displayed in advertising if an AI business is selling only CSS Health Certified Semen. If semen other than CSS Health Certified Semen is marketed, the CSS logo cannot be used in advertising. The same is true for a custom freezing service. All semen frozen by a custom freezing service must be CSS approved in order to utilize the CSS logo when advertising custom freezing services.

Many AI businesses offer a custom freezing service which is separate from their semen marketing business. Understandably, an AI business may be selling semen which meet the CSS requirements from bulls they own or lease, but at the same time custom collect semen from bulls which may not meet the CSS requirements. In this case, the CSS logo may be placed on semen packages containing semen from bulls meeting the requirements. The CSS logo could be used in advertisements for semen marketed by the AI business but not in advertisements for that business's custom freezing service.

Virtually all semen marketed by AI businesses participating in CSS will exceed the CSS Minimum

A typical semen package (0.5 ml straw) imprinted with the CSS logo (arrow) indicating semen is CSS "Health Certified." Proper identification includes a) collection code, b) sire name, c) registry ID, and d) NAAB Uniform Code.

Requirements; however, this is not the case for many of the custom-collected bulls. In most cases, a bull custom collected "on the owner's farm" will not be in compliance with the CSS Minimum Requirements for Disease Control of Semen Produced for AI. This is due to the lack of adequate isolation facilities on the farm.

## FOR MORE INFORMATION

CSS and its participating AI businesses are providing a sire and semen health and identification program to complement and help protect the herd health and breeding program of every dairy and beef producer using AI.

For more detailed information on the programs and guidelines of Certified Semen Services, including the CSS Minimum Requirements for Disease Control of Semen Produced for AI, contact:

Certified Semen Services
P.O. Box 1033
Columbia, MO 65205-1033
Tel: 573/445-4406
Fax: 573/446-2279
E-mail: *naab-css@naab-css.org*
Website: *www.naab-css.org*

# Index

# Index

384